Surgery

PreTest®
Self-Assessment
and Review

Surgery
PreTest®
Self-Assessment
and Review

Seventh Edition

Edited by

Thomas C. King, M.D., M.A.
José M. Ferrer Professor of Surgery
Columbia University College of Physicians and Surgeons
New York, New York

Peter L. Geller, M.D.
Associate Professor of Clinical Surgery
Columbia University College of Physicians and Surgeons
New York, New York

John A. Chabot, M.D.
Assistant Professor of Surgery
Columbia University College of Physicians and Surgeons
New York, New York

McGraw-Hill, Inc.
Health Professions Division/PreTest® Series

New York   St. Louis   San Francisco   Auckland
Bogotá   Caracas   Lisbon   London   Madrid
Mexico City   Milan   Montreal   New Delhi
San Juan   Singapore   Sydney   Tokyo   Toronto

2 3 4 5 6 7 8 9 0   DOCDOC   9 9 8 7 6 5

ISBN 0-07-052065-8

The editors were Gail Gavert and Bruce MacGregor.
The production supervisor was Gyl A. Favours.
R.R. Donnelley & Sons was printer and binder.
This book was set in Times Roman by Compset, Inc.

The illustrations on the inside front and back covers are used with permission from Ben Pansky, *Review of Gross Anatomy,* 5/e. New York, McGraw-Hill, 1982.

Library of Congress Cataloging-in-Publication Data

Surgery : Pretest self-assessment and review / edited by Thomas C.
  King, Peter L. Geller, John A. Chabot.—7th ed.
    p.   cm—(Clinical sciences series)
  Includes bibliographical references and index.
  ISBN 0-07-052065-8
  1. Surgery—Examinations, questions, etc.   I. King, Thomas C.,
  1928–   .   II. Geller, Peter L.   III. Chabot, John A.   IV. Series.
  [DNLM: 1. Surgery—examination questions.   WO 18 S959 1995]
RD37.2.S97   1995
617′.0076—dc20
DNLM/DLC
for Library of Congress   93-42940

Contents

Contributors

Adam L. Basner, M.D.
Clinical Fellow in Plastic and Reconstructive Surgery
New York University Hospital
New York, New York

Steven B. Slovic, M.D.
Attending Surgeon
Southwest Washington Medical Center
Vancouver, Washington

Samuel Weinstein, M.D.
Clinical Fellow in Surgery
Columbia University College of Physicians and Surgeons
New York, New York

Preface

Although the questions and explanations presented in this book are designed chiefly as a review in preparation for certifying examinations, the approach they embody has much to recommend it as a study format in a more general sense. The lives of physicians are made up of a series of real problems, the solutions to which require a series of logical steps: analyzing patient-related data; recalling relevant information, both general and specific; making choices among alternatives; reviewing the consequences of action taken; and making corrections in plans. The problem-solving model, as a stimulus to studying and learning, simulates to a small degree this learning model. It also takes advantage of many of the characteristics recognized by educational psychologists as conducive to efficient learning experiences. Information is gathered in response to a perceived need rather than in anticipation of that need. The learner is actively involved. There is immediate feedback, error correction, and reinforcement. The process can be carried out at the learner's own pace and in a natural setting. The material in this book is an approach to continuing education of student-physicians using methods designed to exploit these characteristics.

No longer can students assume that this kind of continuing education ends with the completion of formal training and the successful completion of licensing or certifying examinations. As of October 1979, all 22 member boards of the American Board of Medical Specialties had committed themselves to the principle of periodic recertification of their members. Despite the Board's recognition that the cognitive skills measured in the objective examination do not assure clinical competence, recertification efforts—insofar as they involve examinations—are based on the assumption that knowledge of current information upon which good clinical decisions should be made is worth cultivating; that, while such information does not guarantee competent practice, lack of it probably impedes competent practice; that this knowledge, unlike technical skills, is reasonably easy to assess; and that it can be acquired by well-motivated physicians. These assumptions all seem reasonable.

The questions presented in this book deal with issues of relative importance to medical students; other problem-oriented materials are becoming available that are aimed at more sophisticated audiences—groups that, within a very few years, will include the present generation of students. Regular review of such material is a habit worth developing. We hope that this edition of *Surgery: PreTest® Self-Assessment and Review* will justify your efforts in working through the problems by providing guidance for further study and by helping you to develop enduring learning habits.

Thomas C. King, M.D.

Introduction

Surgery: PreTest® Self-Assessment and Review, 7/e, has been designed to provide medical students, as well as physicians, with a comprehensive and convenient instrument for self-assessment and review within the field of surgery. The 500 questions provided have the same format and are of the same degree of difficulty as the questions contained in Step 2 of the United States Medical Licensing Examination (USMLE) and will be a useful tool for USMLE Step 3 as well.

Each question in the book is accompanied by an answer, a paragraph explanation, and a specific page reference to either a current journal article, a textbook, or both. A bibliography, which lists all the sources used in the book, follows the last chapter.

Perhaps the most effective way to use this book is to allow yourself one minute to answer each question in a given chapter; as you proceed, indicate your answer beside each question. By following this suggestion, you will be approximating the time limits imposed by the board examinations previously mentioned.

When you have finished answering the questions in a chapter, you should then spend as much time as you need verifying your answers and carefully reading the explanations. Although you should pay special attention to the explanations for the questions you answered incorrectly, you should read every explanation. The authors of this book have designed the explanations to reinforce and supplement the information tested by the questions. If, after reading the explanations for a given chapter, you feel you need still more information about the material covered, you should consult and study the references indicated.

Pre- and Postoperative Care

DIRECTIONS: Each question below contains five suggested responses. Select the **one best** response to each question.

1. The earliest clinical indication of hypermagnesemia is

(A) loss of deep tendon reflexes
(B) flaccid paralysis
(C) respiratory arrest
(D) hypotension
(E) stupor

2. Five days after an uneventful cholecystectomy, an asymptomatic middle-aged woman is found to have a serum sodium level of 120 meq/L. Proper management would be

(A) administration of hypertonic saline solution
(B) restriction of free water
(C) plasma ultrafiltration
(D) hemodialysis
(E) observation

3. A 50-year-old patient presents with symptomatic nephrolithiasis. He reports that he underwent a jejunoileal bypass for morbid obesity when he was 39. One would expect to find

(A) pseudohyperparathyroidism
(B) hyperuric aciduria
(C) "hungry-bone" syndrome
(D) hyperoxaluria
(E) sporadic unicameral bone cysts

4. A 45-year-old woman with Crohn's disease and a small intestinal fistula develops tetany during the second week of parenteral nutrition. The laboratory findings include Ca 8.2 meq/L, Na 135 meq/L, K 3.2 meq/L, Cl 103 meq/L, PO_4 2.4 meq/L, albumin 2.4, pH 7.48, P_{CO_2} 38 torr, P_{O_2} 84 torr, and bicarbonate 25 meq/L. The most likely cause of her tetany is

(A) hyperventilation
(B) hypocalcemia
(C) hypomagnesemia
(D) essential fatty acid deficiency
(E) focal seizure

1

5. All the following preoperative interventions are recommended for cardiac patients who are undergoing noncardiac surgery EXCEPT

(A) administration of antiarrhythmic and antihypertensive medications through the morning of surgery

(B) administration of prophylactic antibiotics, including ampicillin and gentamicin, for patients with valvular heart disease who are undergoing gastrointestinal procedures

(C) control of congestive heart failure with diuretics and digitalis in severe cases

(D) discontinuation of beta-blocking medications the day prior to surgery

(E) postponement of elective surgery for 6 months after a subendocardial myocardial infarction

6. A characteristic finding of prerenal azotemia in a postoperative patient is

(A) urine sodium of 28 meq/L

(B) urine chloride of 15 meq/L

(C) fractional excretion of sodium less than 1

(D) urine/serum creatinine ratio of 20

(E) urine osmolality of 350 mOsm/kg

7. Each of the following methods helps reduce the incidence of wound infection after elective colon surgery EXCEPT

(A) mechanical bowel cleansing

(B) oral antibiotics effective against aerobes and anaerobes

(C) a single preoperative, parenteral dose of antibiotic effective against aerobes and anaerobes

(D) postoperative administration for 2 to 4 days of parenteral antibiotics effective against aerobes and anaerobes

(E) operative time less than 3 h

Questions 8–9

A previously healthy 55-year-old man undergoes elective right hemicolectomy for a Dukes' A cancer of the cecum. His postoperative ileus is somewhat prolonged, and on the fifth postoperative day his nasogastric tube is still in place. Physical examination reveals diminished skin turgor, dry mucous membranes, and orthostatic hypotension. Pertinent laboratory values are as follows:

Arterial blood gases: pH 7.56; P_{O_2} 85 torr; P_{CO_2} 50 torr
Serum electrolytes (meq/L): Na^+ 132; K^+ 3.1; Cl^- 80; HCO_3^- 42
Urine electrolytes (meq/L): Na^+ 2; K^- 5; Cl^- 6

8. The values given above allow the descriptive diagnosis of

(A) uncompensated metabolic alkalosis
(B) respiratory acidosis with metabolic compensation
(C) combined metabolic and respiratory alkalosis
(D) metabolic alkalosis with respiratory compensation
(E) "paradoxical" metabolic respiratory alkalosis

9. The most appropriate therapy for the patient described would be

(A) infusion of 0.9% NaCl with supplemental KCl until clinical signs of volume depletion are eliminated
(B) infusion of isotonic (0.15 N) HCl via a central venous catheter
(C) clamping the nasogastric tube to prevent further acid losses
(D) administration of acetazolamide to promote renal excretion of bicarbonate
(E) intubation and controlled hypoventilation on a volume-cycled ventilator to further increase the P_{CO_2}

Questions 10–11

A 23-year-old woman is brought to the emergency room from a halfway house, where she had apparently swallowed a handful of pills. The patient complains of shortness of breath and tinnitus, but refuses to identify the pills she ingested. Pertinent laboratory values are as follows:

Arterial blood gases: pH 7.45; P_{O_2} 126 torr; P_{CO_2} 12 torr
Serum electrolytes (meq/L): Na^+ 138; K^+ 4.8; Cl^- 102; HCO_3^- 8

10. The patient's acid-base disturbance is best characterized by which of the following descriptions?

(A) Acute respiratory alkalosis, compensated
(B) Chronic respiratory alkalosis, compensated
(C) Metabolic acidosis, compensated
(D) Mixed metabolic acidosis and respiratory alkalosis
(E) Mixed metabolic acidosis and respiratory acidosis

11. The most likely cause of the disturbance in this patient is an overdose of

(A) phenformin
(B) aspirin
(C) barbiturates
(D) methanol
(E) diazepam (Valium)

12. A 65-year-old man undergoes a technically difficult abdomino-perineal resection for a rectal cancer during which he receives three units of packed red blood cells. Four hours later in the intensive care unit he is bleeding heavily from his perineal wound. Emergency coagulation studies reveal normal prothrombin, partial thromboplastin, and bleeding times. The fibrin degradation products are not elevated but the serum fibrinogen content is depressed and the platelet count is 70,000/mm³. The most likely cause of the bleeding is

(A) delayed blood transfusion reaction
(B) autoimmune fibrinolysis
(C) a bleeding blood vessel in the surgical field
(D) factor VIII deficiency
(E) hypothermic coagulopathy

13. A 68-year-old man is admitted to the coronary care unit with an acute myocardial infarction. His postinfarction course is marked by congestive heart failure and intermittent hypotension. On the fourth hospital day, he develops severe midabdominal pain. On physical examination, blood pressure is 90/60 mmHg and the pulse is 110 beats per minute and regular; the abdomen is soft with mild generalized tenderness and distention. Bowel sounds are hypoactive; stool hematest is positive. The next step in this patient's management should be which of the following?

(A) Barium enema
(B) Upper gastrointestinal series
(C) Angiography
(D) Ultrasonography
(E) Celiotomy

14. All the following are risk factors for perioperative myocardial infarction EXCEPT

(A) coronary artery bypass 3 months prior to the current procedure
(B) a third heart sound
(C) old age (in the absence of any history of cardiac disease)
(D) myocardial infarction 1 year prior to the current procedure
(E) a non-Q-wave myocardial infarction 3 weeks prior to emergency surgery

15. A 20-year-old woman is found to have an activated partial thromboplastin time (APTT) of 78/32 on routine testing prior to cholecystectomy. Further investigation reveals a prothrombin time (PT) of 13/12 (patient/control), a template bleeding time of 13 min, and a platelet count of 350 × 100/mm^3. All the following are true of this woman's coagulopathy EXCEPT

(A) infusion of factor VIII concentrate is usually required to normalize concentration prior to surgery
(B) transfusion of cryoprecipitate will be followed by an improvement in coagulation
(C) few of these patients are seropositive for HIV
(D) epistaxis or menorrhagia is common
(E) lack of aggregation in response to ristocetin is a common feature of this disease

16. The chief surgical risk to which patients with polycythemia vera are exposed is that due to

(A) anemic disturbances
(B) hemorrhage
(C) infection
(D) renal dysfunction
(E) cardiopulmonary complications

17. A 30-year-old woman in the last trimester of pregnancy suddenly develops massive swelling of the left lower extremity from the inguinal ligament to the ankle. The correct sequence of workup and treatment should be

(A) venogram, bed rest, heparin
(B) impedance plethysmography, bed rest, heparin
(C) impedance plethysmography, bed rest, vena caval filter
(D) impedance plethysmography, bed rest, heparin, warfarin (Coumadin)
(E) clinical evaluation, bed rest, warfarin

18. Banked blood is deficient in which of the following coagulation factors?

(A) II only
(B) II and VII
(C) V and VIII
(D) IX and X
(E) XI and XII

19. A 65-year-old woman has a life-threatening pulmonary embolus 5 days following removal of a uterine malignancy. She is immediately heparinized and maintained in good therapeutic range for the next 3 days, then passes gross blood from her vagina and develops tachycardia, hypotension, and oliguria. During resuscitation, an abdominal CT scan reveals a major retroperitoneal hematoma. You should now

(A) immediately reverse heparin by a calculated dose of protamine and place vena caval filter (e.g., a Greenfield filter)
(B) reverse heparin with protamine, explore and evacuate hematoma, and ligate vena cava below the renal veins
(C) switch to low-dose heparin
(D) stop heparin and observe closely
(E) stop heparin, give fresh frozen plasma (FFP), and begin warfarin therapy

20. Following celiotomy, normal bowel motility can ordinarily be presumed to have returned

(A) in the stomach in 4 h, the small bowel in 24 h, and the colon after the first oral intake

(B) in the stomach in 24 h, the small bowel in 4 h, and the colon in 3 days

(C) in the stomach in 3 days, the small bowel in 3 days, and the colon in 3 days

(D) in the stomach in 24 h, the small bowel in 24 h, and the colon in 24 h

(E) in the stomach in 4 h, the small bowel immediately, and the colon in 24 h

21. All the following operations are likely to provide acceptable prolongation of life for patients with AIDS EXCEPT

(A) splenectomy for AIDS-related idiopathic thrombocytopenic purpura

(B) colonic resection for perforation secondary to cytomegalovirus infection

(C) cholecystectomy for acalculous cholecystitis

(D) tracheostomy for ventilator-depenent patients with respiratory failure

(E) gastric resection for a bleeding gastric lymphoma or Kaposi's sarcoma

22. An elderly, diabetic, steroid-dependent, bronchospastic woman has had an ileocolectomy for a perforated cecum. She is recovering well in the ICU, intubated on triple antibiotics and a rapid steroid taper, and making adequate urine on renal-dose dopamine. On postoperative day 2 she develops a fever of 39.2°C (102.5°), hypotension, lethargy, and laboratory values remarkable for hypoglycemia and hyperkalemia. The most likely diagnosis of this acute event is

(A) sepsis

(B) hypovolemia

(C) adrenal insufficiency

(D) acute tubular necrosis

(E) diabetic ketoacidosis

23. For a necessary transfusion of fresh frozen plasma in a patient who requires surgery as protection from bleeding in the perioperative period, the most appropriate timing would be

(A) the day before surgery

(B) the night before surgery

(C) on-call to surgery

(D) intraoperatively

(E) none of the above

24. On postoperative day 5 a patient is noted to have serosanguineous drainage from an abdominal incision. All the following measures are appropriate EXCEPT

(A) removal of several sutures and probing of the wound
(B) starting intravenous antibiotics
(C) placing an abdominal binder
(D) operative exploration
(E) bed rest

25. Signs and symptoms of hemolytic transfusion reactions include all the following EXCEPT

(A) fever
(B) hypertension
(C) oliguria
(D) abnormal bleeding
(E) heat and pain at the transfusion site

26. A patient suspected of having a hemolytic transfusion reaction should be treated with all the following EXCEPT

(A) placement of a Foley catheter
(B) fluid resuscitation
(C) bicarbonate infusion
(D) steroids
(E) mannitol

27. Five days after a sigmoid colectomy for cancer, a patient's skin staples are removed and serosanguineous fluid emerges. The most appropriate management is

(A) wide opening of the wound to assure adequate drainage
(B) smear and culture of the fluid and appropriate antibiotics after the smear is reviewed
(C) careful reapproximation of the wound edges with tape
(D) immediate return to the operating room
(E) application of a Scultetus binder

28. The surgeon should be particularly concerned about platelet function in patients receiving any of the following anti-inflammatory or analgesic medications EXCEPT

(A) ibuprofen
(B) aspirin
(C) indomethacin
(D) phenylbutazone
(E) acetaminophen

29. The substrate depleted earliest in the postoperative period is

(A) branched-chain amino acids
(B) non-branched-chain amino acids
(C) ketone
(D) glycogen
(E) glucose

30. Diagnostic abdominal laparoscopy is indicated in each of the following patients EXCEPT

(A) a stable patient with rebound tenderness following a tangential gunshot wound to the abdomen
(B) a stable patient with a stab wound to the lower chest wall
(C) a patient with a mass in the head of the pancreas
(D) a young female with pelvic pain and fever
(E) an elderly patient in the intensive care unit suspected of having intestinal ischemia

DIRECTIONS: Each question below contains four suggested responses of which **one or more** is correct. Select

A	if	**1, 2, and 3**	are correct
B	if	**1 and 3**	are correct
C	if	**2 and 4**	are correct
D	if	**4**	is correct
E	if	**1, 2, 3, and 4**	are correct

31. A 23-year-old woman undergoes total thyroidectomy for carcinoma of the thyroid gland. On the second postoperative day she begins to complain of tingling sensation in her hands. She appears quite anxious and later complains of muscle cramps. Appropriate therapy over the next several days might include administration of

(1) 10 mL of 10% calcium chloride intravenously
(2) continuous infusion of calcium gluconate
(3) oral calcium gluconate
(4) oral vitamin D

32. Hypocalcemia is associated with

(1) alkalosis
(2) prolonged QT interval
(3) hypomagnesemia
(4) myocardial depression

33. Enteric fluids with an electrolyte (Na^+, K^+, Cl^-) content similar to that of Ringer's lactate include

(1) saliva
(2) ileal contents
(3) right colon contents
(4) bile

34. Reduction of an elevated potassium level can be obtained by use of

(1) sodium polystyrene sulfonate (Kayexalate)
(2) sodium bicarbonate
(3) glucose and insulin
(4) calcium gluconate

Questions 35–37

An in-hospital workup of a 78-year-old, steroid-dependent, asthmatic man who is receiving chemotherapy for colon cancer reveals symptomatic gallstones. Preoperative laboratory results are notable for a hematocrit (HCT) of 24 percent and a urinalysis with 8 to 12 WBCs and 3 + bacteria. The night prior to surgery his abdomen is shaved and washed with antiseptic soap. On-call to the operating room he receives intravenous cefoxitin and steroids. Despite lack of indications to explore the common bile duct, a cystic duct cholangiogram was obtained. The wound was closed primarily with a Penrose drain exiting a separate stab wound. To avoid inhibiting his oxygen-dependent respiratory drive postoperatively, the Pa_{O_2} was maintained at 60 mmHg. On postoperative day 3 the patient developed a wound infection.

35. Which of the following changes could make this wound a less favorable environment for infection?

(1) Decreasing the operative time by omitting the cholangiogram
(2) A Jackson-Pratt drain exiting the inferior aspect of the wound
(3) Increasing the patient's HCT and Pa_{O_2}
(4) Leaving a seroma in the wound to prevent desiccation of the tissues

36. Which of the following characteristics of this patient increased the risk of a wound infection?

(1) Age
(2) Steroid dependence
(3) Receipt of chemotherapy
(4) Male sex

37. Which of the following changes in this patient, related to the bacterial inoculum, could decrease the chance of a postoperative wound infection?

(1) Decreasing the length of preoperative hospital stay
(2) Clipping the operative site in the operating room
(3) Successfully treating the urinary infection prior to surgery
(4) Continuing the prophylactic antibiotics for 3 postoperative days

SUMMARY OF DIRECTIONS

A	B	C	D	E
1,2,3 only	1,3 only	2,4 only	4 only	All are correct

Questions 38–39

The two solutions most commonly used to maintain fluid and electrolyte balance in the postoperative management of patients are 5% dextrose in 0.9% sodium chloride and lactated Ringer's solution.

38. Correct statements regarding 5% dextrose in 0.9% saline include which of the following?

(1) It contains the same concentration of sodium ions as does plasma
(2) It can be given in large quantities without seriously affecting acid-base balance
(3) It is isosmotic with plasma
(4) It has a pH of less than 7.0

39. Correct statements regarding lactated Ringer's solution include which of the following?

(1) It contains the same concentration of sodium ions as does plasma
(2) It can be given in large quantities without seriously affecting acid-base balance
(3) It is isosmotic with plasma
(4) It has a pH of less than 7.0

40. Four days after surgical evacuation of an acute subdural hematoma, a 44-year-old man becomes mildly lethargic and develops asterixis. He has received 2400 mL of 5% dextrose in water intravenously each day since surgery, and he appears well hydrated. Pertinent laboratory values are as follows:

Serum electrolytes (meq/L):
Na^+ 118; K^+ 3.4; Cl^- 82; HCO_3^- 24
Serum osmolality:
242 mOsm/L
Urine sodium: 47 meq/L
Urine osmolality:
486 mOsm/L

Correct statements about this patient's fluid and electrolyte status include which of the following?

(1) His low serum sodium indicates sodium deficiency, which should be treated with 3% saline infusion
(2) He probably has the syndrome of inappropriate secretion of antidiuretic hormone
(3) His blood glucose level should be checked since the hyponatremia may be artifactual
(4) Water restriction is the cornerstone of therapy

41. A 43-year-old woman develops acute renal failure following an emergency resection of a leaking abdominal aortic aneurysm. Three days after surgery, the following laboratory values are obtained:

> Serum electrolytes (meq/L):
> Na^+ 127; K^+ 5.9; Cl^- 92;
> HCO_3^- 15
> Blood urea nitrogen:
> 82 mg/dL
> Serum creatinine: 6.7 mg/dL

The patient has gained 4 kg since surgery and is mildly dyspneic at rest. Eight hours after these data are reported, the electrocardiogram shown below is obtained. The initial treatment for this patient should include intravenous administration of

(1) 10% calcium gluconate, 10 mL

(2) digoxin, 0.25 mg every 3 h for three doses

(3) sodium bicarbonate, 44 meq (50 mL)

(4) lidocaine, 100 mg

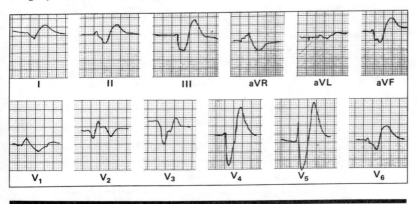

42. Prophylactic regimens of documented benefit in decreasing the risk of postoperative thromboembolism include

(1) early ambulation
(2) external pneumatic compression devices placed on the upper extremities
(3) elastic stockings
(4) low-dose heparin

43. Signs and symptoms associated with early sepsis include

(1) respiratory alkalosis
(2) ongoing requirement of fluid resuscitation
(3) glucose intolerance
(4) narrowed arteriovenous oxygen difference

DIRECTIONS: Each group of questions below consists of lettered headings followed by a set of numbered items. For each numbered item select the **one** lettered heading with which it is **most** closely associated. Each lettered heading may be used **once, more than once, or not at all.**

Questions 44–46

Match the gastrointestinal content at each site with its appropriate ionic composition (meq/L).

	Na	K	Cl	HCO₃
(A)	140	5	104	30
(B)	140	5	75	115
(C)	60	10	130	0
(D)	10	26	10	30
(E)	60	30	40	50

44. Salivary

45. Stomach

46. Small bowel

Questions 47–50

A 42-year-old man has a calculated resting energy expenditure of 1800 kcal/day (basal energy expenditure plus 10 percent). Match the following clinical situations with the appropriate daily energy requirement.

(A) 1600
(B) 2300
(C) 2800
(D) 3600
(E) 4500

47. Sepsis

48. Skeletal trauma

49. Third-degree burns of 60 percent of body surface area (BSA)

50. Prolonged starvation

Pre- and Postoperative Care

Answers

1. The answer is A. *(Schwartz, 6/e, p 74.)* States of magnesium excess are characterized by generalized neuromuscular depression. Clinically, severe hypermagnesemia is rarely seen except in those patients with advanced renal failure treated with magnesium-containing antacids. Hypermagnesemia is produced intentionally, however, by obstetricians who use parenteral magnesium sulfate ($MgSO_4$) to treat preeclampsia. $MgSO_4$ is administered until depression of the deep tendon reflexes is observed, a deficit that occurs with modest hypermagnesemia (over 4 meq/L). Greater elevations of magnesium produce progressive weakness, which culminates in flaccid quadriplegia and in some cases respiratory arrest from paralysis of the chest bellows mechanism. Hypotension may occur because of the direct arteriolar relaxing effect of magnesium. Changes in mental status occur in the late stages of the syndrome and are characterized by somnolence that progresses to coma.

2. The answer is B. *(Hall, pp 1930–1933.)* Acute severe hyponatremia sometimes occurs following elective surgical procedures. It is usually the result of the combination of appropriate postoperative stimulation of antidiuretic hormone and injudicious administration of excess free water in the first few postoperative days. Totally sodium-free intravenous fluids (e.g., dextrose and water) should be given with great caution postoperatively, since occasionally the resulting hyponatremia can be associated with sudden death from a flaccid heart or with severe permanent brain damage. The condition is usually best treated by withholding free water and allowing the patient to reequilibrate. At levels below 115 meq/L seizures or mental obtundation may mandate hypertonic sodium solutions. This must be done with extreme care since the risk of fluid overload with acute pulmonary or cerebral edema is high.

3. The answer is D. *(Way, 9/e, pp 611–612.)* Any patient who has lost much of the ileum—whether from injury, disease, or elective surgery—is at high risk to develop enteric hyperoxaluria if the colon remains intact. Calcium oxalate stones will develop in at least 10 percent of these

15

patients. The condition results from excessive absorption of oxalate from the colon through two related synergistic mechanisms: unabsorbed fatty acids combine with calcium, which prevents the formation of insoluble calcium oxalate and allows oxalate to remain available for colonic absorption; and unabsorbed fatty acids and bile acids also increase the permeability of the colon to the oxalate.

4.   The answer is C. *(Schwartz, 6/e, pp 73–74.)* Magnesium deficiency is common in malnourished patients and patients with large gastrointestinal fluid losses. The neuromuscular effects resemble those of calcium deficiency—namely, paresthesia, hyperreflexia, muscle spasm, and ultimately tetany. The cardiac effects are more like those of hypercalcemia. An electrocardiogram therefore provides a rapid means of differentiating between hypocalcemia and hypomagnesemia. Hypomagnesemia also causes potassium wasting by the kidney. Many hospital patients with refractory hypocalcemia will be found to be magnesium-deficient. Often this deficiency becomes manifest during the response to parenteral nutrition when normal cellular ionic gradients are restored. A normal blood pH and arterial P_{CO_2} rule out hyperventilation. The serum calcium in this patient is normal, when adjusted for the low albumin. Hypomagnesemia causes functional hypoparathyroidism, which can lower serum calcium and thus result in a combined defect.

5.   The answer is D. *(Schwartz, 6/e, pp 670–671.)* There are several recommended interventions in cardiac patients who are undergoing noncardiac surgery. The two factors that correlate best with postoperative life-threatening or fatal cardiac complications are myocardial infarction—transmural or subendocardial—and uncontrolled congestive heart failure. Hence, delay of elective surgery for 6 months after myocardial infarction and preoperative control of congestive heart failure with diuretics and digitalis, in severe cases, will have the greatest effect in decreasing the risks of surgery. A patient's cardiac medications should be continued preoperatively, including during the morning of surgery, to maintain adequate therapeutic levels. This is especially true for beta blockers, which can manifest withdrawal rebound hypertension and tachycardia approximately 24 h after discontinuation. Patients with prosthetic valves or valvular heart disease should be given prophylactic antibiotics to prevent seeding of their valves during episodes of significant bacteremia. This most commonly occurs during gastrointestinal or genitourinary procedures. Ampicillin and gentamicin cover the flora frequently encountered, including enterococci and gram-negative organisms.

6. The answer is C. *(Hall, pp 1902–1904.)* When oliguria occurs postoperatively, it is important to differentiate between low output caused by the physiological response to intravascular hypovolemia and that caused by acute tubular necrosis. The fractional excretion of sodium (FE_{Na}) is an especially useful test to aid in this differentiation. Values of $FE_{Na} <1$ percent in an oliguric setting indicate aggressive sodium reclamation in the tubules; values above this suggest tubular injury. The fractional excretion is a simple calculation: (urine Na × serum creatinine) ÷ (serum sodium × urinary creatinine). In the setting of postoperative hypovolemia, all findings would reflect the kidney's efforts to retain volume: the urine sodium would be below 20 meq/L, the urine chloride would not be helpful except in the metabolically alkalotic patient, the serum osmolality would be over 500 mOsm/kg, and the urine/serum creatinine ratio would be above 40.

7. The answer is D. *(Wilmore, vol 2, sect 6, chap 4, pp 1–10.)* Many clinical and experimental studies have looked at the optimum bowel preparation and preoperative regimen for elective colonic surgery to reduce the postoperative infectious complications of wound infection, intraabdominal abscess, and anastomotic leakage. Currently, a postoperative rate of wound infection of only 5 percent can be attained by combining mechanical cleansing, oral antibiotics, and perioperative parenteral antibiotics. The type of mechanical cleansing does not matter as long as it is effective. Preoperative oral antibiotics should be administered only the day prior to surgery and should cover aerobes and anaerobes (e.g., neomycin-erythromycin). Parenteral antibiotics effective against aerobes and anaerobes (e.g., cefoxitin) should be administered on-call to the operating room as a single dose or no more than 24 h postoperatively. Both antibiotic regimens yield maximum prophylaxis without fostering resistant transformation of microbes. Operative time greater than 3 h and a procedure that is extraperitoneal into the rectum are associated with an increased risk of infectious complications.

8. The answer is D. *(Wilson, 12/e, pp 293–294.)* Both the arterial pH and the P_{CO_2} are elevated in the patient presented in the question; the disturbance is alkalosis with hypoventilation. The P_{CO_2} typically increases by 0.5 to 1.0 torr for each meq/L increase in serum bicarbonate. These findings suggest that the hypoventilation is compensatory rather than a primary phenomenon. This assumption is further supported by the absence of clinical lung disease.

9. The answer is A. *(Wilson, 12/e, pp 293–294.)* The development of a clinically significant metabolic alkalosis in a patient requires not only the loss of acid or addition of alkali, but renal responses that *maintain* the alkalosis. The normal kidney can tremendously augment its excretion of acid or alkali in response to changes in ingested load. However, in the presence of significant volume depletion and consequent avid salt and water retention, the tubular maximum for bicarbonate reabsorption is increased. Correction of volume depletion alone is usually sufficient to correct the alkalosis, since the kidney will then excrete the excess bicarbonate. HCl infusion is usually unnecessary and can be dangerous. Acetazolamide is unlikely to be effective in the face of distal Na^+ reabsorption (in exchange for H^+ secretion). Moreover, to the extent that acetazolamide causes natriuresis, it will exacerbate the volume depletion.

10. The answer is D. *(Wilmore, vol 1, sect 1, chap 5, pp 5–7.)* The patient presented in the question is in a state of metabolic acidosis as shown by a markedly increased anion gap of 28 meq unmeasured anions per liter of plasma. However, the respiratory response is greater than can be explained by a compensatory response, since the patient is mildly alkalemic. The disturbance cannot be a pure respiratory alkalosis, since the serum bicarbonate does not drop below 15 meq/L as a result of renal compensation, and the anion gap does not vary more than 1 to 2 meq/L from its normal value of 12 in response to a respiratory disturbance. The renal response to hyperventilation involves wasting of bicarbonate and compensatory retention of chloride; it does not involve a change in the concentration of "unmeasured" anions.

11. The answer is B. *(Anderson, Ann Intern Med 85:745–748, 1976. Wilson, 12/e, pp 2178–2179.)* The acid-base disturbance in the patient described in the previous question demonstrates the value of extracting all available information from a small amount of rapidly retrievable data—e.g., arterial blood gases. Salicylates directly stimulate the respiratory center and produce respiratory alkalosis. By building up an accumulation of organic acids, salicylates also produce a concomitant metabolic acidosis. Characteristically both disturbances exist simultaneously following massive ingestion of salicylates. If sedative agents have been taken as well, the respiratory alkalosis (and even the respiratory compensation) may be absent. Phenformin and methanol overdoses also produce "high anion-gap" metabolic acidosis, but without the simultaneous respiratory disturbance. In the case presented, the patient's history of tinnitus in conjunction with her mixed metabolic acidosis–respiratory alkalosis is essentially pathognomonic of salicylate intoxication.

12. The answer is C. *(Hall, pp 1818–1825.)* Whenever significant bleeding is noted in the early postoperative period, the presumption should always be that it is due to an error in surgical control of blood vessels in the operative field. Hematologic disorders that are not apparent during the long operation are most unlikely to surface as problems postoperatively. Blood transfusion reactions can cause diffuse loss of clot integrity; the sudden appearance of diffuse bleeding during an operation may be the only evidence of an intraoperative transfusion reaction. In the postoperative period, transfusion reactions usually present as unexplained fever, apprehension, and headache—all symptoms difficult to interpret in the early postoperative period. Factor VIII deficiency (hemophilia) would almost certainly be known by history in a 65-year-old man, but if not, intraoperative bleeding would have been a problem earlier in this long operation. Severely hypothermic patients will not be able to form clots effectively, but clot dissolution does not occur. Care should be taken to prevent the development of hypothermia during long operations through the use of warmed intravenous fluid, gas humidifiers, and insulated skin barriers.

13. The answer is C. *(Schwartz, 6/e, pp 958–961.)* Acute mesenteric ischemia may be difficult to diagnose. The condition should be suspected in patients with either systemic manifestations of arteriosclerotic vascular disease or low cardiac output states associated with a sudden development of abdominal pain that is out of proportion to the physical findings. Lactic acidosis and an elevated hematocrit reflecting hemoconcentration are common laboratory findings. Abdominal films show a nonspecific ileus pattern. The cause may be embolization of thrombosis of the superior mesenteric artery, primary mesenteric venous occlusion, or nonocclusive mesenteric ischemia secondary to low cardiac output states. A mortality of 65 to 100 percent is reported. The majority of affected patients are at high operative risk, but since early diagnosis followed by revascularization or resectional surgery or both is the only hope for survival, celiotomy must be performed once the diagnosis of arterial occlusion or bowel infarction has been made. Initial treatment of nonocclusive mesenteric ischemia includes measures to increase cardiac output and blood pressure and the direct intraarterial superior mesenteric infusion of vasodilators such as papaverine. The patient presented in the question is at risk for both occlusive and nonocclusive mesenteric ischemic disease. If his clinical status permits, angiographic studies should be performed before the operation to establish the diagnosis and to determine whether embolectomy, revascularization, or nonsurgical management is indicated as initial treatment.

14. The answer is A. *(Schwartz, 6/e, pp 670–671.)* The work of Goldman and others has served to identify risk factors for perioperative myocardial infarction. The highest likelihood is associated with recent myocardial infarction: the more recent the event the higher the risk up to 6 months. It should be noted, however, that the risk never returns to normal. A non-Q-wave infarction may not have destroyed much myocardium, but it leaves the surrounding area with borderline perfusion, hence the particularly high risk for subsequent perioperative infarction. Evidence of congestive heart failure, such as jugular venous distention, or S3 gallop also carries a high risk, as does the frequent occurrence of ectopic beats. Old age and emergency surgery are risk factors independent of these others. Coronary revascularization by coronary artery bypass graft (CABG) tends to protect against myocardial infarction. Smoking, diabetes, hypertension, and hyperlipidemia (all of which predispose to coronary artery disease) are surprisingly not independent risk factors, although they may increase the death rate should an infarct occur. The value of this information and data derived from further testing is that it identifies the patient who needs to be monitored invasively with a systemic arterial catheter and pulmonary arterial catheter. Most perioperative infarcts occur postoperatively when the "third-space" fluids return to the circulation, which increases the preload and the myocardial oxygen consumption. This generally occurs around the third postoperative day.

15. The answer is A. *(Schwartz, 6/e, pp 101–102.)* Von Willebrand's disease has an autosomal dominant pattern of inheritance that affects both men and women. The deficiency of factor VIII activity is generally less severe than in classic hemophilia and tends to fluctuate even in an untreated patient. However, the bleeding tendency is compounded by abnormal platelet function. This is responsible for the common occurrence of epistaxis and menorrhagia. In 70 percent of patients, platelets fail to aggregate in response to ristocetin. Transfusion of cryoprecipitate provides factor VIII R:WF (the von Willebrand factor), whereas infusions of high-purity concentrates of factor VIII:C are not effective. These patients do not generally require treatment unless they need surgery or are severely injured; therefore, they have not usually received the contaminated concentrates responsible for the 80 percent prevalence of HIV seropositivity among hemophiliacs.

16. The answer is B. *(Schwartz, 6/e, p 105.)* Intraoperative and postoperative hemorrhage is a significant problem in the patient with polycythemia vera. Despite thrombocytosis, these patients have a hemorrhagic tendency generally ascribed to a qualitative deficiency of the platelets. Elective surgery should be postponed until the hematocrit and platelet count reach normal levels. Alkylating agents, such as busulfan or chlorambucil, are effective in this regard. In the emergency situation, phlebectomy should be performed prior to operation and especially careful hemostatic technique should be employed. Infection also is a problem in patients with polycythemia vera, but hemorrhagic problems are the more frequently encountered complications.

17. The answer is B. *(Schwartz, 6/e, pp 990–1003.)* This patient has a left ileofemoral vein thrombosis, as evidenced by sudden massive swelling of her entire left lower extremity. Noninvasive venous testing should be quite helpful as the venous obstruction extends above the knee and therefore venography and x-ray exposure are unnecessary. Heparin is the preferred agent because it does not cross the placenta. The vena caval filter is not indicated because there is no contraindication to heparin therapy and there has not been any evidence of pulmonary embolus.

18. The answer is C. *(Schwartz, 6/e, pp 111, 113.)* When large amounts of banked blood are transfused, the recipient becomes deficient in factors V and VIII (the "labile" factors) and an acquired coagulopathy ensues. Since banked blood is also deficient in platelets, thrombocytopenia may also develop.

19. The answer is A. *(Hall, pp 1495–1496.)* In a heparinized patient with significant life-threatening hemorrhage, immediate reversal of heparin anticoagulation is indicated. Protamine sulfate is a specific antidote to heparin and should be given as 1 mg for each 100 U heparin if hemorrhage begins shortly after a bolus of heparin. For a patient (such as this) in whom heparin therapy is ongoing, the dose should be based on the half-life of heparin (90 min). Since protamine is also an anticoagulant, only half the calculated circulating heparin should be reversed. The protaminization should be followed by placement of a percutaneous vena caval filter (Greenfield). In this critically ill patient, exploration of the retroperitoneal space would be surgically challenging and meddlesome.

20. The answer is B. (*Hall, pp 1076–1077.*) The misconception that the entire bowel does not function in the early postoperative period is still widely held. Intestinal motility and absorption studies have clarified the patterns by which bowel activity resumes. The stomach remains uncoordinated in its muscular activity and does not empty efficiently for about 24 h after abdominal procedures. The small bowel functions normally within hours of surgery and is able to accept nutrients promptly, either by nasoduodenal or percutaneous jejunal feeding catheters or, after 24 h, by gastric emptying. The colon is stimulated in large measure by the gastrocolic reflex but ordinarily is relatively inactive for 3 to 4 days.

21. The answer is D. (*Diettrich, Arch Surg 126:860–865, 1991.*) Patients who have AIDS frequently present with problems that potentially require surgical care. The involvement of surgeons with these patients will increase as more effective treatments are developed and the AIDS patient's survival is prolonged. AIDS patients not only suffer from common surgical illnesses, they also develop problems especially associated with their altered immune status such as bleeding from gastrointestinal lymphomas or Kaposi's lesions, bowel ischemia, perforation from parasitic or viral infection, acalculous cholecystitis, and retroperitoneal and intraabdominal masses due to massive lymphadenitis. With the exception of tracheostomy, experience has demonstrated that surgery can be performed with acceptable morbidity and mortality and that it seems to provide comfort and prolong quality life. Though it may facilitate nursing care, tracheostomy does not reverse or slow the pulmonary failure once the patient has become ventilator-dependent.

22. The answer is C. (*Schwartz, 6/e, pp 1574–1578.*) Acute adrenal insufficiency is classically manifest as changing mental status, increased temperature, cardiovascular collapse, hypoglycemia, and hyperkalemia. The diagnosis can be difficult to make and requires a high index of suspicion. Its clinical presentation is similar to that of sepsis; however, sepsis is generally associated with hyperglycemia and no significant change in potassium. The treatment for adrenal crisis is hydrocortisone 100 mg intravenously, volume resuscitation, and other supportive measures to treat any new or ongoing stress. Then, hydrocortisone 200 to 400 mg is administered over the next 24 h followed by a taper of the steroid as tolerated.

23. The answer is C. *(Schwartz, 6/e, p 104.)* Transfusions with fresh frozen plasma (FFP) are given to replenish clotting factors. The effectiveness of the transfusion in maintaining hemostasis is dependent on the quantity of each factor delivered and its half-life. The half-life of the most stable clotting factor, factor VII, is 4 to 6 h. A reasonable transfusion scheme would be to give FFP on-call to the operating room. This way the transfusion is complete prior to the incision with circulating factors to cover the operative and immediate postoperative period.

24. The answer is B. *(Wilmore, vol 2, sect 6, chap 7, p 6.)* Serosanguineous drainage is classically associated with fascial dehiscence. A reasonable approach to this problem is to remove several sutures and gently explore the wound to determine the extent of the dehiscence. A small fascial dehiscence, 1 to 2 cm, can be treated conservatively with local wound care and an abdominal binder to support the fascia. A larger dehiscence requires reoperation for formal reclosure of the fascia. High-risk patients with a large fascial dehiscence may be treated with an abdominal binder and modified bed rest, which allows both intraabdominal adhesion formation and local granulation. Although fascial dehiscence can occur from local infection, it is usually not an infectious process and does not require parenteral antibiotic therapy.

25. The answer is B. *(Hardy, 2/e, p 74. Schwartz, 6/e, pp 115–117.)* Allergic and febrile reactions occur in about 1 percent of all transfusions. Hemolytic transfusion reactions are much less common—0.2 percent—with fatal reactions in 1:100,000 transfusions. Hemolytic transfusion reactions are due to the reaction of recipient antibodies against transfused antigens. These reactions can be both immediate and delayed. Symptoms of a hemolytic transfusion reaction include fever, chills, and pain and heat at the infusion site, as well as respiratory distress, anxiety, hypotension, and oliguria. During surgery a hemolytic transfusion reaction can manifest as abnormal bleeding.

26. The answer is D. *(Wilmore, vol 1, sect 1, chap 6, p 11.)* Hemolytic transfusion reactions lead to hypotension and oliguria. The increased hemoglobin in the plasma will be cleared via the kidneys, which leads to hemoglobinuria. Placement of an indwelling Foley catheter with subsequent demonstration of oliguria and hemoglobinuria not only confirms the diagnosis of a hemolytic transfusion reaction but is useful in monitoring corrective therapy. Treatment begins with discontinuation of the transfusion, followed by aggressive fluid resuscitation to support the hypotensive episode and increase urine output. Inducing a diuresis through aggressive fluid resuscitation and osmotic diuretics is important to clear the hemolyzed red cell membranes, which can otherwise collect in glomeruli and cause renal damage. Alkalinization of the urine (pH > 7) helps prevent hemoglobin clumping and renal damage. Steroids do not have a role in the treatment of hemolytic transfusion reactions.

27. The answer is D. *(Way, 9/e, pp 26–27.)* The appearance of a gush of serosanguineous fluid from an abdominal incision is pathognomonic of a disruption of the deep fascia. The source of large amounts of serous fluid is the peritoneum. The temptation to avoid direct reclosure of these wounds should be resisted since delayed resumption of normal ambulation and activity with a late ventral hernia is the best outcome to be hoped for; evisceration, wound infections, or failure-to-thrive convalescence is far more likely. Recurrence of eviscerations following reclosure of these wounds is extremely rare, though 10 to 20 percent will later develop incisional hernias. The Scultetus binder is a corsetlike cloth wrap that was once a favored support to reduce likelihood of evisceration in those wounds in which the fascia was left unrepaired after dehiscence.

28. The answer is A. *(Hall, pp 2074–2075.)* Platelet dysfunction has been associated with a long list of drugs. Among analgesics all the listed agents except ibuprofen have been implicated, along with aminopyrine, codeine, and phenacetin. In addition, many antibiotics, anticonvulsants, and sedatives have been associated with thrombasthenia. Any time platelet abnormalities are suspected, a careful review of the drugs the patient is receiving should be undertaken, and a measurement should be made of the platelet count and bleeding time.

29. The answer is D. *(Way, 9/e, pp 160–162.)* The metabolic response to surgery (and other trauma) is a result of neuroendocrine stimulation that sharply accelerates protein breakdown, stimulates gluconeogenesis, and produces glucose intolerance. The glycogen stores are rapidly depleted because of a fall in insulin and a rise in glucagon levels in the plasma. The peripheral effects of the neuroendocrine secretion result in an increase in plasma levels of amino acids, free fatty acids, lactate, glucose, and glycerol. In the liver, the cortisol and glucagon stimulate glycogenolysis, gluconeogenesis, and increased substrate uptake.

30. The answer is A. *(Berci, Am J Surg 161:332–335, 1991.)* The indications for diagnostic laparoscopic exploration are increasing rapidly as the tools and techniques for such intervention improve. In the stable trauma patient with a tangential gunshot wound or with a stab wound to the lower chest wall or abdomen, laparoscopy may show no actual peritoneal penetration and might make a laparotomy unnecessary. If the peritoneum or diaphragm is injured, subsequent laparotomy and exploration are generally indicated to exclude other possible injuries and to facilitate repair of the diaphragm. All unstable patients or those with signs of peritoneal irritation (e.g., rebound tenderness) should undergo prompt celiotomy. Laparoscopic staging of malignancies allows improved preoperative assessment of the resectability of intraabdominal malignancies. The procedure has proved particularly useful in cases with pancreatic carcinoma. Laparoscopic evaluations may expedite differentiation of competing etiologies of right lower quadrant pain; this would allow appendectomy for appendicitis or appropriate therapy such as intravenous antibiotics for pelvic inflammatory disease and preempt celiotomy. In critically ill patients, the development of low flow or embolic ischemic insults to the bowel can be fatal if not recognized and treated early. Many such patients are already being ventilated in intensive care units; in this setting bedside laparoscopy can ascertain the need for early exploration for bowel revascularization or resection.

31. The answer is B (1, 3). *(Schwartz, 6/e, pp 72–73.* Postthyroidectomy hypocalcemia is usually due to transient ischemia of the parathyroid glands and is self-limited. When it becomes symptomatic it should be treated with intravenous infusions of calcium. In most cases the problem is resolved in several days. If hypocalcemia persists, oral therapy is started with calcium gluconate. Vitamin D preparations are only used if hypocalcemia is prolonged and permanent hypoparathyroidism is suspected.

32. The answer is E (all). *(Schwartz, 6/e, pp 72–73. Wilson, 12/e, pp 1915–1921.)* Hypocalcemia is associated with a prolonged QT interval and may be aggravated by both hypomagnesemia and alkalosis. Serum calcium levels below 7.0 mg/dL, encountered most frequently following parathyroid or thyroid surgery or in patients with acute pancreatitis, should be treated with intravenous calcium gluconate or lactate. The myocardium is very sensitive to calcium levels; therefore calcium is considered a positive inotropic agent. Calcium increases the contractile strength of cardiac muscle as well as the velocity of shortening. In its absence the efficiency of the myocardium decreases.

33. The answer is C (2, 4). *(Schwartz, 6/e, pp 65, 75.)* Bile and the fluids found in the duodenum, jejunum, and ileum all have an electrolyte content similar to that of Ringer's lactate. Saliva and right colon fluids have high K^+ and low Na^+ content. It is important to consider these variations in electrolyte patterns when calculating replacement requirements following gastrointestinal losses.

34. The answer is A (1, 2, 3). *(Schwartz, 6/e, p 71.)* Reduction of an elevated serum potassium level is important to avoid the cardiovascular complications that ultimately culminate in diastolic cardiac arrest. Kayexalate is a cation exchange resin that is instilled into the gastrointestinal tract and exchanges sodium for potassium ions. Its use is limited to semiacute and chronic potassium elevations. Sodium bicarbonate causes a rise in serum pH and shifts potassium intracellularly. Administration of glucose initiates glycogen synthesis and uptake of potassium. Insulin can be used in conjunction with this to aid in the shift of potassium intracellularly. Calcium gluconate does not affect the serum potassium level but rather counteracts the myocardial effects of hyperkalemia.

35–37. The answers are 35-B (1,3); 36-A (1,2,3); 37-A (1,2,3). *(Wilmore, vol 2, sect 9, chap 5, pp 1–10.)* The determinants of a postoperative wound infection include those related to the bacteria, the environment (i.e., the wound), and the host's defense mechanisms. Within this triad there are factors predetermined by the status of the patient (e.g., age, obesity, steroid dependence, multiple diagnoses [more than three], immunosuppression) and by the type of procedure (e.g., contaminated versus clean, emergent versus elective). However, there are several factors that can be optimized by the surgeon. Decreasing the bacterial inoculum and virulence by limiting the patient's prehospital stay, clipping the operative site in the operating room, administering perioperative antibiotics (within a 24-h period surrounding operation), treating remote infections, avoiding breaks in technique, using closed drainage systems (if needed at all), and minimizing the duration of the operation have all been shown to decrease postoperative infection. Making a wound less favorable to infection requires attention to basic Halstedian principles of hemostasis, anatomic dissection, and gentle handling of tissues as well as limiting the amount of foreign body and necrotic tissue in the wound. Although they are the most difficult factors to influence, host defense mechanisms can be improved by optimizing nutritional status, tissue perfusion, and oxygen delivery.

38–39. The answers are 38-D (4), 39-C (2, 4). *(Schwartz, 6/e, p 113.)* Isotonic saline solutions contain 154 meq/L of both sodium and chloride ions. Each ion is in a substantially higher concentration than is found in the normal serum (Na = 142 meq/L; Cl = 103 meq/L). When isotonic solutions are given in large quantities, they overload the kidney's ability to excrete chloride ion, which results in a dilutional acidosis. They also may intensify preexisting acidosis by reducing the base bicarbonate/carbonic acid ratio in the body. Isotonic saline solutions are particularly useful in hyponatremic or hypochloremic states and whenever a tendency to metabolic alkalosis is present, as occurs with significant nasogastric suction losses or vomiting.

Administration of lactated Ringer's solution is appropriate for replacing gastrointestinal losses and correcting extracellular fluid deficits. Containing 130 meq/L sodium, lactated Ringer's is hyposmolar with respect to sodium and provides approximately 150 mL of free water with each liter given. Although ordinarily not a significant load, in some clinical situations it can be. Lactated Ringer's is sufficiently "physiological" to enable administration of large amounts without affecting the body's acid-base balance significantly. It is worth noting that both isotonic saline and lactated Ringer's are acid with respect to the plasma: 0.9% NaCl/5% dextrose has a pH of 4.5; lactated Ringer's has a pH of 6.5.

40. The answer is C (2, 4). *(Schwartz, 6/e, pp 44–45, 78–79.)* The findings in the patient presented in the question are typical of the syndrome of inappropriate antidiuretic hormone secretion (SIADH). Although this syndrome is primarily associated with diseases of the central nervous system or of the chest (e.g., oat cell carcinoma of the lung), excessive amounts of antidiuretic hormone are also present in most postoperative patients. The pathophysiology of SIADH involves an inability to dilute the urine, and administered water is therefore retained, which produces dilutional hyponatremia. Body sodium stores and fluid balance are normal, as evidenced by the absence of the clinical findings suggestive of abnormalities of extracellular fluid volume. While hypertonic saline infusions can transiently improve hyponatremia, the appropriate therapy is to restrict water ingestion to a level below the patient's ability to excrete water. Hypertonic saline may be dangerous, since it can shift accumulated water into the extracellular fluid and precipitate pulmonary edema in the patient who suffers from low cardiac reserves. Hyperglycemia cannot account for the hyponatremia seen in this patient because the serum osmolality, as well as the serum sodium, is depressed. Hyponatremia resulting from hyperglycemia would be associated with an elevated serum osmolality.

41. The answer is B (1, 3). *(Wilson, 12/e, pp 287–289, 858–859.)* The electrocardiogram exhibited in the question demonstrates changes that are essentially diagnostic of severe hyperkalemia. Correct treatment for the affected patient includes administration of a source of calcium ions (which will immediately oppose the neuromuscular effect of potassium) and administration of sodium ions (which, by producing a mild alkalosis, will shift potassium into cells); each will temporarily reduce serum potassium concentration. Infusion of glucose and insulin would also effect a temporary transcellular shift of potassium. However, these maneuvers are only temporarily effective; definitive treatment calls for removal of potassium from the body. The sodium-potassium exchange resin sodium polystyrene sulfonate (Kayexalate) would accomplish this removal but at the price of adding a sodium ion for each potassium ion that is removed. Hemodialysis or peritoneal dialysis is probably required for this patient, since these procedures also rectify the other consequences of acute renal failure. Both lidocaine and digoxin would not only be ineffective but contraindicated, since they would further depress the myocardial conduction system.

42. The answer is C (2, 4). *(Schwartz, 6/e, pp 993–994.)* The problem of deep vein thrombosis and pulmonary embolism is significant in general surgery. There are approximately 2.5 million episodes of deep vein thrombosis and 600,000 pulmonary embolic events that result in 200,000 deaths annually. The problem is exacerbated by the disorder's frequent unheralded progression—only 20 to 25 percent of fatal pulmonary emboli are suspected clinically by the physician or manifest by classic signs or symptoms. The fact that most deaths due to pulmonary embolism occur before effective therapy can be started highlights the importance of preventive measures. Several documented factors help identify those at increased risk, including age greater than 40, obesity, malignancy, venous disease, congestive heart failure and atrial fibrillation, and prolonged bed rest. Virchow initially attributed venous thrombosis to the combination of venous stasis, hypercoagulability, and endothelial injury. The first two conditions are exacerbated by operative positioning and stress such that 25 percent of patients at moderate risk will develop venous thromboembolism, 50 percent within 24 h and 80 percent within 72 h postoperatively. The recommendation for prophylaxis in those at high risk is preoperative anticoagulation with warfarin. No prophylaxis is recommended for those at low risk (e.g., those less than age 40 with normal weight and no venous disease). Prophylactic regimens for those at moderate risk are basically chemical or mechanical, and the best two, which have equivalent effectiveness, are representative of each type. First, low-dose heparin (5000 units) started 2 h preoperatively and continued every 12 h postoperatively will decrease the risk of deep vein thrombosis from 25 to 7 percent and of major pulmonary embolus from 6 to 0.6 percent. External pneumatic compression devices not only obviate venous stasis, but they also have a systemic effect on coagulation, such that use on the arms also significantly reduces venous thromboembolism of the lower extremities. Early ambulation, elastic stockings, leg elevation, and dipyridamole (Persantine) alone have not been documented to be effective.

43. The answer is E (all). *(Wilmore, vol 2, sect 9, chap 1, pp 33–35.)* It is important to identify and treat occult or early sepsis before it progresses to septic shock and the associated complications of multiple organ failure. An immunocompromised host may not manifest some of the more typical signs and symptoms of infection, such as elevated temperature and white count; this forces the clinician to focus on more subtle signs and symptoms. Early sepsis is a physiologically hyperdynamic, hypermetabolic state representing a surge of catecholamines, cortisol, and other stress-related hormones. A changing mental status, tachypnea that leads to respiratory alkalosis, and flushed skin are often the earliest manifestations of sepsis. Intermittent hypotension requiring increased fluid resuscitation to maintain adequate urine output is characteristic of occult sepsis. Hyperglycemia and insulin resistance during sepsis are typical in diabetic as well as nondiabetic patients. This relates to the gluconeogenic state of the stress response. The cardiovascular response to early sepsis is characterized by an increased cardiac output, decreased systemic vascular resistance, and decreased peripheral utilization of oxygen, which yields a decreased arteriovenous oxygen difference.

44–46. (The answers are 44-D, 45-C, 46-A. *(Schwartz, 6/e, p 65.)* One of the commonest causes of dehydration and metabolic disarray in surgical patients is the failure to replace gastrointestinal losses. External losses can often be collected for measurement of volume and ionic composition. Accurate replacement of these measured losses is clearly the best method of avoiding imbalance. However, a knowledge of the ionic composition of the intestinal contents at various sites permits an accurate estimate for early replacement. Most of these secretions start as extracellular fluid (with a composition similar to that of plasma) and are modified by intestinal glands. The stomach substitutes hydrogen ions for sodium and thus eliminates all but a tiny fraction of bicarbonate. The glands of the small intestine secrete various amounts of bicarbonate; the chloride content is depressed to an equivalent degree (to maintain ionic balance). Colonic contents (stool) and saliva are most notable for their potassium content. Stool also has a high bicarbonate content. Severe diarrhea can therefore cause potassium depletion and a metabolic acidosis.

47–50. The answers are 47-C, 48-B, 49-D, 50-A. *(Schwartz, 6/e, pp 633–634.)* Resting energy expenditure in the nonstressed patient is approximately 10 percent greater than basal energy expenditure. The resting energy expenditure increases directly proportional to the degree of stress. Studies by Kinney and associates using indirect calorimetry have documented the relative degree of increase in resting energy expenditure for a variety of clinical situations. The following table summarizes these results:

Clinical Situation	Change in Energy Expenditure
Prolonged starvation	Decreased 10–30%
Skeletal trauma	Increased 10–30%
Sepsis	Increased 30–60%
3rd degree burns over greater than 20% BSA	Increased 50–100%

Critical Care: Anesthesiology, Blood Gases, Respiratory Care

DIRECTIONS: Each question below contains five suggested responses. Select the **one best** response to each question.

51. The most common physiologic cause of hypoxemia is

(A) hypoventilation
(B) incomplete alveolar oxygen diffusion
(C) ventilation-perfusion inequality
(D) pulmonary shunt flow
(E) elevated erythrocyte 2,3-diphosphoglycerate level (2,3-DPG)

52. Generally accepted indications for mechanical ventilatory support include all the following EXCEPT

(A) Pa_{O_2} of less than 60 torr and Pa_{CO_2} of greater than 60 torr while breathing room air
(B) alveolar-arterial oxygen tension difference of 350 torr while breathing 100% O_2
(C) vital capacity of 40 to 60 mL/kg
(D) respiratory rate greater than 35 breaths per minute
(E) a dead space–tidal volume ratio (V_D/V_T) greater than 0.6

53. In a hemolytic reaction caused by an incompatible blood transfusion, the treatment that is LEAST likely to be helpful is

(A) promoting a diuresis with 20 percent mannitol
(B) preventing anuria through fluid and potassium replacement
(C) alkalinizing the urine with sodium bicarbonate
(D) inserting a Foley catheter to monitor hourly urine output
(E) stopping the blood transfusion immediately

54. Which of the following inhalation anesthetics accumulates in air-filled cavities during general anesthesia?

(A) Diethyl ether
(B) Nitrous oxide
(C) Halothane
(D) Methoxyflurane
(E) Trichloroethylene

55. Major alterations in pulmonary function associated with adult respiratory distress syndrome (ARDS) include all the following EXCEPT

(A) hypoxemia
(B) decreased pulmonary compliance
(C) diffuse interstitial pattern on x-ray
(D) increased functional residual capacity
(E) increased dead-space ventilation

56. The curve depicted below plots the normal relationship of arterial P_{O_2} and percentage of hemoglobin saturation with other variables controlled at pH 7.4, Pa_{CO_2} 40 torr, temperature 37°C (98.6°F), and hemoglobin 15 g/dL. All the following statements regarding this oxygen dissociation relationship are true EXCEPT that

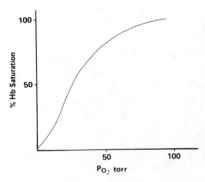

(A) modest decrements of arterial P_{O_2} have little effect on alveolar oxygen uptake
(B) modest decrements of hemoglobin saturation have little effect on tissue oxygen uptake
· (C) the curve shifts to the right with acidosis
(D) the curve shifts to the left following banked blood transfusion
(E) the curve is unaffected by chronic lung disease

57. A 64-year-old man afflicted with severe emphysema, who receives oxygen therapy at home, is admitted to the hospital because of upper gastrointestinal bleeding. The bleeding ceases soon after admission, and the patient becomes agitated and then disoriented; he is given intramuscular diazepam (Valium), 5 mg. Twenty minutes later he is unresponsive. Physical examination reveals a stuporous but arousable man who has papilledema and asterixis. Arterial blood gases are pH 7.17, P_{O_2} 42 torr, P_{CO_2} 95 torr. The best immediate therapy would be to

(A) correct hypoxemia with high-flow nasal oxygen
(B) correct acidosis with sodium bicarbonate
(C) administer intravenous dexamethasone, 10 mg
(D) intubate the patient
(E) call for neurosurgical consultation

58. Dopamine is a frequently used drug in critically ill patients because

(A) at high doses it increases splanchnic flow
(B) at high doses it increases coronary flow
(C) at low doses it decreases heart rate
(D) at low doses it lowers peripheral resistance
(E) it inhibits catecholamine release

59. True statements regarding transmission of viral illness through homologous blood transfusion include all the following EXCEPT

(A) the most common viral agent transmitted via blood transfusion is cytomegalovirus (CMV)
(B) blood is not routinely tested for CMV because CMV infection is endemic in the United States
(C) the most frequent infectious complication of blood transfusion continues to be non-A, non-B hepatitis
(D) up to 10 percent of those who develop posttransfusion hepatitis will develop cirrhosis or hepatoma or both
(E) despite recent identification of the hepatitis C virus and anti-hepatitis C antibody, the etiologic agent in posttransfusion hepatitis remains undiscovered

Questions 60–61

A 68-year-old hypertensive man underwent successful repair of a ruptured abdominal aortic aneurysm. He received 9 L Ringer's lactate solution and 4 units of whole blood during the operation. Two hours after transfer to the surgical intensive care unit, the following hemodynamic parameters are obtained:

Systemic blood pressure (BP): 90/60 mmHg
Pulse rate: 110 beats per minute
Central venous pressure (CVP): 7 mmHg
Pulmonary artery pressure: 28/10
Pulmonary capillary wedge pressure: 8 mmHg
Cardiac output: 1.9 L/min
Systemic vascular resistance: 35 Woods units (normal 24 to 30 Woods units)
Pa_{O_2}: 140 torr (FI_{O_2} 0.45)
Urine output: 15 mL/h (specific gravity 1.029)
Hematocrit: 35 percent

60. Proper management would now call for

(A) administration of a diuretic to increase urine output
(B) administration of a vasopressor agent to increase the systemic blood pressure
(C) administration of a fluid challenge to increase the urine output
(D) administration of a vasodilating agent to decrease the elevated systemic vascular resistance
(E) a period of observation to obtain more data

61. The patient then has an improvement in all hemodynamic parameters. However, 6 h later he develops ST-segment depression, and a 12-lead cardiogram shows anterolateral ischemia. New hemodynamic parameters are obtained:

Systemic BP: 70/40 mmHg
Pulse rate: 100 beats per minute
Central venous pressure (CVP): 18 cmH$_2$O
Pulmonary capillary wedge pressure (PCWP): 25 mmHg
Cardiac output: 1.5 L/min
Systemic vascular resistance: 25 Woods units

The single best pharmacological intervention would be

(A) sublingual nitroglycerin
(B) intravenous nitroglycerin
(C) a short-acting beta blocker
(D) sodium nitroprusside
(E) dobutamine

62. A 56-year-old man undergoes a left upper lobectomy. An epidural catheter is inserted for postoperative pain relief. Ninety minutes after the first dose of epidural morphine the patient complains of itching and is becoming increasingly somnolent. Blood gas measurement reveals the following: pH 7.24, Pa_{CO_2} 58, Pa_{O_2} 100, and HCO_3^- 28. Initial therapy should include

(A) endotracheal intubation
(B) intramuscular diphenhydramine (Benadryl)
(C) epidural naloxone
(D) intravenous naloxone
(E) alternative analgesia

63. If end-diastolic pressure is held constant, increasing which of the following will increase the cardiac index?

(A) Peripheral vascular resistance
(B) Pulmonary wedge pressure
(C) Heart rate
(D) Systemic diastolic pressure
(E) Viscosity of the blood

64. A 73-year-old woman with a long history of heavy smoking undergoes femoral artery–popliteal artery bypass for resting pain in her left leg. Because of serious underlying respiratory insufficiency, she continues to require ventilatory support for 4 days after her operation. As soon as her endotracheal tube is removed, she begins complaining of vague upper abdominal pain. She has daily fever spikes to 39°C (102.2°F) and a leukocyte count of 18,000/mm^3. An upper abdominal ultrasonogram reveals a dilated gallbladder, but no stones are seen. A presumptive diagnosis of acalculous cholecystitis is made. You would recommend

(A) nasogastric suction and broad-spectrum antibiotics
(B) immediate cholecystectomy with operative cholangiogram
(C) percutaneous drainage of the gallbladder
(D) endoscopic retrograde cholangiopancreatography (ERCP) to visualize and drain the common bile duct
(E) provocation of cholecystokinin release by cautious feeding of the patient

Questions 65–67

A 32-year-old man undergoes a distal pancreatectomy, splenectomy, and partial colectomy for a gunshot wound to the left upper
quadrant of the abdomen. One week later he develops a shaking chill
in conjunction with a temperature spike to 39.44°C (103°F). His blood
pressure is 70/0 mmHg with a pulse of 140 beats per minute and his
respiratory rate is 45 breaths per minute. He is transferred to the ICU
where he is intubated and a Swan-Ganz catheter is placed.

65. Which of the following would be most consistent with this
patient's preintubation arterial blood gas measurement?

	pH	Pa_{CO_2}	Pa_{O_2}
(A)	7.31	48	61
(B)	7.52	28	76
(C)	7.45	40	77
(D)	7.40	30	72
(E)	7.40	48	94

66. All the following are consistent with the initial Swan-Ganz catheter readings EXCEPT

(A) cardiac output: 9.0 L/min
(B) peripheral vascular resistance: 1660 dynes
(C) pulmonary artery pressure: 33/3 mmHg
(D) pulmonary capillary wedge pressure: 3 mmHg
(E) central venous pressure: 12 mmHg

67. Initial therapy for this patient would include all the following
EXCEPT

(A) fluid replacement
(B) dopamine
(C) clindamycin
(D) laparotomy
(E) gentamicin

68. The preoperative characteristics of patients likely to experience postoperative ischemia after noncardiac surgery include all the following EXCEPT

(A) angina
(B) previous infarction
(C) dyspnea on exertion
(D) mitral regurgitation
(E) age greater than 70 years

69. True statements regarding perioperative risk of stroke in patients with a past history of stroke include all the following EXCEPT

(A) patients with a past history of stroke who undergo surgery have a low risk of new cerebral infarction
(B) elapsed time from the patient's last stroke to subsequent surgery bears no relationship to the risk of recurrent stroke
(C) the risk of postoperative stroke continues late into the convalescent period
(D) general state of health and severity of illness as measured by ASA classification are significant predictors of recurrent stroke
(E) age and sex are not significant predictors of recurrent stroke

70. The correlation between pulmonary capillary wedge pressure (PCWP) and left ventricular end-diastolic pressure (LVEDP) as measured by pulmonary artery catheterization may be adversely affected by all the following EXCEPT

(A) mitral stenosis
(B) mitral regurgitation
(C) pulmonary vasoocclusive disease
(D) positive-pressure ventilation with positive end-expiratory pressure/continuous positive airway pressure (PEEP/CPAP)
(E) aortic stenosis

71. Compensatory mechanisms during acute hemorrhage include all the following EXCEPT

(A) decreased cerebral and coronary blood flow
(B) vasopressin/angiotensin release
(C) adrenergic discharge
(D) increased respiratory rate
(E) increased renal sodium resorption

72. True statements regarding local anesthetics include all the following EXCEPT

(A) when used for infiltration anesthesia, the maximal safe total dose of lidocaine is 4.5 mg per kilogram of body weight

(B) addition of epinephrine (1:200,000) to the solution of lidocaine, procaine, or bupivacaine does not increase the maximal safe total dose but increases the duration of the block

(C) rare individuals are hypersensitive to local anesthetics

(D) a local anesthetic in contact with a nerve trunk can cause both sensory and motor paralysis in the area innervated

(E) rapid systemic administration of local anesthetics may produce death without signs of CNS stimulation

73. An 18-year-old woman develops urticaria and wheezing after an injection of penicillin. Her blood pressure is 90/60 mmHg, heart rate is 115 beats per minute, and respiratory rate is 30 breaths per minute. Immediate therapy should include all the following EXCEPT

(A) intubation
(B) epinephrine
(C) H_1 and H_2 blockers
(D) aminophylline
(E) hydrocortisone

74. Transfusion hemolysis is associated with all the following EXCEPT

(A) ABO incompatibility
(B) minor blood group incompatibility
(C) transfusion through 5% dextrose and water
(D) transfusion through Ringer's lactate
(E) delayed transfusion reactions

75. When an arterial blood gas determination of P_{CO_2} of 40 torr is obtained

(A) there is probably a paradoxical aciduria
(B) alveolar ventilation is adequate
(C) arterial P_{O_2} will indicate the adequacy of alveolar ventilation
(D) arterial P_{O_2} indicates the degree of ventilation-perfusion mismatch
(E) arterial P_{O_2} can be safely predicted to exceed 90 torr on room air

76. An obese 50-year-old woman undergoes a laparoscopic chole-cystectomy. In the recovery room she is found to be hypotensive and tachycardic. Her arterial blood gases reveal a pH of 7.29, partial pressure of oxygen is 60 torr, and the partial pressure of CO_2 is 54 torr. The most likely cause of this woman's problem is

(A) acute pulmonary embolism
(B) CO_2 absorption from induced pneumoperitoneum
(C) alveolar hypoventilation
(D) pulmonary edema
(E) atelectasis from high dia-phragm

77. Among patients who require nutritional resuscitation in an intensive care unit, the best evidence that nutritional support is adequate is

(A) urinary nitrogen excretion levels
(B) total serum protein level
(C) serum albumin level
(D) serum transferrin levels
(E) respiratory quotient

78. Paradoxical aciduria (the excretion of acid urine in the presence of metabolic alkalosis) may occur in the presence of

(A) release of inappropriate anti-diuretic hormone
(B) severe crush injury
(C) acute tubular necrosis
(D) gastric outlet obstruction
(E) an eosinophilic pituitary ade-noma

79. If a patient suffered a pulmonary arterial air embolism during an open thoracotomy, the anes-thesiologist's most likely observation would be

(A) unexpected systemic hyper-tension
(B) rising right atrial filling pres-sures
(C) reduced systemic arterial ox-ygen saturation
(D) rising systemic CO_2 partial pressures
(E) falling end-tidal CO_2

80. A 72-year-old man undergoes resection of an abdominal aneurysm. He arrives in the ICU with a core temperature of 33°C (91.4°F) and shivering. The physiological consequence of the shivering is

(A) rise in mixed venous oxygen saturation
(B) increased production of carbon dioxide
(C) decreased consumption of oxygen
(D) rising base excess
(E) decreased minute ventilation

81. To prepare for operation a patient with a bleeding history diagnosed as von Willebrand's disease (recessive), you would give

(A) high-purity factor VIII:C concentrates
(B) low-molecular-weight dex-tran
(C) fresh frozen plasma (FFP)
(D) cryoprecipitate
(E) whole blood

82. Each of the following clinical situations are indications for treatment with extracorporeal membrane oxygenation (ECMO) EXCEPT

(A) a 1-day-old, full-term, 4-kg male suffering from meconium aspiration syndrome and hypoxia
(B) a postoperative cardiac transplant patient with pneumonia and elevated pulmonary arterial pressure
(C) a neonate with a diagnosis of severe pulmonary hypoplasia who is in respiratory failure
(D) as a bridge to cardiac transplantation in a 5-year-old girl
(E) preoperatively in a 3-day-old male with a congenital diaphragmatic hernia

DIRECTIONS: Each question below contains four suggested responses of which **one or more** is correct. Select

A	if	**1, 2, and 3**	are correct
B	if	**1 and 3**	are correct
C	if	**2 and 4**	are correct
D	if	**4**	is correct
E	if	**1, 2, 3, and 4**	are correct

83. The accidental aspiration of gastric contents into the tracheobronchial tree should be treated by

(1) tracheal suctioning
(2) bronchial lavage
(3) ventilatory support
(4) antibiotic administration to cover oropharyngeal anaerobes

84. In performing a tracheostomy, authorities agree that

(1) the strap muscles should be preserved and retracted
(2) the thyroid isthmus may be divided
(3) the trachea should be entered at the second or third cartilaginous ring
(4) only horizontal incisions should be used

85. In patients with a history of malignant hyperthermia who require another operation, one should

(1) pretreat with dantrolene
(2) use depolarizing muscle relaxants
(3) premedicate heavily
(4) acidify the urine

86. Characteristics of continuous arteriovenous hemofiltration (CAVH) in the treatment of surgical patients with acute renal failure include

(1) CAVH is useful only in hemodynamically stable patients
(2) CAVH requires placement of large-bore (8 French) arterial and venous catheters, usually in the femoral vessels
(3) CAVH results in clearance of solutes (such as urea, creatinine, or potassium), but is not effective in treating hypervolemia
(4) continuous heparinization of the patient who undergoes CAVH is necessary, which increases the potential for bleeding complications

87. Noncardiac factors that can increase central venous pressure (CVP) include

(1) hypervolemia
(2) positive pressure ventilation
(3) pneumothorax
(4) flail chest

SUMMARY OF DIRECTIONS

A	B	C	D	E
1,2,3 only	1,3 only	2,4 only	4 only	All are correct

88. Signs and symptoms of un-suspected Addison's disease include

(1) hypothermia
(2) hypokalemia
(3) hyperglycemia
(4) hyponatremia

89. Correct statements concerning managing the airway in the severely traumatized patient include which of the following?

(1) Awake intubation is contraindicated in patients with penetrating ocular injuries
(2) Awake intubation or rapid-sequence induction of anesthesia with intravenous thiobarbiturate followed by succinylcholine is the method of choice if intubation is deemed necessary
(3) Steroids have not been shown to be of value in the management of aspiration of acidic gastric secretions
(4) Prior to endotracheal intubation, it is safe to assume that the patient's stomach is empty if a reliable history is obtained indicating that the last ingestion of food or liquid occurred 8 h before arrival in the emergency room

90. Treatment for clostridial myonecrosis (gas gangrene) includes which of the following measures?

(1) Administration of penicillin
(2) Administration of hyperbaric oxygen
(3) Wide debridement
(4) Administration of antitoxin

91. An abnormal ventilation-perfusion ratio (Qs/Qr) in the postoperative patient can result from

(1) a supine position
(2) obesity
(3) atelectasis
(4) reduced cardiac output

92. Correct statements concerning drowning or near-drowning include which of the following?

(1) The prognosis for recovery of cerebral function in affected persons is better if submersion occurs in cool water rather than extremely cold water
(2) The presence of a significant metabolic acidosis in affected persons frequently requires the administration of intravenous sodium bicarbonate
(3) Prompt administration of corticosteroids to affected persons has been shown to decrease the extent of pulmonary membrane damage
(4) Renal damage may occur in affected persons as a result of hemoglobinuria

93. Etiologic factors implicated in the development of posttraumatic pulmonary insufficiency include

(1) increase of vasoactive substances
(2) microembolization of platelet aggregates
(3) fluid overload
(4) increased pulmonary surfactant

94. Spontaneous retroperitoneal hemorrhage during anticoagulant therapy

(1) is best confirmed by computed tomography (CT scan)
(2) is equally likely with parenteral and oral anticoagulants
(3) may mimic an acute surgical abdomen
(4) frequently requires laparotomy for ligation of the bleeding site

95. Correct statements concerning smoke inhalation ("smoke poisoning") include which of the following?

(1) "Smoke poisoning" is a chemical rather than thermal injury
(2) Carbon monoxide levels are usually elevated
(3) Chest x-rays during the early postinhalation period are usually normal
(4) Visible damage to the respiratory tract is commonly found

96. The number of drug smugglers has increased considerably over the past decade. Indications for surgical intervention to remove drug packets that have been ingested include

(1) bowel obstruction or perforation
(2) failure of endoscopic retrieval
(3) signs of toxicity from leaking drug packets
(4) intraintestinal drug packets evident on abdominal x-ray in an asymptomatic smuggler

DIRECTIONS: The group of questions below consists of four lettered headings followed by a set of numbered items. For each numbered item select

A	if the item is associated with	(A) **only**
B	if the item is associated with	(B) **only**
C	if the item is associated with	**both** (A) and (B)
D	if the item is associated with	**neither** (A) nor (B)

Each lettered heading may be used **once, more than once, or not at all.**

Questions 97–99

    (A) Normovolemic gram-negative sepsis
    (B) Hypovolemic gram-negative sepsis
    (C) Both
    (D) Neither

97. High cardiac output

98. Increased peripheral vascular resistance

99. Respiratory alkalosis

DIRECTIONS: Each group of questions below consists of lettered headings followed by a set of numbered items. For each numbered item select the **one** lettered heading with which it is **most** closely associated. Each lettered heading may be used **once, more than once, or not at all.**

Questions 100–102

Match the side effects below with the appropriate anesthetic.

(A) Nitrous oxide (N_2O)
(B) Halothane
(C) Methoxyflurane
(D) Enflurane
(E) Morphine

100. Seizures

101. Decreased peripheral resistance

102. Possible worsening of distention in bowel obstruction

Questions 103–105

Match the tests below with the coagulation system they evaluate.

(A) Intrinsic pathway
(B) Fibrinogen function
(C) Platelet function
(D) Extrinsic pathway
(E) None of the above

103. Bleeding time

104. Partial thromboplastin time

105. Prothrombin time

Critical Care: Anesthesiology, Blood Gases, Respiratory Care

Answers

51. The answer is C. *(Hall, pp 7–9.)* Although hypoventilation, incomplete oxygen diffusion, and pulmonary shunts all are causes of hypoxemia, the most common cause is ventilation-perfusion inequality. The mismatch of ventilation and blood flow occurs to some degree in the normal upright lung but may become extreme in the diseased lung. The three indices used to measure ventilation-perfusion inequality are alveolar-arterial P_{O_2} difference, physiologic shunt (venous-admixture), and alveolar dead space. Elevated 2,3-diphosphoglycerate (2,3-DPG) levels shift the oxygen dissociation curve to the right and thereby augment tissue oxygenation. This elevation does not result in hypoxemia.

52. The answer is C. *(Schwartz, 6/e, p 468.)* Anticipation and early aggressive treatment of pulmonary insufficiency by mechanical ventilatory support are critical in managing the seriously ill patient. Readily measured changes that can be used to determine either the need for intubation or the appropriate time for weaning from mechanical respiratory support include arterial blood gas levels, dead space–tidal volume ratio (V_D/V_T), alveolar-arterial oxygen tension difference (A-a)D_{O_2}, vital capacity, and respiratory rate. Indications for mechanical ventilation include a respiratory rate over 35 breaths per minute, vital capacity less than 15 mL/kg, (A-a)D_{O_2} greater than 350 torr after 15 min on 100% oxygen, V_D/V_T greater than 0.6, Pa_{O_2} less than 60 torr, and a Pa_{CO_2} greater than 60 torr.

53. The answer is B. *(Schwartz, 6/e, pp 115–117.)* Whenever a hemolytic reaction caused by an incompatible blood transfusion is suspected, the transfusion should be stopped immediately. A Foley catheter should be inserted, and hourly urine output should be monitored. Renal damage caused by precipitation of hemoglobin in the renal tubules is the major serious consequence of the hemolysis. This precipitation is inhibited in an alkaline environment and is promoted in an acid environment. Stimulating diuresis with 100 mL of 20% mannitol and alkalinizing the urine with 45 meq sodium bicarbonate intravenously are indicated procedures. Fluid and potassium intake should be restricted in the presence of severe oliguria or anuria.

54. The answer is B. *(Hardy, 2/e, pp 252–253.)* Nitrous oxide (N_2O) has a low solubility compared with other inhalation anesthetics. Its blood:gas partition coefficient is 0.47, and it is 30 times more soluble in blood than is nitrogen (N_2). N_2O is also the only anesthetic gas less dense than air. As a result of these properties, N_2O may cause progressive distention of air-filled spaces during prolonged anesthesia. This can lead to undesirable situations whenever there is a pneumothorax or intestinal obstruction or when procedures like pneumoventriculography (in which the intracranial air space is not free to expand in response to the diffusion of gas into the ventricles) are performed. In each of these cases the N_2O diffuses into the gas-filled compartment faster than N_2 can diffuse out. Since the typical mixture of ingested air (or pneumothorax air) is 80% N_2 and the usual mixture of nitrous oxide anesthetic gas is 80% N_2O, rapid increase in the size of gas-filled chambers with potentially serious consequences may occur.

55. The answer is D. *(Schwartz, 6/e, pp 123–130.)* Adult respiratory distress syndrome (ARDS) has been called "shock lung" or "traumatic wet lung" and occurs under a variety of circumstances. Clinically, its manifestations can range from minimal dysfunction to unrelenting pulmonary failure. Three major physiologic alterations include (1) hypoxemia usually unresponsive to elevations of inspired oxygen concentration; (2) decreased pulmonary compliance, as the lungs become progressively "stiffer" and harder to ventilate; and (3) decreased functional residual capacity. Progressive alveolar collapse occurs owing to leakage of protein-rich fluid into the interstitium and the alveolar spaces with the subsequent radiologic picture of diffuse, fluffy infiltrates bilaterally. Ventilatory abnormalities develop that result in shunt formation, decreased resting lung volume, and increased dead-space ventilation.

56. The answer is E. *(Hall, pp 6–9.)* The shape of the oxygen dissociation curve translates into several physiologic advantages. The relatively flat slope above a P_{O_2} of 50 torr means that, in this region of the curve, hemoglobin saturation decreases slightly with decrements in P_{O_2}; loading of oxygen at the alveolar level is therefore affected minimally with mild-to-moderate degrees of hypoxemia. The steeper slope at the lower end of the curve means that, as the hemoglobin becomes desaturated, arterial P_{O_2} drops only minimally, and a gradient that favors oxygen diffusion into tissue cells is maintained. Acidosis, a rise in Pa_{CO_2}, and elevation of temperature all shift the curve to the right, which enhances tissue oxygen uptake. Red blood cell organic phosphates, particularly 2,3-diphosphoglycerate (DPG), also affect the dissociation curve. Banked blood, low in 2,3-DPG, shifts the curve to the left and therefore decreases tissue oxygen uptake. 2,3-DPG levels increase with chronic hypoxia. Chronic lung disease, therefore, results in a shift of the curve to the right, which enhances oxygen delivery to peripheral tissues.

57. The answer is D. *(Schwartz, 6/e, pp 467–468.)* The patient presented in the question is suffering from acute, life-threatening respiratory acidosis that has been compounded, if not produced, by the injudicious administration of a central nervous system depressant. While hypoxemia must also be corrected, the immediate task is to correct the acidosis caused by carbon dioxide accumulation. Both disturbances can be resolved by skillful endotracheal intubation and by ventilatory support. Sodium bicarbonate and high-flow nasal oxygen would both be inappropriate. Bicarbonate should not be administered because buffer reserves already are adequate (serum bicarbonate is still 34 meq/L based on the Henderson-Hasselbalch equation). Nasal oxygen administration is not warranted because both acidemia and hypoxemia are themselves potent stimulants to spontaneous ventilation. Headache, confusion, and papilledema are all signs of acute carbon dioxide retention and do not imply the presence of a structural intracranial lesion.

58. The answer is B. *(Tintinalli, 3/e, pp 112–115.)* Dopamine has a variety of pharmacological characteristics that make it useful in critically ill patients. In low doses (1 to 5 μg/kg/min), dopamine affects primarily the dopaminergic receptors. Activation of these receptors causes vasodilation of the renal and mesenteric vasculature and mild vasoconstriction of the peripheral bed, which thereby redirects blood flow to kidneys and bowel. At these low doses the net effect on the overall vascular resistance may be slight. As the dose rises (2 to 10 μg/kg/min), *beta*$_1$-receptor activity predominates and the inotropic effect on the myocardium leads to increased cardiac output and blood pressure. Above 10 μg/kg/min *alpha*-receptor stimulation causes peripheral vasoconstriction, shifting of blood from extremities to organs, decreased kidney function, and hypertension. At all doses, the diastolic blood pressure can be expected to rise; since coronary perfusion is largely a result of the head of pressure at the coronary ostia, coronary blood flow should be increased.

59. The answer is E. *(Goodnough, Am J Surg 159:602–609, 1990.)* Cytomegalovirus (CMV) is harbored in blood leukocytes. CMV infection is endemic in the United States, and its prevalence increases steadily with age. While acute CMV infection may cause transient fever, jaundice, and hepatosplenomegaly in cases of large blood donor exposures, posttransfusion CMV infection (seroconversion) is not a significant clinical problem in immunocompetent recipients, and therefore blood is not routinely tested for the presence of CMV. Posttransfusion non-A, non-B hepatitis, however, represents not only the most frequent infectious complication of transfusion, but is associated with an incidence of chronic active hepatitis up to 16 percent and an 8 to 10 percent incidence of cirrhosis or hepatoma or both. The etiologic agent in over 90 percent of cases of posttransfusion hepatitis has been identified as hepatitis C.

60. The answer is C. *(Schwartz, 6/e, pp 65–66.)* A ruptured abdominal aneurysm is a surgical emergency often accompanied by serious hypotension and vascular collapse before surgery and massive fluid shifts with renal failure after surgery. In this case, all the hemodynamic parameters indicate inadequate intravascular volume, and the patient is therefore suffering from hypovolemic hypotension. The low urine output indicates poor renal perfusion, while the high urine specific gravity indicates adequate renal function with compensatory free water conservation. The administration of a vasopressor agent would certainly raise the blood pressure, but it would do so by increasing peripheral vascular resistance and thereby further decrease tissue perfusion. The deleterious effects of shock would be increased. A vasodilating agent to lower the systemic vascular resistance would lead to profound hypotension and possibly complete vascular collapse because of pooling of an already depleted vascular volume. This patient's blood pressure is critically dependent on an elevated systemic vascular resistance. To properly treat this patient, rapid fluid infusion and expansion of the intravascular volume must be undertaken. This can be easily done with lactated Ringer's solution or blood (or both) until improvements in such parameters as the pulmonary capillary wedge pressure, urine output, and blood pressure are noted.

61. The answer is E. *(Schwartz, 6/e, p 140.)* This patient has developed pump failure due to a combination of preexisting coronary artery occlusive disease and high preload following a fluid challenge; afterload remains moderately high as well because of systemic vasoconstriction in the presence of cardiogenic shock. Poor myocardial performance is reflected in the low cardiac output and high pulmonary capillary wedge pressure. Therapy must be directed at increasing cardiac output without creating too high a myocardial oxygen demand on the already-failing heart. Administration of nitroglycerin could be expected to reduce both preload and afterload, but if it is given without an inotrope it would create unacceptable hypotension. Nitroprusside similarly would achieve afterload reduction but would result in hypotension if it was not accompanied by an inotropic agent. A beta blocker would act deleteriously by reducing cardiac contractility and slowing the heart rate in a setting in which cardiac output is likely to be rate-dependent. Dobutamine is a synthetic catecholamine that is becoming the inotropic agent of choice in cardiogenic shock. As a beta$_1$-adrenergic agonist, it improves cardiac performance in pump failure both by positive inotropy and peripheral vasodilation. With minimal chronotropic effect, dobutamine only marginally increases myocardial oxygen demand.

62. The answer is D. *(Miller, 3/e, pp 1103–1107. Thoren, Anesth Analg 67:687, 1988.)* Thoracic epidural narcotics have become an increasingly popular means of postoperative pain relief in thoracic and upper abdominal surgery. Local action on gamma opiate receptors ensures pain relief and consequent improvement in respiration without vasodilation or paralysis. The less lipid-soluble opiates are effective for long periods. Their slow absorption into the circulation also ensures a low incidence of centrally mediated side effects, such as respiratory depression or generalized itching. When these do occur, the intravenous injection of an opiate antagonist is an effective antidote. The locally mediated analgesia is not affected. One poorly understood side effect, which is apparently unrelated to systemic levels, is a profound reduction in gastric activity. This may be an important consideration after thoracic surgery when an early resumption of oral intake is anticipated.

63. The answer is C. *(Schwartz, 6/e, p 496.)* The cardiac index is computed by dividing the cardiac output by the body surface area; the cardiac output is the product of the stroke volume and the heart rate (CI = CO/BSA; CO = SV × HR; therefore, CI = [SV × HR]/BSA).

Therefore an increased heart rate will directly increase the cardiac output and cardiac index. The remaining choices in the question will either decrease or not affect the stroke volume and consequently will not increase the cardiac index.

64. The answer is C. *(Boland, New Horizons 2:246–260, 1993.)* The development of acute postoperative cholecystitis is an increasingly recognized complication of the severe illnesses that precipitate admissions to the intensive care unit. The causes are obscure but probably lead to a common final pathway of gallbladder ischemia. The diagnosis is often extremely difficult because the signs and symptoms may be those of occult sepsis. Moreover, the patients are often intubated, sedated, or confused as a consequence of the other therapeutic or medical factors. Biochemical tests, though frequently revealing abnormal liver function, are nonspecific and nondiagnostic. Bedside ultrasonography is usually strongly suggestive of the diagnosis when a thickened gallbladder wall or pericholecystic fluid is present, but radiological findings may also be nondiagnostic. If the diagnosis is delayed, mortality and morbidity are very high. Percutaneous drainage of the gallbladder is usually curative of acalculous cholecystitis and affords stabilizing palliation if calculous cholecystitis is present. Some authors have recommended prophylactic percutaneous drainage of the gallbladder under CT guidance in any ICU patient who is failing to thrive or has other signs of low-grade sepsis after appropriate therapy of the primary illness has been provided. The distractor items in the question are all either too aggressive to be safely done in critically ill patients or too cautious for a patient with a potentially fatal complication.

65–67. The answers are 65-B, 66-B, 67-D. *(Schwartz, 6/e, pp 140–143.)* The case presented is most consistent with septic shock from a postoperative intraabdominal abscess. In the early phase of septic shock the respiratory profile is characterized by mild hypoxia with a compensatory hyperventilation and respiratory alkalosis. Hemodynamically a hyperdynamic state is seen with an increase in cardiac output and a decrease in peripheral vascular resistance in the face of relatively normal central pressures. Initial therapy is aimed at resuscitation and stabilization. This includes fluid replacement and vasopressors as well as antibiotic therapy aimed particularly at gram-negative rods and anaerobes for patients with presumed intraabdominal collections, especially after bowel surgery. Laparotomy and drainage of a collection is the definitive therapy but should await stabilization of the patient and confirmation of the presence and location of such a collection.

68. The answer is A. *(Charlson, Ann Surg 210:637–648, 1989.)* The landmark study by Goldman in 1978 identified cardiac risk factors in noncardiac surgical patients that included previous infarction (particularly infarction within 6 months, but with increased risk continuing for life), functional impairment such as dyspnea on exertion, age over 70 years, mitral regurgitation, more than five premature ventricular contractions (PVCs) per minute, and a tortuous or calcified aorta. Angina alone was not a risk factor. Subsequent studies by others have differed regarding the importance of several of these factors, which probably reflects different comorbid characteristics in the study populations (e.g., diabetes and hypertension). Additional predictors of perioperative cardiac risk that achieved significance in some studies but not in others include cardiomegaly, upper abdominal or intrathoracic surgery, and intraoperative hypotension.

69. The answer is D. *(Landercasper, Arch Surg 125:986–989, 1990.)* In an 8-year, retrospective study of 173 consecutive patients with a documented medical history of stroke who underwent subsequent general anesthesia and surgery (excluding cardiac, cerebrovascular, and neurological surgery), 5 patients (2.9 percent) had documented postoperative strokes from 3 to 21 days (mean 12.2 days) after surgery. The risk of stroke did not correlate with age, sex, history of multiple strokes or poststroke transient ischemic attacks (TIAs), ASA classification, aspirin use, coronary artery disease, peripheral vascular disease, intraoperative blood pressure, time since previous stroke, or cause of previous stroke. The risk of recurrent stroke appears to be comparable with that of surgical patients who do not have a history of prior stroke and are undergoing cardiac and peripheral vascular surgery. Most recurrent strokes occur many hours to days following surgery and do not appear directly related to operative events. The mortality after postoperative stroke is high.

70. The answer is E. *(Hall, pp 334–336.)* When a Swan-Ganz pulmonary artery catheter is in the wedge position, i.e., isolating the pulmonary arterial system from the pulmonary capillaries, the measured pulmonary capillary wedge pressure (PCWP) is usually equivalent to both the left atrial pressure (LAP) and the left ventricular end-diastolic pressure (LVEDP). Pathological processes in the pulmonary vasculature and heart valves, however, may alter this relationship. Pulmonary vasoocclusive disease may elevate the PCWP independently of the LAP or LVEDP. Mitral stenosis and regurgitation cause increased LAP and

PCWP, which results in an overestimated LVEDP. However, aortic stenosis elevates the PCWP, LAP, and LVEDP equally. Accurate measurement of PCWP by a Swan-Ganz catheter may not be possible in the presence of positive airway pressure with PEEP/CPAP; transmission of the positive airway pressure to the pulmonary microvasculature via the alveolus, especially in the upper lung zones, results in measurement of alveolar pressure rather than LAP or LVEDP.

71. The answer is A. *(Schwartz, 6/e, pp 119–120.)* Acute hemorrhage triggers the potent vasopressor activity of both angiotensin and vasopressin to increase blood flow to the heart and brain via selective vasoconstriction of the skin, kidneys, and splanchnic organs. Adrenergic discharge also results in selective vasoconstriction of skin, renal, and splanchnic vessels. Myocardial contractility and heart rate are increased, with a resultant increased cardiac output. Hyperventilation is the typical response to the metabolic (lactic) acidosis associated with hemorrhagic shock and hypoperfusion. Aldosterone release, with subsequent increased renal sodium resorption, is mediated by angiotensin II and ACTH, which prevents further intravascular depletion.

72. The answer is B. *(Hall, pp 1509–1510.)* The maximal safe total dose of lidocaine administered to a 70-kg man is 4.5 mg/kg, or approximately 30 to 35 mL of a 1% solution. The addition of epinephrine to lidocaine, procaine, or bupivacaine not only doubles the duration of infiltration anesthesia, but increases by one-third the maximal safe total dose by decreasing the rate of absorption of drug into the bloodstream. Epinephrine-containing solutions should not, however, be injected into tissues supplied by end arteries (e.g., fingers, toes, ears, nose, penis). Hypersensitivity to local anesthetics is uncommon and occurs most prominently with anesthetics of the ester type (procaine, tetracaine). While small nerve fibers seem to be most susceptible to the action of local anesthetics, these agents act on any part of the nervous system and on every type of nerve fiber. CNS toxicity usually appears as stimulation followed by depression, probably because of an early selective depression of inhibitory neurons; with a massive overdose, all neurons may be depressed simultaneously.

73. The answer is A. *(Hall, pp 1047–1056, 2072–2073.)* This patient is having an anaphylactoid reaction with destabilization of the cardiovascular and respiratory systems. Anaphylactoid reactions are most commonly caused by iodinated contrast media, β-lactam antibiotics (e.g., penicillin), and Hymenoptera stings. Manifestations of anaphylactoid reactions include both the lethal (bronchospasm, laryngospasm, hypotension, dysrhythmia) and the nonlethal (pruritus, urticaria, syncope, weakness, and seizure). Epinephrine is the initial treatment for laryngeal obstruction and bronchospasm, followed by histamine antagonists, aminophylline, and hydrocortisone. Vasopressors and fluid challenges may be given for shock. Conscious patients are usually stabilized with injected or inhaled epinephrine, while unconscious patients and those with refractory hypotension or hypoxia should be intubated.

74. The answer is D. *(Hall, pp 459–461, 1051.)* Most hemolytic transfusion reactions are due to clerical errors that result in administration of blood with major (ABO) and minor antigen incompatibility. Interestingly, Rh incompatibility is not associated with intravascular hemolysis. Administration of blood through hypotonic solutions such as 5% dextrose and water results in swelling of the erythrocytes and hemolysis. Calcium-containing solutions such as Ringer's lactate cause clotting within the intravascular line rather than hemolysis and may lead to pulmonary embolism. Delayed transfusion reactions, caused by a presumed anamnestic immune response that occurs 3 to 21 days after blood is infused, result in a hemolytic anemia.

75. The answer is B. *(Hall, pp 200–202.)* Because of the highly efficient diffusion characteristics of the gas carbon dioxide, Pa_{CO_2} levels are reliable indicators of adequacy of alveolar ventilation. A Pa_{CO_2} of 40 torr is the normal value. Paradoxical aciduria occurs when hypokalemic metabolic alkalosis is present as the kidney excretes hydrogen ion in an effort to conserve potassium ion. Though a Pa_{CO_2} of 40 torr is not incompatible with metabolic alkalosis, it would ordinarily be higher as the patient tries to conserve carbolic acid by hypoventilating to compensate. Pa_{O_2} levels are influenced by so many other variables (e.g., age, concentration of inspired O_2, altitude) that no inferences can be made about adequacy of alveolar ventilation from Pa_{O_2} alone, nor can Pa_{O_2} be safely predicted by the presence of normocarbia. The ventilation-perfusion mismatch is a reflection of the gradient between alveolar and arterial oxygen tension in relationship to percentage of inspired O_2.

76. The answer is C. *(Hall, pp 984–985.)* Because of the ease with which carbon dioxide diffuses across the alveolar membranes, the Pa_{CO_2} is a highly reliable indicator of alveolar ventilation. In this postoperative patient with respiratory acidosis and hypoxemia, the hypercarbia is diagnostic of alveolar hypoventilation. Acute hypoxemia can occur with pulmonary embolism, pulmonary edema, and significant atelectasis, but in all those situations the CO_2 partial pressures should be normal or reduced as the patient hyperventilates to improve oxygenation. The absorption of gas from the peritoneal cavity may affect transiently the Pa_{CO_2}, but should have no effect on oxygenation.

77. The answer is C. *(Way, 9/e, pp 152–155.)* The serum albumin level provides a rough estimate of protein nutritional adequacy. The accuracy of this estimate is affected by the long half-life of albumin (3 weeks) and vagaries of hemodilution. The acute-phase serum proteins have a very short half-life (hours) and may also provide good short-term indications of nutritional status. Transferrin is one of these acute-phase proteins, but unfortunately its levels too are influenced by changes in intravascular volume and, along with the other acute-phase reactants, rise nonspecifically during acute illness. All the listed responses provide some useful information about nutrition and adequacy of replacement.

78. The answer is D. *(Way, 9/e, pp 148–152.)* The body has elaborate mechanisms to compensate for metabolic acidosis. Not only do most body functions work better in an acidotic state, the patient is able to move toward correction of the pH by excreting acid urine and by hyperventilating to "blow off" carbonic acid. On the other hand, we are poorly equipped to deal with metabolic alkalosis. We cannot hold our breath to save acid since the respiratory center overrides our efforts as the Pa_{CO_2} rises and the Pa_{O_2} falls. The kidney cannot make urine under any circumstance that is very far above normal pH. In the subtraction alkalosis that accompanies gastric outlet obstruction with loss of gastric acid by vomiting or suction, the potassium depletion and volume deficits provoke exchange of sodium for hydrogen ion in the distal tubule with resultant exacerbation of the metabolic alkalosis. All the other conditions listed would be expected to produce acidosis; consequently, acid urine would not be paradoxical.

79. The answer is E. *(Hall, pp 1486–1487.)* Air carried into the pulmonary arterial vasculature creates an abnormal blood-air interface that leads to denaturing of plasma proteins and creates amorphous proteinaceous and cellular debris and endothelial injury. The ensuing increased capillary permeability results in alveolar flooding. The occlusion of pulmonary vessels increases the proportion of ventilated but underperfused alveoli. The increment in dead space results in a drop in end-tidal carbon dioxide.

80. The answer is B. *(Hall, pp 2242–2244.)* Shivering is the physiological effort of the body to generate heat to maintain the core temperature. In healthy persons, shivering will increase the metabolic rate by 3 to 5 times and result in increased oxygen consumption and carbon dioxide production. In critically ill patients these metabolic consequences are almost always counterproductive and should be prevented with other means employed to correct systemic hypothermia. In the presence of vigorous shivering, oxygen debt in the muscles and lactic acidemia develop.

81. The answer is D. *(Hall, p 1826. Schwartz, 6/e, p 522.)* Von Willebrand's disease is similar to true hemophilia in frequency of occurrence. It is being diagnosed more commonly today because of more reliable assays for factor VIII. This autosomally dominant disorder (recessive transmission can occur) is characterized by a diminution in factor VIII:C (procoagulant) activity. The reduction in activity is not as great as that in classic hemophilia, and the clinical manifestations are more subtle. These manifestations are often overlooked until an episode of trauma or surgery makes them apparent. Treatment requires correcting the bleeding time and providing factor VIII R:WF (the von Willebrand factor). Only cryoprecipitate is reliably effective. High-purity factor VIII:C concentrates, effective in hemophilia, lack the von Willebrand factor and are, consequently, undependable.

82. The answer is C . *(Hall, pp 374–382.)* Extracorporeal membrane oxygenation (ECMO) is a form of cardiopulmonary support that is useful in the setting of potentially reversible pulmonary or cardiac disease. Treatment of meconium aspiration syndrome, sepsis, pneumonia, and congenital diaphragmatic hernia (pre- or postoperatively) are thus appropriate uses. The technique is also applicable in some circumstances as a bridge to cardiac or lung transplantation since the outlook for survival is quite good if the child can be maintained in a good physiological state until donor organs are available. Hypoplastic lungs do not have enough surface area to perform adequate gas exchange and are unlikely to mature to a point where they can sustain life. Babies with hypoplastic lungs will be bypass-dependent for life and, consequently, are not candidates for institution of ECMO therapy.

83. The answer is B (1, 3). *(Schwartz, 6/e, p 464.)* Gastric aspiration is best treated by tracheal suctioning, oxygen, and positive pressure ventilation. Bronchoscopy is helpful if particulate matter is causing bronchial obstruction or if the vomitus is found to contain particulate material. Bronchial lavage is no longer recommended, and steroids and prophylactic antibiotics have not been shown to be of value.

84. The answer is A (1, 2, 3). *(Hall, pp 136–138.)* Although tracheostomy is occasionally an emergency procedure, it can be more effectively performed in an operating room where hemostasis and antisepsis are readily achieved. Most authorities recommend a horizontal incision; however, limited direct midline incisions have the advantage of not opening any unnecessary tissue planes and perhaps reducing the incidence of bleeding complications. Both approaches have advocates. In either case, the incision is made just below the cricoid cartilage, the strap muscles are spared and retracted, the thyroid isthmus is divided, if necessary, and the trachea is entered at the second tracheal ring. The second and third tracheal rings are incised vertically, allowing placement of the tracheostomy tube. The first tracheal ring and the cricoid cartilage must be left intact.

85. The answer is B (1, 3). *(Larew, Postgrad Med 85:117–118, 1989. Melton, Anesth Analg 69:437–443, 1989.)* The cause of malignant hyperthermia is unknown; it may develop in an otherwise healthy young man who has tolerated previous surgery without incident. It should be suspected in the presence of a history of unexplained fever, muscle or connective tissue disorder, or a positive family history (evidence suggests an autosomal dominant inheritance pattern). In addition to fever during anesthesia, the syndrome includes tachycardia, increased O_2 consumption, increased CO_2 production, increased serum K^+, myoglobinuria, and acidosis. Rigidity rather than relaxation following succinylcholine injection may be the first clue to its presence. Investigations have shown excess calcium in myoplasm in patients with the disorder.

If reoperation is necessary, one should premedicate heavily, alkalinize the urine, and avoid depolarizing agents such as succinylcholine. Pretreatment for 24 h with dantrolene is helpful; it is thought to act directly on muscle fiber to attenuate calcium release.

86. The answer is C (2, 4). *(Hall, pp 1923–1924.)* Continuous arteriovenous hemofiltration (CAVH) is a relatively new method of therapy for acute renal failure in the intensive care unit. Continuous blood flow is maintained by the hydrostatic pressure gradient between an inflowing arterial cannula and the venous cannula that returns blood to the patient. The blood passes through an extracorporeal membrane, which clears an ultrafiltrate up to 12 L per day. This volume is replaced with an intravenous solution at a rate that achieves the desired fluid balance. CAVH in the surgical patient with acute renal failure allows a slow and continuous removal of fluid and is particularly advantageous in the volume-overloaded patient. Unlike traditional hemodialysis, it can be used over a wide range of blood pressures in the unstable patient. Solutes (such as urea nitrogen and potassium) that are not in the replacement intravenous fluid are also cleared. The main complications associated with CAVH relate to vascular access problems: arterial thrombosis, aneurysm, fistula formation, and infection. Anticoagulation, with the concomitant bleeding risks, must be maintained to prevent thrombosis of the filter and cannulae. The potential for electrolyte imbalance during long-term CAVH requires careful monitoring.

87. The answer is E (all). *(Schwartz, 6/e, p 491.)* Determination of CVP is an integral part of the overall hemodynamic assessment of the patient. This pressure can be affected by a variety of factors including those of cardiac, noncardiac, and artifactual origin. Venous tone, right ventricular compliance, intrathoracic pressure, and blood volume all influence CVP. Vasoconstrictor drugs, positive pressure, ventilation (with and without PEEP), mediastinal compression, and hypervolemia all increase CVP.

88. The answer is D (4). *(Schwartz, 6/e, pp 1574–1576.)* Clinical manifestations of adrenocortical insufficiency include hyperkalemia, hyponatremia, hypoglycemia, fever, weight loss, and dehydration. There is excessive sodium loss in the urine, contraction of the plasma volume, and perhaps hypotension or shock. Classic hyperpigmentation is present in *chronic* Addison's disease only. Addison's disease may present in newborns as a congenital atrophy, as an insidious chronic state often due to tuberculosis, as an acute dysfunction secondary to trauma or adrenal hemorrhage, or as a semiacute adrenal insufficiency seen during stress or surgery. In this last instance, signs and symptoms include nausea, lassitude, vomiting, fever, progressive salt wasting, hyperkalemia, and hypoglycemia. It may be confirmed by measurements of urinary Na^+ loss and absence of response to ACTH.

89. The answer is A (1, 2, 3). *(Hardy, 2/e, pp 147–149.)* Securing a stable airway is one of the most fundamental and important aspects of the management of the severely injured patient. The level of control required will vary from a simple oropharyngeal airway to tracheostomy, depending on the clinical situation. Full control of the airway should be secured in the emergency room if the patient is unstable. Endotracheal intubation will usually be the method chosen, but one should be prepared to do a tracheotomy if attempts at peroral or pernasal intubation are failing or are impractical because of maxillofacial injuries. The most dangerous period is just prior to and during the initial attempts to get control of the airway. Manipulation of the oronasopharynx may provoke combative behavior or vomiting in a patient already confused by drugs, alcohol, hypoxia, or cerebral trauma. The risk of aspiration is high during these initial attempts, and one should make no assumptions about the state of the contents of the patient's stomach. Antacids are recommended just prior to the intubation attempt, if feasible. Although steroids have been recommended in the past, they are no longer considered of value in the management of aspiration of acidic gastric juice. The best management requires prevention of the complication of aspiration. In a reasonably cooperative patient awake intubation with topical anesthesia may help to avoid some of the risks of hypotension, arrhythmia, and aspiration associated with the induction of anesthesia. If awake intubation is inappropriate, then an alternative is rapid-sequence induction with a thiobarbiturate followed by muscle paralysis with succinylcholine. If elevated intracranial pressure is suspected, or in the presence of a penetrating eye injury, awake intubation is contraindicated.

90. The answer is A (1, 2, 3). *(Schwartz, 6/e, p 149.)* The most clinically significant clostridial organism is *Clostridium perfringens*. Muscles infected by this organism undergo myonecrosis owing to the action of a necrotizing, hemolytic exotoxin. Treatment consists of rapid incision and drainage of involved areas and penicillin in large doses. Good results have been obtained with the use of hyperbaric oxygen as an adjunct to surgical and antimicrobial therapies. Antitoxin is of no benefit either prophylactically or therapeutically.

91. The answer is E (all). *(Schwartz, 6/e, pp 201–202.)* Abnormalities of ventilation-perfusion ratio result from the shunting of blood to a hypoventilated lung or from the ventilation of hypoperfused regions of lung tissue. Common predisposing factors in the postoperative patient that contribute to this maldistribution include the assumption of a supine position, thoracic and upper abdominal incisions, obesity, atelectasis, and reduced cardiac output.

92. The answer is C (2, 4). *(Shoemaker, 2/e, pp 39–41.)* The metabolic and physiologic effects of drowning and near-drowning depend upon variables that include fluid temperature, extent of aspiration, and whether the aspirate is fresh water or sea water. Cold-water submersion decreases oxygen consumption and results in preferential shunting of blood flow to the heart and brain. This shunting prolongs the period of submersion that can be endured without irreversible cerebral damage. Return of normal cerebral function after as long as 40 min of submersion in extremely cold water has been reported. One should also remember that cooling below 30°C (86°F) will often cause cardiac arrhythmias. Ten percent of affected patients do not aspirate fluid but succumb to asphyxia because of breath holding or laryngospasm. Seventy percent have a significant metabolic acidosis requiring administration of sodium bicarbonate. Significant electrolyte and blood volume changes may or may not be present, depending on the degree of aspiration and toxicity of the fluid medium. Renal damage may occur as a result of hemoglobinuria (from hemolysis), acidosis, hypoxia, or changes in renal blood flow. The most important initial treatment of drowning victims is ventilation. Mouth-to-mouth or mouth-to-nose ventilation should be begun as soon as possible. Corticosteroids and prophylactic antibiotics are not recommended for the prevention of pulmonary complications. However, some workers feel that steroids may be of value in managing the complication of cerebral edema.

93. The answer is A (1, 2, 3). *(Schwartz, 6/e, p 684.)* Many factors are responsible for those lung changes that lead to pulmonary insufficiency in nonthoracic trauma. Among these factors are microembolization of platelet aggregates, fat particles or debris from infused blood, oxygen toxicity, loss of pulmonary surfactant with subsequent alveolar collapse, sepsis, fluid overload, aspiration, and release of vasoactive substances into the pulmonary circulation. Treatment and prophylaxis include the use of micropore filters, diuretics, positive end-expiratory pressure ventilation (PEEP), holding inspired $F_{I_{O_2}}$ to less than 0.45, treatment of sepsis, and early use of corticosteroids for aspiration and fat embolization.

94. The answer is B (1, 3). *(Hall, p 1497.)* Major hemorrhage that requires the termination of anticoagulant therapy occurs in up to 15 percent of anticoagulated patients. Spontaneous retroperitoneal hemorrhage constitutes a small subset of such cases and can be a fatal complication. Heparin is much more frequently associated with spontaneous retroperitoneal hemorrhage than are oral agents. Advanced patient age and poor regulation of coagulation times also increase the likelihood of bleeding complications. Most cases of retroperitoneal hemorrhage present with flank pain and signs of peritoneal irritations suggestive of an acute intraabdominal process. CT scans are most useful in confirming the diagnosis and following the course of the bleeding. Successful management is usually nonoperative and consists of the discontinuation of anticoagulants, administration of vitamin K or protamine, possible transfusion of clotting factors, and repletion of intravascular volume with intravenous fluids.

95. The answer is A (1, 2, 3). *(Pruitt, J Trauma 30:363–368, 1990.)* Smoke inhalation injuries ("smoke poisoning") and asphyxia account for almost one-third of all fire fatalities. As opposed to respiratory burns, which are thermal injuries of the upper respiratory tract, smoke inhalation is a chemical injury to the distal tracheobronchial tree and alveoli. Most patients admitted for this injury have elevated carbon monoxide levels, but a minority will have physical evidence of skin burns (20 percent) or of oropharyngeal burns (25 percent). Visible damage to the respiratory tract is not a frequent finding. Chest films initially are often negative even in those patients who subsequently develop respiratory failure from pulmonary edema or pneumonitis. Patients with elevated carboxyhemoglobin levels or evidence of smoke inhalation should be hospitalized for a minimum of 24 h for observation regardless of normal arterial blood gases and chest x-ray.

96. The answer is B (1, 3). *(Robinson, Surgery 113:709–711, 1993.)* Some drug smugglers, often called "body packers" or "mules," ingest cocaine or heroin-filled packets and retrieve them at a later date from their stools. The drugs are usually contained in latex or plastic packets. Rupture or leakage of even one bag carries the risk of severe toxicity and death. Although conservative medical management with moderate doses of laxatives is usually safe in stable body packers, close physiological monitoring is necessary until all packets are passed. High doses of laxatives, digital rectal disimpaction, or endoscopic removal create a high risk of rupture of the bags and therefore are generally discouraged. Emergency surgery is indicated when complications develop.

97–99. The answers are 97-A, 98-B, 99-C. *(Schwartz, 6/e, pp 140–143.)* The initial profile of gram-negative sepsis is dependent on the patient's volume status. The normovolemic patient will enter a hyperdynamic state characterized by a high cardiac output with a decreased peripheral vascular resistance, while the hypovolemic patient will maintain a low cardiac output with increased peripheral vascular resistance. Hypotension is present in both situations as is an early respiratory alkalosis secondary to hyperventilation, which is replaced by a metabolic acidosis if the septic state goes untreated. Treatment centers around resolving the sepsis either with antibiotics or antibiotics in conjunction with surgical drainage. Aggressive fluid replacement and pulmonary support are also extremely important.

100–102. The answers are 100-D, 101-E, 102-A. *(Hardy, 2/e, pp 250–255.)* Nitrous oxide (N_2O) is a frequently used inhalation analgesic. However, because the MAC (minimum alveolar anesthetic concentration) is so high (over 100), true anesthesia at one atmosphere pressure cannot be obtained without compromising oxygen delivery to the patient. Since nitrous oxide is thirty times more soluble than nitrogen in blood, it enters a collection of trapped air at a rate faster than nitrogen leaves the collection. Thus, the trapped air will increase in volume. If the trapped air is a result of bowel obstruction, intestinal distention will increase.

Halothane is a very potent inhalation anesthetic with an MAC of 0.75. Cardiovascular depression results from a number of different mechanisms. Hypotension and decreased cardiac output have been associated with a direct depression of myocardial muscle fibers and peripheral vascular smooth muscle fibers. An effect on the medullary vasomotor centers as well as on sympathetic ganglionic transmissions to the heart has been reported.

Enflurane is a halogenated inhalation anesthetic with an MAC of 1.2. It is similar to halothane in its anesthetic characteristics. However, in a small number of normal patients it may induce electroencephalographic changes similar to those seen in epilepsy.

Methoxyflurane is the most potent and least volatile halogenated inhalation anesthetic with an MAC of 0.16. Its clinical use has been curtailed because of the high risk of nephrotoxicity of the free fluoride ions released during its biodegradation.

Morphine is a potent narcotic agent. Its use during general anesthesia can potentiate the analgesic effects of the inhalation agents. It causes histamine release with the risk of hypotension if given in a large bolus dose.

103–105. The answers are 103-C, 104-A, 105-D. *(Schwartz, 6/e, pp 103–108.)* Prothrombin time measures the speed of coagulation in the extrinsic pathway. A tissue source of procoagulant (thromboplastin) with calcium is added to plasma. The test will detect deficiencies in factors II, V, VII, X, and fibrinogen and is used to monitor patients receiving coumarin derivatives. However, even small amounts of heparin will artificially prolong the clotting time so that accurate prothrombin times can only be obtained when the patient has not received heparin for at least 5 h.

The intrinsic pathway is measured by the partial thromboplastin time. This test is sensitive for defects in factors VIII, IX, XI, XII, and all the factors of the extrinsic pathway and is used to monitor the status of patients on heparin.

The bleeding time assesses the interaction of platelets and the formation of the platelet plug. Therefore it will pick up deficiencies in both qualitative and quantitative platelet function. Ingestion of aspirin within 1 week of the test will alter the result.

The thrombin time assesses qualitative abnormalities in fibrinogen and the presence of inhibitors to fibrin polymerization. A standard amount of fibrin is added to a fixed volume of plasma and clotting time is measured.

Skin: Wounds, Infections, Burns; Hands; and Plastic Surgery

DIRECTIONS: Each question below contains five suggested responses. Select the **one best** response to each question.

106. Wasting of the intrinsic muscles of the hand can be expected to follow injury of the

(A) ulnar nerve
(B) radial nerve
(C) brachial nerve
(D) axillary nerve
(E) thenar and hypothenar nerves

107. Although wide surgical excision is the traditional treatment for malignant melanoma, narrow excision of thin (less than 1 mm deep) stage I melanomas has been found to be equally safe and effective when the margin of resection is as small as

(A) 3 mm
(B) 5 mm
(C) 1 cm
(D) 3 cm
(E) 5 cm

108. All the following statements are true EXCEPT

(A) a dehisced wound that is resutured gains strength faster than a primary wound
(B) wounds heal faster at 39°C (102.2°F) than at 37°C (98.6°F)
(C) wound healing is accelerated in an environment of low tissue oxygen
(D) synthesis of new collagen is blocked during periods of deficiency of ascorbic acid
(E) wound healing will not occur normally in the absence of monocytes

Questions 109–110

109. While you are on duty in the emergency room, a 12-year-old boy arrives with pain and inflammation over the ball of his left foot and red streaks extending up the inner aspect of his leg. He remembers removing a wood splinter from the sole of his foot on the previous day. The most likely infecting organism is

(A) *Clostridium perfingens*
(B) *Clostridium tetanus*
(C) *Staphylococcus*
(D) *Escherichia coli*
(E) *Streptococcus*

110. The appropriate antibiotic to prescribe while awaiting specific culture verification is

(A) penicillin
(B) erythromycin
(C) tetracycline
(D) azathioprine
(E) cloxacillin

111. Proper treatment for frostbite consists of

(A) debridement of the affected part followed by silver sulfadiazine dressings
(B) administration of corticosteroids
(C) administration of vasodilators
(D) immersion of the affected part in water at 40 to 44°C (104 to 111.2°F)
(E) rewarming of the affected part at room temperature

112. True statements regarding tendon injuries in the hand include all the following EXCEPT

(A) flexor digitorum superficialis inserts on the middle phalanx
(B) flexor digitorum profundus inserts on the distal phalanx
(C) the tendons of flexor digitorum profundus arise from a common muscle belly
(D) the best results for repair of a flexor tendon are obtained with injuries in the fibroosseous tunnel (zone 2)
(E) the process of healing involves formation of a tenoma

DIRECTIONS: Each question below contains four suggested responses of which **one or more** is correct. Select

A	if	**1, 2, and 3**	are correct
B	if	**1 and 3**	are correct
C	if	**2 and 4**	are correct
D	if	**4**	is correct
E	if	**1, 2, 3, and 4**	are correct

113. Correct statements regarding pyomyositis include

(1) its victims live in the tropics or are immunocompromised
(2) it is a mycobacterial infection
(3) septic complications such as endocarditis, brain abscess, or septic arthritis can occur in advanced cases
(4) abscess formation is rare and most cases can be cured with antibiotics

114. True statements regarding the management of biliary ascaris infections include

(1) hepatobiliary ultrasonography is the mainstay of diagnosis
(2) patients may present with biliary colic, acute cholecystitis, pancreatitis, or liver abscesses
(3) ova and fragments of ascaris serve as nidi for stone formation
(4) endoscopic removal through the ampulla is the treatment of choice

115. A 60-year-old woman presents with the skin lesion shown below, which had been present for 10 years. She reported a history of radiation treatments to that hand for "eczema." Correct statements concerning this lesion include

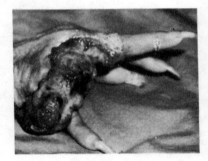

(1) it is more malignant than basal cell carcinoma
(2) it occurs more frequently in blondes
(3) it often metastasizes to regional lymph nodes
(4) it should be treated by radiation therapy

Questions 116–117

A 25-year-old man is brought to the emergency room after sustaining burns during a fire in his apartment. He has blistering and erythema of his face, left upper extremity, and chest with frank charring of his right upper extremity. He is agitated, hypotensive, and tachycardiac.

116. Initial management would include which of the following?

(1) Measurement of arterial blood gas and carboxyhemoglobin level and administration of 100% oxygen

(2) Aggressive intravenous resuscitation with crystalloid for the first 24 h, followed by colloid in accordance with the Parkland formula

(3) Nasogastric decompression and administration of antacids

(4) Prophylactic administration of high-dose penicillin

117. Appropriate initial management of his wounds would include

(1) debridement of blisters in areas of second-degree burn and application of topical antibiotics

(2) immediate deep excision of areas of third-degree burn

(3) elevation of the right arm with application of topical antibiotics and performance of an escharotomy at the first sign of vascular insufficiency

(4) immediate application of split-thickness skin grafts over the eschar of areas of third-degree burn to prevent fluid loss

---

118. True statements regarding squamous cell carcinoma of the lip include

(1) it is the most common cancer of the lip

(2) more than 90 percent of cases occur on the upper lip

(3) the lesion often arises in areas of persistent hyperkeratosis

(4) radiotherapy is considered inappropriate treatment for these lesions

119. Correct statements regarding the carpal tunnel syndrome include which of the following?

(1) It is often secondary to a wrist fracture

(2) It may be associated with pregnancy

(3) it may cause nocturnal dysesthesia

(4) It is often associated with vascular compromise

SUMMARY OF DIRECTIONS

A	B	C	D	E
1,2,3	1,3	2,4	4	All are
only	only	only	only	correct

120. True statements regarding wound healing and wound strength include which of the following?

(1) Initial tensile strength (days 1 to 5) in a wound is due to vascular ingrowth, epithelialization, and accumulation of aggregate proteins
(2) Wound tensile strength continues to increase slowly for approximately 2 years by the slow, on-going deposition of collagen
(3) The major increase in wound tensile strength occurs from days 5 to 17
(4) After approximately 2 years, the scar attains the same tensile strength as that of the surrounding tissue

121. Management of leukoplakia of the oral cavity includes

(1) excisional biopsy of all lesions
(2) improvement of oral hygiene
(3) low-dose radiation therapy
(4) ascertaining that dentures fit properly

122. An 8-lb infant, born following uncomplicated labor and delivery, is noted to have a unilateral cleft lip and palate. The parents should be advised that

(1) the child almost certainly has other congenital anomalies
(2) rehabilitation requires adjunctive speech and hearing therapy
(3) lip repair is indicated at 1 year of age
(4) palate repair is indicated between 1 and 1½ years of age

123. A 40-year-old woman undergoes wide excision of a pigmented lesion of her thigh. Pathologic examination reveals malignant melanoma that is Clark's level IV. Findings on examination of the groin are normal. The patient should be advised that

(1) radiotherapy will be an important part of subsequent therapy
(2) the likelihood of groin node metastases is remote
(3) immunotherapy is an effective form of adjunctive treatment for metastatic malignant melanoma
(4) groin dissection is not indicated unless and until groin nodes become palpable

DIRECTIONS: Each group of questions below consists of four lettered headings followed by a set of numbered items. For each numbered item select

A	if the item is associated with	(A) **only**	
B	if the item is associated with	(B) **only**	
C	if the item is associated with	**both** (A) and (B)	
D	if the item is associated with	**neither** (A) nor (B)	

Each lettered heading may be used **once, more than once, or not at all.**

Questions 124–125

   (A) Basal cell carcinoma
   (B) Squamous cell carcinoma
   (C) Both
   (D) Neither

124. Predominant occurrence in exposed areas, most frequently in weather-beaten skin

125. Improved survival when excision is accompanied by prophylactic lymph node dissection

Questions 126–128

   (A) Port wine stain
   (B) Strawberry hemangioma
   (C) Both
   (D) Neither

126. Flat lesion with uniform color whose growth parallels that of the involved tissue

127. A lesion that grows rapidly during infancy but regresses by age 10 in more than 90 percent of patients

128. Treatment with laser or surgical excision

Questions 129–131

   (A) Clostridial cellulitis
   (B) Clostridial myonecrosis
   (C) Both
   (D) Neither

129. Crepitus

130. Usually mild systemic effects

131. Rapid invasion of uninjured tissue

Skin: Wounds, Infections, Burns; Hands; and Plastic Surgery

Answers

106. The answer is A. *(Way, 9/e, pp 1138–1140.)* The ulnar nerve innervates 15 of the 20 intrinsic muscles of the hand. The musculocutaneous, radial, ulnar, and median nerves are all important to hand function. The musculocutaneous and radial nerves allow forearm supination; the radial nerve alone innervates the extensor muscles. The median nerve is the "eye of the hand" because of its extensive contribution to sensory perception; it also maintains most of the long flexors, the pronators of the forearm, and the thenar muscles.

107. The answer is C. *(Schwartz, 6/e, pp 526–527.)* Wide excision of melanomas, with margins of 3 to 5 cm beyond the lateral edges of tumor, has traditionally been considered mandatory. A 5-year prospective multicenter study of over 600 randomly assigned patients with thin stage I melanomas, however, showed that local recurrence rates, as well as the subsequent development of metastatic disease, were not different when margins of 1 cm or 3 cm were taken, provided that tumor thickness did not exceed 1 mm.

108. The answer is C. *(Davis, pp 461–504.)* Wound healing is decreased, both in rate and in tensile strength, by a decrease in oxygen tension. Therefore, it is important for the patient to have good oxygenation and an adequate hemoglobin. When a normally healing wound is disrupted and resutured, the return of tensile strength is so rapid that the burst strength is nearly what it would have been had the dehiscence not occurred. Wounds heal faster at higher temperatures because of increased blood flow and metabolic rate. Scars appear to undergo remodeling as long as 30 years after injury. There exists an equilibrium between collagen synthesis and collagen destruction that results in this remodeling process. Vitamin C deficiency blocks the synthesis of new collagen and thus destroys the equilibrium and causes disruption of wounds that had healed perfectly months before. Inflammation is necessary for wound healing. The release of various amines from mast cells, the perfusion of capillaries, and accumulation of white cells, especially monocytes and macrophages, are important in providing the best milieu for repair to proceed.

109–110. The answers are 109-E, 110-A. *(Schwartz, 6/e, pp 148–149, 157–158, 165.)* The significant observation in this question is the description of lymphangitic inflammatory streaking up the inner aspect of the patient's leg. This is highly suggestive of a streptococcal infection and the presumptive therapy should be high doses of a bactericidal antibiotic. Penicillin remains the mainstay of therapy against presumed streptococcal infections. Most streptococcal cellulitis is adequately treated by penicillin, elevation of the infected extremity, and attention to the local wound to ascertain adequate local drainage and absence of any persisting foreign body. However, the clinician must be alert to the possibility of a more fulminant and life- or limb-threatening infection by clostridia, micro-aerophilic streptococcus, or other potentially synergistic organisms that can produce rapidly progressive deep infections in fascia of muscle. Smears and cultures of drainage fluid or aspirates should be taken. Close observation of the wound is essential, and aggressive debridement in the operating room is mandatory at the slightest suggestion that fasciitis or myonecrosis may be ensuing.

111. The answer is D. *(Davis, pp 2929–2933.)* Many methods of treating frostbite have been tried throughout the years. These include massage, warm-water immersion, or covering the affected area. Rapid warming by immersion in water slightly above normal body temperature (40 to 44°C) is the most effective method, however, Because the frostbitten region is numb and especially vulnerable, it should be protected from trauma or excessive heat during treatment. Further treatment may include elevation to minimize edema, administration of antibiotics and tetanus toxoid, and debridement of necrotic skin as needed.

112. The answer is D. *(Schwartz, 6/e, pp 1997–2001.)* Each digit has two long flexors, named *superficial* and *deep* according to the relative position of the muscle bellies. In the fingers each superficial flexor tendon divides around the corresponding deep tendon to reach its insertion on the base of the middle phalanx. The deep flexor tendon continues to its insertion on the base of the distal phalanx. Only the deep flexors can flex the distal interphalangeal joint. Since the tendons of the deep flexors share a common muscle belly, only the superficial flexors can move a finger when the adjacent fingers are immobilized. These tendons are prevented from bowstringing across the joints by the flexor retinaculum of the wrist and the fibroosseous tunnels, which extend from the distal palmar crease to the middle phalanx. They run within synovial sheaths and are nourished by vincula tendinum (short mesenteries). The process of healing a tendon injury involves the formation of a tenoma, which tends to become adherent to the surrounding sheath. A difficult balance has to be struck between the desire to prevent adhesions by early mobilization and the risk of rupturing an unhealed tendon. Verdan has divided the hand into six regions according to the anatomy surrounding the tendons. Zone 2, sometimes referred to as "no-man's land," refers to the fibroosseous tunnels. Repair in this region is fraught with difficulty.

113. The answer is B (1, 3). *(Blumberg, South Med J 83:1092–1095, 1990.)* Pyomyositis is a bacterial infection of skeletal muscle, usually caused by *Staphylococcus aureus*. The disease is endemic in tropical areas such as those of South America, Asia, and Africa, but it has recently been increasingly encountered elsewhere in immunocompromised patients, particularly those with HIV infection. The infection tends to involve large skeletal muscles such as the thigh and gluteal muscles. If diagnosed early, it can be cured with antibiotics alone. The majority of cases, however, progress to abscess development and require surgical drainage. Rarely, more serious complications can occur including endocarditis, brain abscess, or septic arthritis, though more commonly the infection responds well to treatment even in immunosuppressed patients, and aggressive treatment with curative intent is warranted.

114. The answer is A (1, 2, 3). *(Khuroo, Br J Surg 79:1335–1338, 1992.)* *Ascaris lumbricoides* is one of the most common helminthic diseases in humans; one-fourth of the world's population harbors ascarides in their gastrointestinal tract. The hepatobiliary tree is the most common ectopic site of infestation. In patients from endemic areas (primarily underdeveloped areas), one needs to be suspicious of ascaris as the etiologic factor in pancreatic or biliary disease. Ultrasound is very successful (approximately 90 percent) in diagnosing ascaris in the biliary system. ERCP is also useful in establishing the diagnosis, but endoscopic removal of the worms should be avoided because of their friability. Treatment depends primarily on the administration of antispasmodic and antihelminthic medications. Surgical exploration and extraction of the worms is necessary in patients who fail to respond to conservative treatment or who develop complications such as deepening jaundice, cholecystitis, associated gallstones, or peritonitis.

115. The answer is A (1, 2, 3). *(Schwartz, 6/e, pp 522–524.)* Squamous cell carcinoma occurs in people who have had chronic sun exposure, chronic ulcers or sinus tracts (draining osteomyelitis), and a history of radiation or thermal injury (Margolin's ulcer). It is more malignant than basal cell carcinoma, grows more rapidly, and metastasizes. The lesions occur more frequently in blondes. A radiation-induced carcinoma, or one arising in a burn scar, should not be treated with radiation therapy for fear of further damage.

116. The answer is A (1, 2, 3). *(Schwartz, 6/e, pp 240–243.)* Initial management of burns is similar to that of all traumatic injuries with attention directed toward maintaining an airway and gas exchange along with cardiovascular support. Burn victims are at risk for both carbon monoxide poisoning and thermal injury to the airways. It is necessary to determine carboxyhemoglobin levels and closely monitor the patient for evidence of developing airway edema, which may necessitate intubation. Carbon monoxide has a greater affinity for hemoglobin than does oxygen; therefore 100% oxygen is given to help displace the carbon monoxide from the hemoglobin molecule. Massive fluid shifts are characteristic of burns and aggressive fluid resuscitation is essential to avoid hypovolemic shock. The Parkland formula or similar formulas are used to guide hydration based on the total body surface area (TBSA) burned. Crystalloid is given during the first 24 h with half of the calculated volume given in the first 8 h. Colloid is used in the second 24 h to maintain circulating volume and to help prevent increased edema. It is important to remember that these are only guidelines and must be modified according to changes in the patient's hemodynamic parameters and urine output. Patients with burns of greater than 20 percent of their TBSA frequently develop a reflex ileus and require nasogastric decompression to avoid vomiting and aspiration. Antacids and H_2 blockers should be given as prophylaxis for stress gastritis. Administration of prophylactic penicillin or other systemic antibiotics is no longer encouraged. The eschar that becomes colonized is avascular; thus intravenous antibiotics are ineffective. In addition, the use of intravenous antibiotics tends to select out resistant organisms and to increase the colonization of the gastrointestinal tract with yeast. It should be remembered that tetanus prophylaxis is indicated in burn patients.

117. The answer is B (1, 3). *(Schwartz, 6/e, pp 244–248.)* Initial management of second-degree burns consists of debriding ruptured and intact vesicles and application of topical antibiotics. Care must be taken to prevent bacterial infection, which can convert second- to third-degree burns. Areas of third-degree burn have an eschar, which initially is very adherent to the underlying tissues. After 48 to 72 h the eschar begins to separate as a result of proteases elaborated by bacteria. The eschar must be meticulously debrided at this time to prevent abscess formation and systemic sepsis. Homo- or heterografts are then placed over the debrided wounds. Immediate deep excision is rarely performed and only when burns greater than 60 to 70 percent of TBSA are present. Massive bleeding can occur with this procedure and it is practiced only at specialized burn centers. Tangential excision is currently favored as a means of early debridement, especially for areas at risk for loss of function. No skin grafting can be performed over eschar. Skin grafts require a vascularized bed with bacterial counts less than 10^5 colonies per gram of tissue. Third-degree burns cause loss of tissue elasticity, which in conjunction with soft tissue edema beneath the eschar can cause vascular compromise in circumferentially burned limbs. Escharotomy is essential to allow adequate arterial inflow and venous return. It should not be performed, however, until the patient's hypovolemia and hypotension have been corrected.

118. The answer is B (1, 3). *(Schwartz, 6/e, pp 600–603.)* Squamous cell carcinoma of the lip is the most common malignant tumor of the lip and constitutes 15 percent of all malignancies of the oral cavity. Basal cell carcinomas do occur on the lip, but much less frequently. There is a strong association between squamous cell tumors of the lip and sun exposure. Therefore, these lesions are more common in the southern United States and in occupational groups who work out of doors. Because of its greater sun exposure, the lower lip is the site of more than 90 percent of such lesions. Persistent hyperkeratosis precedes 35 to 40 percent of these lesions. The incidence of metastases increases with the size of the lesion, and spread is usually via lymphatics to the ipsilateral submental node. Contralateral nodal metastases are rare unless the lesion crosses the midline. Approximately 10 to 15 percent of all patients have metastases at the time of diagnosis. These lip tumors are very responsive to radiotherapy, which works well for small- to medium-sized lesions. Large lesions treated with radiotherapy usually require surgical reconstruction. Radiotherapy should not be used in patients who will have ongoing sun exposure to the area since radiation therapy sensitizes the tissues to solar trauma.

119. The answer is A (1, 2, 3). *(Davis, pp 2348–2349.)* Signs and symptoms of the carpal tunnel syndrome are related to the distribution of the median nerve. This nerve, which passes through the carpal tunnel in the wrist with the finger flexor tendons, may suffer compression from fibrous scarring or malalignment following a fracture of the wrist. Nerve compression may also occur in patients with rheumatoid arthritis who develop flexor tenosynovitis. In women, the syndrome frequently first appears during pregnancy and recurs during the premenstrual phase of subsequent menstrual cycles. In these cases, symptoms are presumably the result of the effects of fluid retention and pressure on the median nerve owing to tissue swelling. In many instances, symptoms are limited to nocturnal pain and paresthesias.

120. The answer is B (1, 3). *(Schwartz, 6/e, pp 297–298.)* Wound healing is initiated by an inflammatory response. Various amines released from connective tissue mast cells cause increased capillary permeability and extravasation of leukocytes, enzymes, fluid, and proteins. A clot of platelets, red cells, and fibrin forms quickly and creates a protective barrier under which epithelialization from the wound edges begins. In addition there is a rapid proliferation of capillary loops that creates a bed of granulation tissue. The combination of the agglutinated proteins, clot, and new capillaries provides enough strength to coapt the skin edges for the first 5 days if there is no significant tension. From days 5 through 17 there is rapid deposition of new collagen and the tensile strength of the wound rapidly increases almost to its maximum attainable strength. Over the next 2 years the wound strength increases slightly as the result of collagen remodeling, not further deposition. Even with remodeling the wounded tissue never regains the strength of normal tissue.

121. The answer is C (2, 4). *(Davis, pp 2458–2459.)* White patches in the oral cavity (leukoplakia) sometimes are incorrectly interpreted as a premalignant condition. Microscopic examination of leukoplakia may in fact reveal hyperplasia, keratosis, or dyskeratosis, of which the last finding is the most serious because of its association with malignancy. Only about 5 percent of patients with leukoplakia develop cancer. A suggested treatment protocol for patients with thin lesions advocates a program of strict oral hygiene and avoidance of alcohol and tobacco. Biopsy is reserved only for those with thick lesions (since carcinoma in situ may be present). Radiation therapy is contraindicated. Approximately 50 percent of all oral cancers occur in patients who have associated areas of hyperkeratosis and dyskeratosis.

122. The answer is C (2, 4). *(Davis, pp 3160–3162.)* Clefts of the lip and palate occur relatively frequently (1 in 750 live births); they may be unilateral or bilateral and can vary from a small notch to a complete cleft of the lip and palate. Most clefts occur as isolated anomalies but occasionally are associated with neurologic, orthopedic, or cardiac anomalies. A frequently recommended protocol for management is lip repair in the first 3 months of life and palate repair at 12 to 18 months. Other cosmetic procedures can be performed late in childhood and adolescence. Palate repair after 2 years of age is associated with a high incidence of speech impairment; repair in the early months of life can lead to a hazardous loss of blood that is poorly tolerated by the infant. Repair of the lip usually should be accomplished as soon as the infant is sufficiently stabilized to tolerate anesthesia with reasonable safety. Ten to twelve weeks is often recommended as the time for lip repair. At this age, the affected baby usually can be converted to dropper or cup feedings in the postoperative period, which thereby facilitates healing of the lip by reducing the need for suckling with the freshly wounded tissues.

123. The answer is D (4). *(Schwartz, 6/e, pp 526–527.)* The survival of patients with malignant melanoma correlates with the depth of invasion (Clark) and the thickness of the lesion (Breslow). It is widely held that patients with thin lesions (<0.76 mm) and Clark's level I and II lesions are adequately managed by wide local excision. The incidence of nodal metastases rises with increasing Clark's level of invasion such that a level IV lesion has a 30 to 50 percent incidence of nodal metastases. The assumption that removal of microscopic foci of disease is beneficial, in conjunction with retrospective data indicating improved survival in patients who have undergone removal of clinically negative but pathologically positive nodes, has led to the widely held belief that prophylactic node dissections are indicated for melanoma. Prospective data have challenged this concept. Veronesi and Sim have found that patients undergoing prophylactic node dissections survived no longer than those who were followed closely and underwent node dissections only after nodes became palpable. The subject remains controversial and further study and follow-up are necessary. Immunotherapy has not been successful in controlling widespread metastatic melanoma even when added to chemotherapy. Intralesional administration of BCG has been demonstrated to control local skin lesions in only 20 percent of patients. Dinitrochlorobenzene (DNCB) can also be used.

124–125. The answers are 124-C, 125-D. *(Davis, pp 2408–2418.)* Basal and squamous cell carcinomas are the two most common cancers in humans. Both occur predominantly in areas of chronic inflammation or trauma. Consequently, weather-beaten, irradiated, burned, or tobacco-irritated areas of the head, neck, lips, limbs, and hands are sites of most frequent occurrence. Squamous cell cancers with high-risk features (larger than 2 cm in diameter, poorly differentiated, or present in un-healing wounds such as burn scars) have a 21 to 35 percent incidence of lymph node metastasis when first seen. Otherwise, nodal involve-ment is unusual and lymph node dissection should be reserved for pal-pable nodes. Basal cell cancers, by contrast, are extremely low-grade malignancies that rarely metastasize.

126–128. The answers are 126-A, 127-B, 128-C. *(Schwartz, 6/e, pp 521, 2060–2061.)* Port wine stains and strawberry hemangiomas are both capillary hemangiomas frequently seen in the pediatric population. They result from abnormal proliferation of small vessels in the subepi-dermal and deep dermal layers but have very distinct appearances and clinical courses. Port wine stains are present at birth and are flat with a homogeneous, dark-red coloration. These lesions grow with the sur-rounding tissues and do not regress; treatment options include excision (if small), laser cauterization, tattooing, or make-up. In contradistinc-tion, strawberry hemangiomas are frequently not prominent at birth but can grow rapidly during the first 6 to 12 months of life. They tend to be raised and irregular with bright-red areas. Initial therapy consists merely of observation since greater than 90 percent will regress spon-taneously by age 7 to 10 years. These lesions may ulcerate with trauma or become secondarily infected, but this is rare and bleeding is easily controlled with pressure. Rapidly enlarging lesions affecting the eyes or aerodigestive tract are treated with high-dose steroids, excision, or laser cauterization.

129–131. The answers are 129-C, 130-A, 131-B. *(Schwartz, 6/e, pp 149, 158, 165.)* Clostridial cellulitis results from infection of devitalized tis-sue by predominantly nontoxigenic clostridia species. Subcutaneous gas may be present and spread dramatically along fascial planes; how-ever, uninjured tissue is not invaded, and toxemia is not characteristic of this type of wound infection. Treatment is open drainage, debride-ment, and anticlostridial antibiotics.

Clostridial myonecrosis, or "gas gangrene," is a life-threatening, invasive infection, usually caused by *C. perfringens* and additional synergistic aerobic and anaerobic bacteria. Crepitus and severe toxemia are common. Extensively contaminated traumatic injuries, including neglected skin lesions in diabetic extremities, are frequent sites of involvement. When no portal of entry can be found, gastrointestinal (especially colonic) neoplasms have been implicated. Treatment consists of aggressive debridement or amputation, high-dose anticlostridial antibiotics, and hyperbaric oxygen in selected cases.

Trauma and Shock

DIRECTIONS: Each question below contains five suggested responses. Select the **one best** response to each question.

132. A teenaged boy falls from his bicycle and is run over by a truck. On arrival in the emergency room, he is awake, alert, and appears frightened but in no distress. The chest radiograph suggests an air fluid level in the left lower lung field and the nasogastric tube seems to coil upward into the left chest. The next best step in management is

(A) placement of a left chest tube
(B) immediate thoracotomy
(C) immediate celiotomy
(D) esophagogastroscopy
(E) removal and replacement of the nasogastric tube; diagnostic peritoneal lavage

133. Which of the following abdominal lesions is LEAST likely to follow a rapid-deceleration injury?

(A) Renal vascular injury
(B) Superior mesenteric thrombosis
(C) Mesenteric vascular injury
(D) Avulsion of the splenic pedicle
(E) Diaphragmatic hernia

134. A 65-year-old man who smokes cigarettes and has chronic obstructive pulmonary disease falls and fractures the 7th, 8th, and 9th ribs in the left anterolateral chest. Chest x-ray is otherwise normal. Appropriate treatment might include all the following EXCEPT

(A) strapping the chest with adhesive tape
(B) postural drainage physiotherapy
(C) intercostal nerve block
(D) abdominal paracentesis
(E) hospitalization

135. Blunt trauma to the abdomen most commonly injures which of the following organs?

(A) Liver
(B) Kidney
(C) Spleen
(D) Intestine
(E) Pancreas

136. Repair of injured peripheral veins is preferable to ligation for all the following reasons EXCEPT that

(A) in popliteal injuries, ligation leads to an increased amputation rate despite successful arterial reconstruction
(B) ligation leads to an increased incidence of chronic venous insufficiency
(C) ligation leads to an increased incidence of pulmonary embolization
(D) in the presence of extensive associated soft tissue injury, venous return already is significantly impaired
(E) even though repaired veins thrombose, they often recanalize

137. A 27-year-old man sustains a single gunshot wound to the left thigh. In the emergency room he is noted to have a large hematoma of his medial thigh. He complains of paresthesias in his foot. On examination there are weak pulses palpable distal to the injury and he is unable to move his foot. The appropriate initial management of this patient would be

(A) angiography
(B) immediate exploration and repair
(C) fasciotomy of anterior compartment
(D) observation for resolution of spasm
(E) local wound exploration

Questions 138–139

A 25-year-old woman arrives in the emergency room following an automobile accident. She is acutely dyspneic with a respiratory rate of 60 breaths per minute. Breath sounds are markedly diminished on the right side.

138. The first step in managing the patient should be to

(A) take a chest x-ray
(B) draw arterial blood for blood gas determination
(C) decompress the right pleural space
(D) perform pericardiocentesis
(E) administer intravenous fluids

139. A chest x-ray of this woman before therapy would probably reveal all the following EXCEPT

(A) air in the right pleural space
(B) shifting of the mediastinum toward the left
(C) compression of the left lung
(D) shifting of the trachea toward the left
(E) fluid in the left pleural cavity

140. Among the physiological responses to acute injury is

(A) increased secretion of insulin
(B) increased secretion of thyroxine
(C) decreased secretion of vasopressin (ADH)
(D) decreased secretion of glucagon
(E) decreased secretion of aldosterone

141. The management of a complete transection of the common bile duct distal to the insertion of the cystic duct may include all the following EXCEPT

(A) ligation of the common duct, cholecystojejunostomy
(B) loop choledochojejunostomy
(C) primary end-to-end anastomosis
(D) Roux-en-Y choledochojejunostomy
(E) bridging the injury with a T-tube

142. Although nonoperative management of penetrating neck injuries has been advocated as an alternative to mandatory exploration in asymptomatic patients, all the following findings would necessitate formal neck exploration EXCEPT

(A) expanding hematoma
(B) dysphagia
(C) dysphonia
(D) pneumothorax
(E) hemoptysis

143. Following blunt abdominal trauma, a 12-year-old girl develops upper abdominal pain, nausea, and vomiting. An upper gastrointestinal series reveals a total obstruction of the duodenum with a "coiled spring" appearance in the second and third portions. Appropriate management is

(A) gastrojejunostomy
(B) nasogastric suction and observation
(C) duodenal resection
(D) TPN to increase size of retroperitoneal fat pad
(E) duodenojejunostomy

144. Following traumatic peripheral nerve transection, regrowth usually occurs at which of the following rates?

(A) 0.1 mm per day
(B) 1 mm per day
(C) 5 mm per day
(D) 1 cm per day
(E) None of the above

Questions 145–147

A 28-year-old man is brought to the emergency room for a severe head injury after a fall. Initially lethargic, he becomes comatose and does not move his right side. His left pupil is dilated and responds only sluggishly.

145. The most common initial manifestation of increasing intracranial pressure in the victim of head trauma is

(A) change in level of consciousness
(B) ipsilateral (side of hemorrhage) pupillary dilatation
(C) contralateral pupillary dilatation
(D) hemiparesis
(E) hypertension

146. Initial emergency reduction of intracranial pressure is most rapidly accomplished by

(A) saline-furosemide (Lasix) infusion
(B) urea infusion
(C) mannitol infusion
(D) intravenous dexamethasone (Decadron)
(E) hyperventilation

147. In the patient described, compression of the affected nerve is produced by

(A) infection within the cavernous sinus
(B) herniation of the uncal process of the temporal lobe
(C) laceration of the corpus callosum by the falx cerebri
(D) occult damage to the superior cervical ganglion
(E) cerebellar hypoxia

148. A 30-year-old man is stabbed in the arm. There is no evidence of vascular injury, but he cannot flex his three radial digits. He has injured the

(A) flexor pollicis longus and flexor digitus medius tendons
(B) radial nerve
(C) median nerve
(D) thenar and digital nerves at the wrist
(E) ulnar nerve

149. A 31-year-old man is brought to the emergency room following an automobile accident in which his chest struck the steering wheel. Examination reveals stable vital signs but the patient exhibits multiple palpable rib fractures and paradoxical movement of the right side of the chest. Chest x-ray shows no evidence of pneumothorax or hemothorax, but a large pulmonary contusion is developing. Proper treatment would consist of which of the following?

(A) Tracheostomy, mechanical ventilation, and positive-end-expiratory pressure
(B) Stabilization of the chest wall with sandbags
(C) Stabilization with towel clips
(D) Immediate operative stabilization
(E) No treatment unless signs of respiratory distress develop

150. Following a 2-h fire-fighting episode, a 36-year-old fireman begins complaining of a throbbing headache, nausea, dizziness, and visual disturbances. He is taken to the emergency room where his carboxyhemoglobin (COHb) level is found to be 31 percent. Appropriate treatment would be to

(A) begin an immediate exchange transfusion
(B) transfer the patient to a hyperbaric oxygen chamber
(C) begin bicarbonate infusion and give 250 mg acetazolamide (Diamox) IV
(D) administer 100% oxygen by mask
(E) perform flexible bronchoscopy with further therapy determined by findings

151. An elderly pedestrian collides with a bicycle-riding pizza delivery man and suffers a unilateral fracture of his pelvis through the obturator foramen. You would manage this injury by

(A) external pelvic fixation
(B) angiographic visualization of the obturator artery with surgical exploration if the artery is injured or constricted
(C) direct surgical approach with internal fixation of the ischial ramus
(D) short-term bed rest with gradual ambulation as pain allows after 3 days
(E) hip spica

152. A 23-year-old, previously healthy man presents to the emergency room after sustaining a single gunshot wound to the left chest. The entrance wound is 3 cm inferior to the nipple and the exit wound just below the scapula. A chest tube is placed and drains 400 mL of blood and continues to drain 50 to 75 mL/h during the initial resuscitation. Initial blood pressure of 70/0 mmHg responds to 2 L crystalloid and is now 100/70 mmHg. Abdominal examination is unremarkable. Chest x-ray reveals a reexpanded lung and no free air under the diaphragm. The next management step should be

(A) admission and observation
(B) peritoneal lavage
(C) exploratory thoracotomy
(D) exploratory celiotomy
(E) local wound exploration

153. All the following fractures and dislocations of the extremities induced by blunt trauma are associated with significant vascular injuries EXCEPT

(A) knee dislocation
(B) closed anterior elbow dislocation
(C) open elbow dislocation
(D) supracondylar humerus fracture
(E) tibial plateau fracture

154. A patient who has sustained a severe high-voltage electrical burn to the right upper extremity may require each of the following EXCEPT

(A) emergent surgical debridement, skin grafting, fasciotomy, or amputation
(B) anticlostridial prophylaxis with large doses of penicillin and application of topical antimicrobial agents
(C) intravenous fluid replacement based upon the percentage of body surface area burned
(D) evaluation for fracture of the other extremities and visceral injury
(E) continuous ECG monitoring for ectopy or cardiac conduction abnormalities

155. A patient is brought to the emergency room after a motor vehicle accident. He is unconscious and has a deep scalp laceration and one dilated pupil. His heart rate is 120 beats per minute, blood pressure 80/40 mmHg, and respiratory rate 35 breaths per minute. Despite rapid administration of 2 L normal saline, his vital signs do not change significantly. The injury likely to explain this patient's hypotension is

(A) epidural hematoma
(B) subdural hematoma
(C) intraparenchymal brain hemorrhage
(D) basilar skull fracture
(E) none of the above

156. Regarding myocardial contusion from blunt chest trauma, which of the following statements is correct?

(A) Elevated cardiac isoenzyme levels sensitively identify patients at risk for life-threatening arrhythmias

(B) The majority of patients will have abnormalities on the initial ECG post injury

(C) First-pass radionuclide angiography (RNA) and echocardiography are considered "the gold standard" for diagnosis

(D) RNA and echocardiography are good predictors of subsequent cardiac complications such as arrhythmias and pump failure

(E) All patients diagnosed with myocardial contusion should be monitored in an intensive care unit setting for 72 h

157. All the following statements regarding repair of civilian colon injuries are correct EXCEPT

(A) a colostomy should be performed for colonic injury in the presence of gross fecal contamination

(B) the presence of shock on admission or more than two associated intraabdominal injuries is an absolute contraindication to primary colonic repair

(C) distal sigmoidal injuries may be repaired primarily with the formation of a protective proximal colostomy

(D) primary repair for small right- and left-sided colonic wounds can be performed safely in the absence of major fecal spillage

(E) early administration of intravenous antibiotics with aerobic and anaerobic coverage decreases the incidence of wound infections after repair of colonic injuries

158. A 34-year-old prostitute with a history of long-term intravenous drug use is admitted with a 48-h history of pain in her left arm. Physical examination is remarkable for crepitus surrounding needle track marks in her antecubital space with a serous exudate. The plain x-ray of her arm is shown below. Which of the following organisms is LEAST likely to be responsible for this condition?

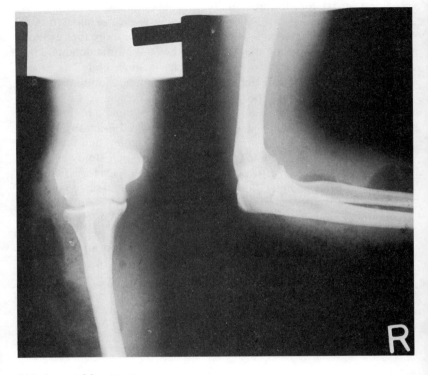

(A) Anaerobic streptococcus
(B) *Staphylococcus aureus*
(C) *Pseudomonas aeruginosa*
(D) *Clostridium perfringens*
(E) *Escherichia coli*

159. Protein metabolism after trauma is characterized by all the following EXCEPT

(A) increased liver gluconeogenesis
(B) inhibition of skeletal muscle breakdown by interleukin 1 and tumor necrosis factor (TNF, cachectin)
(C) increased urinary nitrogen loss
(D) hepatic synthesis of acute-phase reactants
(E) increased glutamine consumption by fibroblasts, lymphocytes, and intestinal epithelial cells

DIRECTIONS: Each question below contains four suggested responses of which **one or more** is correct. Select

A	if	**1, 2, and 3**	are correct
B	if	**1 and 3**	are correct
C	if	**2 and 4**	are correct
D	if	**4**	is correct
E	if	**1, 2, 3, and 4**	are correct

160. A 36-year-old man sustains a gunshot wound to the left buttock. He is hemodynamically stable. There is no exit wound and an x-ray of the abdomen shows the bullet to be located in the right lower quadrant. Proctoscopic examination in the emergency room reveals fresh blood and clots in the rectal ampulla and a through-and-through injury to the rectum at 6 cm from the anal verge. Appropriate management would include

(1) diverting colostomy
(2) irrigation of distal rectum
(3) debridement and closure of rectal injuries
(4) presacral drainage

161. Correct statements regarding blunt trauma to the liver include which of the following?

(1) Hepatic artery ligation for control of bleeding is associated with decreased morbidity and mortality
(2) The incidence of intraabdominal infections is significantly lower in patients with abdominal drains
(3) Intracaval shunting has dramatically improved survival among patients with hepatic vein injuries
(4) Nonanatomic hepatic debridement, with removal of the injured fragments only, is preferable to resection along anatomic planes

162. If traumatic injury to an artery in a major extremity is suspected by clinical or angiographic examination, surgical exploration should be carried out regardless of the presence of palpable pulses distal to the injury. The rationale for this procedure includes which of the following statements?

(1) Subsequent development of arteriovenous fistulae and false aneurysms can be avoided
(2) The presence of palpable distal pulses does not reliably exclude significant arterial trauma
(3) Intimal injuries can lead to delayed arterial occlusion
(4) Prophylactic fasciotomy should be performed to avert an anterior compartment syndrome

163. The response to shock includes which of the following metabolic effects?

(1) Sodium and water retention
(2) Shift to anaerobic metabolism
(3) Hyperkalemia
(4) Hyperglycemia

164. Appropriate treatment for an acute stable hematoma of the pinna of the ear includes which of the following measures?

(1) Ice packs and prophylactic antibiotics
(2) Excision of the hematoma
(3) Needle aspiration
(4) Incision, drainage, and pressure bandage

165. Animal and clinical studies have shown that administration of lactated Ringer's solution to patients with hypovolemic shock may

(1) decrease serum lactate concentration
(2) avert the need for transfusion of whole blood
(3) improve hemodynamics by alleviating the deficit in the interstitial fluid compartment
(4) increase metabolic acidosis

SUMMARY OF DIRECTIONS

A	B	C	D	E
1,2,3	1,3	2,4	4	All are
only	only	only	only	correct

Questions 166–167

An 18-year-old high school football player is kicked in the left flank. Three hours later he develops hematuria. His vital signs are stable.

166. Initial diagnostic tests in the emergency room should include which of the following?

(1) Retrograde urethrography
(2) Retrograde cystography
(3) Arteriography
(4) High-dose infusion urography

167. The diagnostic tests performed reveal extravasation of contrast into the renal parenchyma. Treatment should consist of

(1) increased fluid intake and antibiotics
(2) exploration and suture of laceration
(3) serial monitoring of blood count and vital signs
(4) nephrostomy

168. True statements concerning penetrating pancreatic trauma include

(1) the major cause of death is exsanguination from associated vascular injuries
(2) management of a ductal injury to the left of the mesenteric vessels is distal pancreatectomy
(3) small peripancreatic hematomas should be explored to search for pancreatic injury
(4) management of a ductal injury to the right of the mesenteric vessels is pancreaticoduodenectomy

169. Rapid fluid resuscitation of the hypovolemic patient after abdominal trauma is significantly enhanced by which of the following?

(1) Placement of long, 18-gauge subclavian vein catheters
(2) Infusion of warmed, diluted blood
(3) Bilateral saphenous vein cutdowns
(4) Placement of short, large-bore percutaneous peripheral intravenous catheters

170. True statements regarding the use of the pneumatic anti-shock garment (PASG) include

(1) use of the PASG may delay assessment of injuries in the trauma patient
(2) use of the PASG is recommended for control of persistent bleeding in the setting of severe pelvic fracture
(3) irreversible hypotension may follow deflation of the PASG
(4) the PASG elevates blood pressure by an "autotransfusion" effect, with augmentation of venous return and cardiac output

171. Which of the following situations would be an indication for performance of a thoracotomy in the emergency room?

(1) Massive posttraumatic intraabdominal bleeding
(2) Multiple organ system blunt trauma with obtainable vital signs in the field but none on arrival in the emergency room
(3) Rapidly deteriorating patient with cardiac tamponade from penetrating thoracic trauma
(4) Penetrating thoracic trauma and no signs of life in the field

172. A 22-year-old man sustains a gunshot wound to the abdomen. At exploration, an apparently solitary distal small-bowel injury is treated with resection and primary anastomosis. On postoperative day 7, he drains small-bowel fluid through his operative incision. The fascia remains intact. The fistula output is 300 mL/day and there is no evidence of intraabdominal sepsis. Correct treatment includes

(1) percutaneous intubation of the fistula tract
(2) barium swallow with small-bowel follow-through
(3) total parenteral nutrition
(4) somatostatin

173. A 26-year-old man sustains a gunshot wound to the left thigh. Exploration reveals that a 2-cm portion of superficial femoral artery is destroyed. Appropriate management may include

(1) debridement and end-to-end anastomosis
(2) debridement and repair with interposition Goretex graft
(3) debridement and repair with interposition vein graft
(4) ligation and observation

SUMMARY OF DIRECTIONS

A	B	C	D	E
1,2,3	1,3	2,4	4	All are
only	only	only	only	correct

174. The patient illustrated on the chest x-ray film and contrast study (on the following page) was hospitalized after being assaulted. He sustained several left rib fractures, but was hemodynamically stable. True statements about the injury demonstrated in the films include

(1)   delayed operative repair is indicated after allowing patient's rib fractures to stabilize

(2)   surgical treatment of this injury is indicated during this hospitalization

(3)   repair of this injury is preferably accomplished through a left posterolateral thoracotomy

(4)   if this injury is identified during a laparoscopic exploration for trauma, it should be repaired acutely

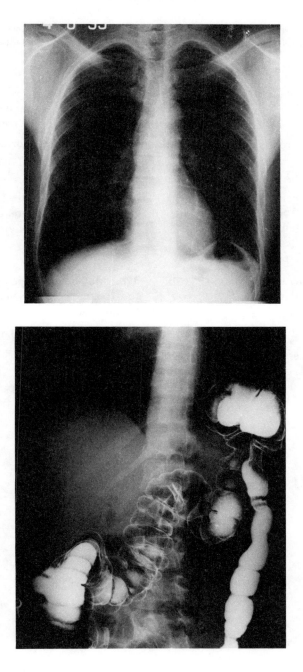

DIRECTIONS: Each group of questions below consists of four lettered headings followed by a set of numbered items. For each numbered item select

A	if the item is associated with	(A) **only**
B	if the item is associated with	(B) **only**
C	if the item is associated with	**both** (A) and (B)
D	if the item is associated with	**neither** (A) nor (B)

Each lettered heading may be used **once, more than once, or not at all.**

Questions 175–177

(A) Peritoneal lavage
(B) Abdominal computed tomography
(C) Both
(D) Neither

175. Useful in evaluating retroperitoneal injury

176. Useful in evaluating intraperitoneal injury

177. Useful in detecting as little as 20 mL of intraperitoneal blood

Questions 178–180

(A) Splenectomy with autotransplantation of spleen
(B) Splenorrhaphy
(C) Both
(D) Neither

178. May be safely performed at low risk in properly selected trauma patients

179. May result in radiographically demonstrable viability of remnant

180. May result in impaired splenic immunological function

DIRECTIONS: The group of questions below consists of lettered headings followed by a set of numbered items. For each numbered item select the **one** lettered heading with which it is **most** closely associated. Each lettered heading may be used **once, more than once, or not at all.**

Questions 181–185

For each of the immediately life-threatening injuries of the chest listed below, select the proper intervention.

(A) Endotracheal intubation
(B) Cricothyroidotomy
(C) Subxiphoid window
(D) Tube thoracostomy
(E) Occlusive dressing

181. Laryngeal obstruction

182. Open pneumothorax

183. Flail chest

184. Tension pneumothorax

185. Pericardial tamponade

Trauma and Shock

Answers

132. The answer is C. *(Schwartz, 6/e, pp 675–677.)* The finding of an air-fluid level in the left lower chest with a nasogastric tube entering it after blunt trauma to the abdomen is diagnostic of diaphragmatic rupture with gastric herniation into the chest. This lesion needs to be fixed immediately. With continuing negative pressure in the chest, each breath sucks more of the abdominal contents into the chest and increases the likelihood of vascular compromise of the herniated viscera. While the diaphragm is easily fixed from the left chest, this injury should be approached from the abdomen. The possibility of injury below the diaphragm after sufficient blunt injury to rupture the diaphragm mandates examination of the intraabdominal solid and hollow viscera; adequate exposure of the diaphragm to allow secure repair is possible from this approach.

133. The answer is E. *(Shires, 3/e, pp 291–340.)* In the rapid-deceleration injury associated with automobile crashes, the abdominal viscera tend to continue moving anteriorly after the body wall has been stopped. These organs exert great stress upon the structures anchoring them to the retroperitoneum. Intestinal loops stretch and may tear their mesenteric attachments, injuring and thrombosing the superior mesenteric artery; kidneys and spleen may similarly shear their vascular pedicles. In these injuries, however, ordinarily the intraabdominal pressure does not rise excessively and diaphragmatic hernia is not likely. Diaphragmatic hernia is primarily associated with compression-type abdominal or thoracic injuries that increase intraabdominal or intrathoracic pressure sufficiently to tear the central portion of the diaphragm.

134. The answer is A. *(Schwartz, 6/e, pp 677–680.)* The preeminent concern in treatment of rib fractures is the prevention of pulmonary complications (atelectasis and pneumonia), particularly for patients with preexisting pulmonary disease, who are in danger of progressing to respiratory failure. Attempts to relieve pain by immobilization or splinting, such as strapping the chest, merely compound the problem of inadequate ventilation. Mild pain may be controlled with oral analgesics, and patients with minor fracture injuries, if they can be closely monitored, may be managed at home with appropriate instructions for coughing and deep breathing. Patients with significant fractures or severe pain should be hospitalized. Rib fractures in the elderly are particularly treacherous. Intercostal nerve blocks often provide prolonged periods of pain relief and, together with appropriate pulmonary physiotherapy, will inhibit development of respiratory complications. Rib fractures are often associated with either intrathoracic or intraabdominal injuries. In particular, fractures of the left chest wall should arouse suspicion of splenic trauma. In equivocal cases, abdominal paracentesis will often be diagnostic.

135. The answer is C. *(Schwartz, 6/e, pp 175–219. Shires, 3/e, pp 291– 340. Walt, 3/e, pp 142–159.)* The diagnosis of injuries resulting from blunt abdominal trauma is difficult; injuries often are masked by associated injuries. Thus, trauma to the head or chest, together with fractures, frequently conceals intraabdominal injury. Apparently trivial injuries may rupture abdominal viscera in spite of the protection offered by the rib cage. The structures most likely to be damaged in blunt abdominal trauma are, in order of frequency, spleen, kidney, intestine, liver, abdominal wall, mesentery, pancreas, and diaphragm. Abdominal paracentesis is a rapid, sensitive diagnostic test for patients with suspected intraabdominal injury and may be extremely helpful in the management of patients with associated head, thoracic, or pelvic trauma in whom signs and symptoms of the abdominal injuries may be masked or overlooked. Abdominal CT scans, which should be done promptly and rapidly, are being used more frequently to evaluate these injuries.

136. The answer is C. *(Zuidema, 4/e, pp 631–655.)* Ligation rather than repair of large veins in the extremities has, in the past, been advocated in patients with multiple injuries or severe trauma. Venous repair adds to the operative time, often results in thrombosis and occlusion, and was thought to lead to an increased incidence of pulmonary embolization. Recent studies, including reviews of the Viet Nam Vascular Registry, indicate that the risk of pulmonary embolization is *not* increased with repair and that vein repair, in conjunction with arterial repair, increases limb salvage, particularly in popliteal injuries. Venous repair may also be necessary in the presence of extensive soft tissue trauma and an already severely compromised venous return. Long-term followup reveals that the sequelae of chronic venous insufficiency are developing with increasing frequency in those patients who have had ligations of lower extremity veins. Morbidity from chronic deep venous occlusion may be diminished even in those patients who develop thrombosis following repair, since recanalization often occurs. For these reasons, it is currently recommended that large veins be repaired whenever clinically feasible.

137. The answer is B. *(Schwartz, 6/e, pp 942–945.)* The five *p*'s of arterial injury include pain, paresthesias, pallor, pulselessness, and paralysis. In the extremities the tissue most sensitive to anoxia are the peripheral nerves and striated muscle. The early developments of paresthesias and paralysis are signals that there is significant ischemia present and immediate exploration and repair are warranted. The presence of palpable pulses does not exclude an arterial injury as this presence may represent a transmitted pulsation through a blood clot. When severe ischemia is present the repair must be completed within 6 to 8 h to prevent irreversible muscle ischemia and loss of limb function. Delay to obtain an angiogram or to observe for change needlessly prolongs the ischemic time. Fasciotomy may be required but should be done in conjunction with and after reestablishment of arterial flow. Local wound exploration is not recommended because brisk hemorrhage may be encountered without the securing of prior vascular control.

138–139. The answers are 138-C, 139-E. *(Schwartz, 6/e, pp 673–674.)* Tension pneumothorax is a life-threatening problem requiring immediate treatment. A lung wound that behaves as a ball or flap valve allows escaped air to build up pressure in the intrapleural space. This causes collapse of the ipsilateral lung and shifting of the mediastinum and trachea to the contralateral side, in addition to compression of the vena cava and contralateral lung. Sudden death may ensue because of a decrease in the cardiac output, hypoxemia, and ventricular arrhythmias. To accomplish rapid decompression of the pleural space, a large-gauge needle should be passed into the intrapleural cavity through the second intercostal space at the midclavicular line. This may be attached temporarily to an underwater seal with subsequent insertion of a chest tube after the life-threatening urgency has been relieved.

Tension pneumothorax produces characteristic x-ray findings of ipsilateral lung collapse, mediastinal and tracheal shift, and compression of the contralateral lung. Occasionally, adhesions prevent complete lung collapse, but the tension pneumothorax is evident because of the mediastinal displacement. A pleural effusion would not be expected acutely in the absence of associated intrapleural blood.

140. The answer is A. *(Schwartz, 6/e, pp 81–82.)* Though the immediate release of catecholamines causes a transient drop in the insulin levels, shortly thereafter there is a significant rise in plasma insulin levels in injured humans. Since injured patients are highly hypermetabolic, it might be expected that the activity of the thyroid hormones would be increased following injury. This is not the case, however, and increased levels of the thyroid hormones are not seen. Vasopressin (ADH) is regulated by the serum osmolality. In the postinjury period many factors are at play that provoke the excretion of vasopressin. Glucagon secretion is normal or increased after injury and the aldosterone levels are not only elevated, but the diurnal fluctuations ordinarily seen are lost.

141. The answer is C. *(Schwartz, 6/e, pp 208–209, 2089.)* Traumatic injury to the common bile duct must be considered in two separate categories. Complete transection of the common bile duct can be handled in many ways. If the patient is unstable and time is limited, simply placing a T-tube in either end of the open common bile duct and staging the repair is the treatment of choice. In a stable patient a biliary enteric bypass is preferred. This can be accomplished by Roux-en-Y choledochojejunostomy or cholecystojejunostomy. The jejunum is favored over the duodenum because if the anastomosis leaks a lateral duodenal fistula is avoided. For similar reasons the defunctionalizing of the jejunal limb is also preferable. This can be accomplished by creating a Roux-en-Y limb or by performing an enteroenterostomy distal to an anastomosis created with a loop of jejunum. Primary end-to-end repair of a completely transected common bile duct is not recommended because of the high incidence of stricture and need for reoperation and creation of a biliary enteric bypass. However, primary repair is the procedure of choice if the common bile duct is lacerated or only partially transected.

142. The answer is D. *(Davis, pp 2768–2821.)* Reports of a more than 50 percent incidence of negative explorations of the neck, iatrogenic complications, and serious injuries overlooked at operation have caused a reassessment of the dictum that all penetrating neck wounds that violate the platysma must be explored. Stable patients with high (zone III) or low (zone I) injuries, or multiple neck wounds, should undergo initial angiography irrespective of the ultimate treatment plan. Algorithms exist for nonoperative management of asymptomatic patients that employ observation alone or combinations of vascular and aerodigestive contrast studies and endoscopy. Nevertheless, recognition of acute signs of airway distress (stridor, hoarseness, dysphonia), visceral injury (subcutaneous air, hemoptysis, dysphagia), hemorrhage (expanding hematoma, unchecked external bleeding), or neurologic symptoms referable to carotid injury (stroke or altered mental status) or lower cranial nerve or brachial plexus injury requires formal neck exploration. Pneumothorax would mandate a chest tube; the necessity for exploration, additional studies (such as angiography in a stable zone I injury), or observation alone would depend on clinical judgment and institutional policy.

143. The answer is B. *(Schwartz, 6/e, pp 199–201.)* Duodenal hematomas result from blunt abdominal trauma. They present as a high bowel obstruction with abdominal pain and occasionally a palpable right upper quadrant mass. An upper gastrointestinal series is almost always diagnostic with the classic coiled spring appearance of the second and third portions of the duodenum secondary to the crowding of the valvulae conniventes (circular folds) by the hematoma. Nonsurgical management is the mainstay of therapy as the vast majority of duodenal hematomas resolve spontaneously. Simple evacuation of the hematoma is the operative procedure of choice. However, bypass procedures and duodenal resection have been performed for this problem. In patients with duodenal obstruction from the superior mesenteric artery syndrome, the obstruction is usually the result of a marked weight loss and, in conjunction with this, loss of the retroperitoneal fat pad that elevates the superior mesenteric artery from the third and fourth portions of the duodenum. Nutritional repletion and replenishment of this fat pad will elevate the artery off the duodenum and relieve the obstruction.

144. The answer is B. *(Schwartz, 6/e, pp 1838–1839. Shires, 3/e, pp 257–263.)* Transection of a peripheral nerve results in hemorrhage and in retraction of the severed nerve ends. Almost immediately, degeneration of the axon distal to the injury begins. Degeneration also occurs in the proximal fragment back to the first node of Ranvier. Phagocytosis of the degenerated axonal fragments leaves a neurilemmal sheath with empty cylindrical spaces where the axons had been. Several days following the injury, axons from the proximal fragment begin to regrow. If they make contact with the distal neurilemmal sheath, regrowth occurs at about the rate of 1 mm per day. However, if associated trauma, fracture, infection, or separation of neurilemmal sheath ends precludes contact between axons, growth is haphazard and a traumatic neuroma is formed. When neural transection is associated with widespread soft tissue damage and hemorrhage (with increased probability of infection), many surgeons choose to delay reapproximation of the severed nerve end for 3 to 4 weeks.

145–147. The answers are 145-A, 146-E, 147-B. *(Shires, 3/e, pp 232–236. Walt, 3/e, pp 184–190.)* Closed head injuries may result in cerebral concussion from depression of the reticular formation of the brainstem. This type of injury is usually reversible.

Local bleeding and swelling (intracranial or extracranial) produce an increase in the intracranial pressure. A characteristic symptom pattern occurs initiated by progressive depression of mental status. Increasing intracranial pressure tends to displace brain tissue away from the source of the pressure; if the pressure is sufficient, herniation of the uncal process through the tentorium cerebri occurs.

Pupillary dilatation is caused by compression of the ipsilateral oculomotor nerve and its parasympathetic fibers. If the pressure is not relieved, the contralateral oculomotor nerve will become involved and, ultimately, the brainstem will herniate through the foramen magnum and cause death. Hypertension and bradycardia are preterminal events.

Emergency measures to reduce intracranial pressure while preparing for localization of the clot or for a craniotomy or both include hyperventilation, dexamethasone (Decadron), and mannitol infusion. Of these, hyperventilation produces the most rapid decrease in brain swelling.

148. The answer is C. *(Way, 9/e, pp 1140–1141.)* The motor components of the median nerve maintain the muscular function of most of the long flexors of the hand as well as the pronators of the forearm and the thenar muscles. It is also an extremely important sensory innervator of the hand and commonly described as the "eye of the hand" since the palm, the thumb, and the index and middle fingers all receive their sensation via the median nerve.

149. The answer is A. *(Hardy, 2/e, pp 166–171.)* Flail chest is diagnosed in the presence of paradoxical respiratory movement in a portion of the chest wall. At least two fractures in each of three adjacent rib or costal cartilages are required to produce this condition. Complications of flail chest include segmental pulmonary hypoventilation with subsequent infection and ultimately respiratory failure. Management of flail chest should be individualized. If adequate pain control and pulmonary toilet can be provided, patients may be managed without stabilization of the flail. Often intercostal nerve blocks and tracheostomy aid in this form of management. If stabilization is required, external methods such as sandbags or towel clips are no longer used. Surgical stabilization with wires is used if thoracotomy is to be performed for another indication.

If this is not the case, "internal" stabilization is performed by placing the patient on mechanical ventilation with positive end-expiratory pressure. Tracheostomy is recommended because these patients usually require 10 to 14 days to stabilize their flail segment and postventilation pulmonary toilet is simplified by tracheostomy. Indications for mechanical ventilation include significant impedance to ventilation by the flail segment, large pulmonary contusion, an uncooperative patient (e.g., owing to head injury), general anesthesia for another indication, greater than five ribs fractured, and the development of respiratory failure.

150. The answer is D. *(Tintinalli, 3/e, pp 703–706.)* Carbon monoxide (CO) is the leading cause of toxin-related death in the U.S. It is produced by the incomplete combustion of fossil fuels and is emitted by virtually all gas-powered engines and appliances that burn fossil fuel, e.g., home furnaces, water heaters, stoves, pool heaters, kerosene heaters, and charcoal fires. Tobacco smoke—particularly smoke released from the tip of the cigarette, which has 2.5 times more CO than inhaled smoke—produces a significant amount of the gas; nonsmokers working in closed quarters with smokers may have carboxyhemoglobin (COHb) levels as high as 15 percent, easily enough to cause headache and some impairment of judgment. Fire fighters are at particularly high risk for CO intoxication. The pathophysiology of CO poisoning is unclear. It is known to cause an adverse shift in the oxygen-hemoglobin dissociation curve, to cause direct cardiovascular depression, and to inhibit cytochrome A_3. Tissue hypoxia is the result. Treatment is directed toward increasing the partial pressures of O_2 to which the transalveolar hemoglobin is exposed. In most cases, administering 100% oxygen through a tightly fitted face mask will result in a serum elimination half-life of COHb of 80 min (compared with 520 min when one breathes room air). In severe cases, where coma, seizures, or respiratory failure are present, the partial pressure of O_2 is increased by administering it in a hyperbaric chamber with the atmospheric pressure of 2.8. In this situation the serum elimination half-life is reduced to 23 min. In any case, the oxygen therapy should continue until the COHb levels reach 10 percent.

151. The answer is D. *(Tintinalli, 3/e, pp 987–993.)* Most pelvic fractures are the result of automobile-pedestrian accidents and are a frequent cause of death. The pelvis is extremely vascular with a diffuse blood supply that makes hemorrhage common and surgical control of bleeding difficult. This patient has a type II fracture (single break in pelvic ring) through a non-weight-bearing portion of the pelvis. These fractures are best treated by bed rest until hemodynamic stability is assured and thereafter by gentle ambulation as pain permits. The clinician must watch carefully for associated injuries to bladder, urethra, and colon and be alert to the many other possible concurrent injuries to an elderly patient who has suffered a collision, even a low-velocity attack from a pizza man.

152. The answer is D. *(Schwartz, 6/e, pp 196–198.)* Gunshot wounds to the lower chest are often associated with intraabdominal injuries. The diaphragm can rise to the level of T4 during maximal expiration. Therefore, any patient with a gunshot wound below the level of T4 should be subjected to abdominal exploration. Exploratory thoracotomy is not indicated because most parenchymal lung injuries will stop bleeding and heal spontaneously with the use of tube thoracostomy alone. Indication for thoracic exploration for bleeding is usually in the range of 100 to 150 mL/h over several hours. Peritoneal lavage is not indicated even though the abdominal examination is unremarkable. As many as 25 percent of patients with negative physical findings and negative peritoneal lavage will have significant intraabdominal injuries in this setting. These injuries include damage to the colon, kidney, pancreas, aorta, and diaphragm. Local wound exploration is not recommended because the determination of diaphragmatic injury with this technique is unreliable.

153. The answer is E. *(Bunt, Am J Surg 160:226–228, 1990.)* In a 4-year retrospective study of 569 at-risk parajoint fractures or dislocations resulting from blunt trauma, there was only a 1.5 percent incidence of associated vascular injury. Angiograms and vascular surgical consultations were obtained when vascular compromise was suspected by clinical examination or Doppler confirmation of flow abnormalities. While vascular injuries due to fractures on either side of a joint (e.g., supracondylar femur fracture or tibial plateau fracture) were uncommon, major joint dislocations were more commonly associated with vascular injury. An exception to this rule is the type III supracondylar humerus fracture, where displacement of bone may injure or entrap the tethered brachial artery. The highest rate of vascular injury occurs with knee dislocations because of the extreme force required to dislocate the joint. In open elbow dislocations, the brachial artery is often disrupted by forcible hyperextension of the joint; closed elbow dislocations are rarely associated with vascular injury unless the dislocation is anterior.

154. The answer is C. *(Trunkey, 2/e, pp 395–396.)* The treatment of electrical injury should be modified from that of thermal burns because tissue damage is much deeper than is apparent at first inspection. The heat generated is proportional to the resistance to the flow of current. Bone, fat, and tendons offer the greatest resistance. Therefore, the tissue deep within the center of an extremity may be injured while more superficial tissues are spared. For this reason, the quantification of fluid requirements cannot be based on the percentage of body surface area involved, as in the Parkland, Brooke, or Baxter formulas, which are used to calculate fluid replacement after thermal burns. Massive fluid replacement is usually essential. A brisk urine output is desirable because of the likelihood of myonecrosis with consequent myoglobinuria and renal damage. As with deep thermal burns, debridement, skin grafting, and amputation of extremities may be required following electrical injury. However, fasciotomy is more frequently required than escharotomy with electrical injury since deep myonecrosis results in increased intracompartmental pressures and compromised limb perfusion. In addition, distant fractures may result owing to vigorous muscle contraction during the accident or if subsequent falls occur. Cardiac or respiratory arrest may occur if the pathway of the current includes the heart or brain. An electrical current can also damage the pulmonary alveoli and capillaries and lead to respiratory infections, a major cause of death in these victims. Owing to the deep myonecrosis that often accompanies high-voltage injury, prophylaxis for clostridia with high-dose penicillin may be considered. Mafenide acetate is preferred over other topical antimicrobials because of its deeper penetration of eschar.

155. The answer is E. (*Schwartz, 6/e, pp 176–178.*) Loss of consciousness following head trauma should be assumed to be due to intracranial hemorrhage until proved otherwise. However, a thorough evaluation of the head-injured patient includes assessment for other potentially life-threatening injuries. Rarely, a patient may have sufficient hemorrhage from a scalp laceration to cause hypotension. In the patient described, hypotension and tachycardia should not be uncritically attributed to the head injury, since these findings in the setting of blunt trauma are suggestive of serious thoracic, abdominal, or pelvic hemorrhage. When cardiovascular collapse occurs as a result of rising intracranial pressure, it is generally accompanied by hypertension, bradycardia, and respiratory depression.

156. The answer is C. (*Dubrow, Surgery 106:267–273, 1989. Miller, Arch Surg 124:805–807, 1989.*) The spectrum of blunt cardiac injuries includes myocardial contusion, rupture, and internal (chamber and septal) disruptions such as traumatic septal defects, papillary muscle tears, and valvular tears. Myocardial contusions are by far the most common of these injuries. They usually occur in persons who sustain a direct blow to the sternum, as seen in a driver whose sternum is forcibly compressed by the steering column in a deceleration injury. Over 50 percent of patients with myocardial contusion demonstrate external signs of thoracic trauma, including sternal tenderness, abrasions, ecchymosis, palpable crepitus, rib fractures, or flail segments. Overall, less than 10 percent of patients have conduction abnormalities, dysrhythmias, or ischemic patterns on their initial ECG. Elevated cardiac isoenzyme levels are specific for myocardial injury, but they lack clinical significance in patients without ECG abnormalities or hemodynamic instability. First-pass radionuclide angiography (RNA) and echocardiography provide sensitive assessment of ventricular wall motion and ejection fraction after blunt chest trauma and are currently viewed as "the gold standard" for the diagnosis of myocardial contusion. But while RNA and echocardiography sensitively detect small abnormalities in myocardial function, they are poor predictors of the significant cardiac complications of pump failure and arrhythmia. Traditionally, management of patients with myocardial contusion has included continuous ECG monitoring in an intensive care unit for 48 to 72 h, even in hemodynamically stable patients without other injuries. Because of the large number of patients with blunt chest trauma from automobile accidents, however, this policy has been scrutinized. Virtually all patients who develop cardiac complications will have ECG abnormalities present on arrival in the emergency room or within the first 24 h. Since an abnormal ECG is a good predictor of subsequent complications, stable patients with possible myocardial contusions but with a normal ECG tracing may be placed on telemetry for 24 h, rather than monitored in an ICU.

157. The answer is B. (*Schwartz, 6/e, pp 202–204. Trunkey, 2/e, pp 297–298.*) Because of the colon's poor blood supply and its fecal content, colon injuries are more difficult to manage than small-bowel injuries. Recently the necessity of mandatory colostomy for civilian colon injuries has been questioned. About 85 percent of civilian colon injuries are small wounds from low- or medium-velocity gunshots or stab wounds, which are less likely to produce gross fecal spillage. These injuries can be repaired primarily in the absence of gross contamination, regardless of the right- or left-sided location of injury. Shock on admission and multiple associated injuries are not universally viewed as absolute contraindications to primary repair in such cases. Gross contamination or large amounts of hard intraluminal feces remain generally accepted contraindications to primary repair. Alternatives include end colostomy with mucous fistula or Hartmann's pouch, exteriorization of a primary repair, and protection of a primary repair in the distal colon by formation of a proximal colostomy. In all cases in which traumatic colon injury is suspected, the early administration of broad-spectrum intravenous antibiotics seems to reduce the incidence of postoperative infectious complications.

158. The answer is C. *(Hall, pp 1327–1328.)* Because they are so often malnourished and at high risk for other conditions that alter their immunocompetence, the drug addict has an extraordinary susceptibility to infections of the type that can quickly progress to threaten life and limb. Among the most virulent are those that give rise to anaerobic cellulitis. Terms sometimes used for these infections are *gas abscess, gangrenous cellulitis, localized gas gangrene,* and *epifascial gangrene.* Suppuration and extensive gas formation are common and usually localized, unlike the infections associated with myonecrosis. These lesions may be clostridial or nonclostridial. *Clostridium perfringens* is the most common culprit but anaerobic cellulitis and gas formation have been associated with a variety of obligate anaerobes including *Bacteroides* species, *Peptostreptococcus,* and *Peptococcus,* as well as the gram-negative enteric bacilli *(E. coli, Klebsiella),* staphylococci, and streptococci. *Pseudomonas aeruginosa* is not implicated in these aggressive infections. Since the progressive injury results from liberation of bacterial exotoxins, antitoxin administration at this stage is futile. Treatment is determined by immediate inspection of a Gram stain of the thin, dark, malodorous wound drainage or a needle aspirate of the crepitant area: if large, "boxcar-shaped" gram-positive bacilli are present, it is a clostridial infection and high doses of parenteral penicillin G (20 million U/day) are indicated; if a polymicrobial Gram stain is seen, clindamycin-aminoglycoside should be added until specific sensitivities are known. Aggressive debridement is always indicated.

159. The answer is B. *(Weissman, Anesthesiology 73:308–327, 1990.)* Injury and sepsis result in accelerated protein breakdown with increased urinary nitrogen loss and increased peripheral release of amino acids. The negative nitrogen balance represents the net result of breakdown and synthesis (with breakdown increased and synthesis increased or diminished). Amino acids such as alanine are released by muscle and transported to the liver for incorporation into acute-phase proteins including fibrinogen, complement, haptoglobin, and ferritin. The amino acids also undergo gluconeogenesis to glucose, which is utilized primarily by the brain and other glycolytic tissues such as peripheral nerve, erythrocytes, and bone marrow. Other tissues receive energy from fat in the form of fatty acids or ketone bodies during starvation following major trauma; this helps to conserve body protein. Glutamine is the most abundant amino acid in the blood and its levels in muscle and blood decrease following injury and sepsis as it is consumed rapidly by replicating fibroblasts, lymphocytes, and intestinal endothelial cells. The use of glutamine may decrease protein catabolism in the intestine and may help prevent atrophy of the gastrointestinal tract in starved and parenterally nourished patients. Along with the counter-regulatory hormones (glucagon, epinephrine, cortisol), interleukin 1 appears to mediate muscle breakdown. Recent studies have indicated that TNF (also called cachectin because of the role it plays in muscle wasting in septic or oncologic patients) also may be a principal catabolic cytokine in the traumatized patient. This protein is secreted by macrophages and further affects metabolism by inducing secretion of interleukin 1 and inhibiting synthesis and activity of lipogenic enzymes.

160. The answer is E (all). *(Schwartz, 6/e, pp 202–204.)* Traumatic perforations of the extraperitoneal rectum can lead to devastating infectious complications if mishandled. The principles of management are similar to those for intraperitoneal injuries to the large intestine; that is, the wound should be debrided and closed if easily accessible. In all cases of rectal injury a diverting colostomy and presacral drainage are mandatory. Failure to accomplish fecal diversion and drainage can result in perineal sepsis, which can spread through fascial planes involving the lower extremities and trunk with devastating consequences. Finally, irrigation of the distal rectum to remove fecal material is often advocated to maintain low rates of infectious complications.

161. The answer is D (4). *(Schwartz, 6/e, pp 204–207, 1323–1326.)* The overwhelming majority of patients explored for blunt trauma to the liver sustain their injuries in motor vehicle accidents. In a large consecutive series of patients (n = 323) with blunt hepatic trauma who were explored for the finding of hemoperitoneum on peritoneal lavage, the mortality was 31 percent. Forty-two percent of the deaths, due primarily to liver injury, occurred intraoperatively during the initial operation following admission. All operations were performed at a regional trauma center by staff trauma surgeons. Their findings included the following observations; (1) intraoperative deaths were due to uncontrolled hemorrhage; (2) patients with major hepatic injuries who survived operation but nevertheless died appeared to succumb either to sepsis or to associated injuries, usually involving the head or chest; (3) hepatic artery ligation for control of bleeding yielded dismal results; of the three surviving patients who underwent hepatic artery ligation (an additional 11 died), two required reoperation for continued bleeding; (4) the use of drains (passive and active) was associated with a significantly greater incidence of intraabdominal infectious complications; (5) intracaval shunting was used in seven severely injured patients without a survivor; (6) while minor hepatic injuries required little or no treatment, major lacerations could usually be controlled with simple absorbable sutures placed 2 to 3 cm from the fracture edge, without occurrence of subsequent intrahepatic hematoma, hemobilia, or bile fistulae; (7) hepatic fragmentation may be treated by nonanatomic debridement, with suture ligation of individual bleeding points; of nine attempts at formal anatomic resection in stable patients, all ended in uncontrollable hemorrhage and death.

162. The answer is A (1, 2, 3). *(Zuidema, 4/e, pp 631–636.)* The presence of ischemic changes following vascular trauma is an indication for emergency exploration and repair. Nonsurgical management of arterial trauma when distal pulses are palpable may lead to delayed sequelae of embolization, occlusion, secondary hemorrhage, false aneurysm, and traumatic arteriovenous fistula. The presence of palpable pulses does not reliably exclude significant arterial injury. Injuries that may be missed if exploration is not performed include lacerations and partial transections containing hematomas, intramural or intraluminal thromboses, and intimal disruptions or tears. Prophylactic fasciotomy is not routinely performed for all arterial injuries but is indicated in the presence of an ischemic period exceeding 4 to 6 h, combined arterial and major venous injury, prolonged periods of hypotension, massive associated soft tissue trauma, and massive edema.

163. The answer is E (all). *(Hardy, 2/e, pp 36–38.)* The biochemical changes associated with shock result from tissue hypoperfusion, endocrine response to stress, and specific organ system failure. During shock, the sympathetic nervous system and adrenal medulla are stimulated to release catecholamines. Renin, angiotensin, antidiuretic hormone, adrenocorticotropin, and cortisol levels increase. Resultant changes include sodium and water retention and increase in potassium excretion, protein catabolism, and gluconeogenesis. Potassium levels rise as a result of increased tissue release, anaerobic metabolism, and decreased renal perfusion. If renal function is maintained, potassium excretion is high and normal plasma potassium levels are restored.

164. The answer is D (4). *(Tintinalli, 3/e, pp 841–842.)* A subperichondrial hematoma in the pinna of the ear may lead to avascular necrosis of the cartilage with shriveling of the pinna and fibrosis and calcification of the hematoma. The result is the deformity known as "cauliflower ear." Appropriate treatment consists of evacuation of the hematoma by incision and tight packing of the skin and perichondrium onto the cartilage with a pressure dressing. Needle aspiration does not affect adequate drainage. Ice packs may be helpful early, but are not sufficient to prevent the deformity; antibiotics are not indicated for this lesion. Since the hematoma is subperichondrial, excision of the hematoma would remove the perichondrium and lead to cartilage deformities.

165. The answer is A (1, 2, 3). *(Schwartz, 6/e, p 135. Shires, 3/e, pp 16–17.)* Infusion of lactated Ringer's solution is an effective immediate step, both clinically and experimentally, in managing hypovolemic shock. Use of this balanced salt solution helps correct the fluid deficit (in the extracellular, extravascular compartment) resulting from hypovolemic shock. This procedure may decrease requirements for whole blood in patients with hemorrhagic shock. If blood loss has been minimal and is controlled, whole blood transfusion may be avoided entirely. The theoretical objection to infusion of lactated Ringer's solution is that it will increase lactate levels and compound the problem of lactic acidosis. This has not been borne out in animal or clinical studies. Along with the hemodynamic improvement that follows volume restitution, liver function improves, lactate metabolism is improved, excess lactate levels drop, and metabolic acidosis improves.

166–167. The answers are 166-D (4), 167-B (1, 3). *(Cass, Urol Clin North Am 16:213–220, 1989. Zuidema, 4/e, pp 528–534.)* In stable patients with suspected genitourinary tract injury, the first urologic study other than a urinalysis should be the intravenous urogram. The technique of high-dose drip infusion is desirable because the high concentration of contrast achieved greatly facilitates interpretation in an unprepared patient. Intravenous urography should be performed before retrograde cystography to avoid obscuring visualization of the lower ureteral tract. The study also may preclude the need for retrograde urethrography in cases where, unlike the case presented, there is a suspicion of urethral injury. Renal arteriography is not indicated routinely but should be performed to rule out renal pedicle injury when no kidney function is demonstrated by drip infusion urography.

Seventy to eighty percent of patients with blunt renal trauma are successfully treated nonsurgically. Bed rest may reduce the likelihood of secondary hemorrhage; antibiotics may reduce the chance of infection's developing in a perirenal hematoma. Failure of conservative treatment is indicated by rising fever, increasing leukocytosis, evidence of secondary hemorrhage, and persistent or increasing pain and tenderness in the region of the kidney.

168. The answer is A (1, 2, 3). *Schwartz, 6/e, pp 209–212, 1429–1430.*) The majority of penetrating pancreatic injuries can be managed with simple drainage. Injury to the major pancreatic duct to the left of the mesenteric vessels is effectively treated with a distal pancreatectomy. The high morbidity and mortality of a pancreaticoduodenectomy for trauma limit its use to extensive blunt injuries to both pancreatic head and duodenum. For ductal injury in the region of the head of the pancreas, a Roux-en-Y limb of jejunum should be brought up and used to drain the transected duct. The proximity of the pancreas to many other major structures makes combined injuries frequent (90 percent). Complications of pancreatic injury include fistula, pseudocyst, and abscess, but the cause of death in patients with pancreatic injury is most frequently exsanguination from associated injury to major vascular structures such as the splenic vessels, mesenteric vessels, aorta, or inferior vena cava. Finally, however small, all peripancreatic hematomas should be explored to search for pancreatic injury. Simple drainage is usually adequate treatment in such cases but failure to recognize a pancreatic injury can have catastrophic sequelae.

169. The answer is C (2, 4). *(Dutky, J Trauma 29:856–860, 1989.)* Rapid fluid administration is often the key to successful trauma resuscitation. Some of the important factors affecting the rate of fluid resuscitation include the diameter of the intravenous tubing, the size and length of the venous cannulae, the fluid viscosity, and the site of administration. According to Poiseuille's law, flow is proportional to the fourth power of the radius of a catheter and inversely proportional to its length. Therefore, the shorter a catheter and the larger its diameter, the faster one can infuse a solution through it. Central venous placement alone does not assure rapid flow. Importantly, the diameter of the intravenous tubing employed may be the rate-determining factor in fluid delivery: blood-infusion tubing allows twice the flow of standard intravenous tubing and should be used when rapid fluid resuscitation is needed. Any patient who is suspected of having a major abdominal injury should immediately have at least two short, large-bore (16-gauge or larger) intravenous cannulae placed in peripheral veins. Longer, smaller catheters, such as standard 18-gauge central venous catheters, may take more time to place and will have lower flow rates. Once fluid resuscitation is underway, one may elect to place an 8- or 9-French pulmonary artery catheter-introducer via a central venous approach for further volume administration, as well as for measurement of central venous pressure or for Swan-Ganz catheter insertion. Lower extremity venous cannulae, placed by saphenous vein cutdown or percutaneously into the femoral veins, are no longer advised as primary access for patients with abdominal trauma, since possible disruption of iliac veins or the inferior vena cava will render volume infusion ineffective. Studies have demonstrated that the flow rate of cold whole blood is roughly two-thirds that of whole blood at room temperature. Diluting and warming the blood by "piggybacking" it into infusion lines that are delivering crystalloid will decrease the blood's viscosity, enhance flow, and minimize hypothermia.

170. The answer is A (1, 2, 3). (*Flint, Ann Surg 211:703–707, 1990. Trunkey, Can J Surg 27:479–486, 1984.*) The pneumatic antishock garment (PASG) is composed of inflatable overalls with three compartments, two for the legs and one for the abdomen. It has now been convincingly demonstrated that the PASG elevates blood pressure by increasing peripheral vascular resistance rather than by an "autotransfusion" effect on venous return and increased cardiac output. The PASG is beneficial for controlling bleeding from pelvic fractures by reduction of pelvic volume and immobilization to restrict fracture movement. The suit pressure must be released very slowly since rapid deflation can lead to sudden, irreversible hypotension. This is probably due to sudden decrease in peripheral vascular resistance and to the effects of vasodilation and wash-out of accumulated metabolites of capillary beds under the suit. Upon reperfusion of the lower body, a systemic metabolic acidemia with hyperkalemia may result and must be closely monitored. For these reasons satisfactory intravenous volume must be attained prior to decompression of the PASG, a delay that may prevent adequate early evaluation of concealed injuries to the lower body.

171. The answer is B (1, 3). (*Schwartz, 6/e, p 675.*) Although indications for thoracotomy in the emergency room are controversial, the procedure appears to be most beneficial when it is employed to (1) release cardiac tamponade in patients with penetrating thoracic trauma who are deteriorating too rapidly for a subxiphoid pericardial window to be created; (2) allow cross-clamping of the descending aorta in patients with intraabdominal bleeding for whom other measures are not effective in maintaining blood pressure; and (3) allow effective internal cardiac massage in patients who arrive in the emergency room with faint or absent pulses and distant heart sounds, and for whom other resuscitative efforts are unsuccessful. By contrast, existing evidence suggests that patients who are unsalvageable and do not benefit from emergency room thoracotomy include (1) those with no vital signs (pulse, pupillary reaction, spontaneous respiration) in the field; and (2) those with multiple organ system blunt trauma and absent vital signs upon arrival in the emergency room.

172. The answer is A (1, 2, 3). *(Schwartz, 6/e, pp 1181–1182.)* Most enterocutaneous fistulas result from trauma sustained during surgical procedures. Irradiated, obstructed, and inflamed intestine is prone to fistulization. Complications of fistulas include fluid and electrolyte depletion, skin necrosis, and malnutrition. Fistulas are classified according to their location and the volume of output, as these factors influence prognosis and treatment. When the patient is stable, a barium swallow is obtained to determine (1) the location of the fistula, (2) the relation of the fistula to other hollow intraabdominal organs, and (3) whether there is distal obstruction. Proximal small-bowel fistulas tend to produce a high output of intestinal fluid and are less likely to close with conservative management than are distal, low-output fistulas. Small-bowel fistulas that communicate with other organs, particularly the ureter and bladder, may need aggressive surgical repair because of the risk of associated infections. The presence of obstruction distal to the fistula (e.g., an anastomotic stricture) can be diagnosed by barium contrast study and mandates correction of the obstruction. The patient in the question appears to have a low-output, distal enterocutaneous fistula. Control of the fistulous drainage should be provided by percutaneous intubation of the tract with a soft catheter. This is usually accomplished under fluoroscopic guidance. Somatostatin has not been proved effective; it has been used with mixed success in the setting of high-output (greater than 500 mL/day) fistulas. Total parenteral nutrition (TPN) is given to maintain or restore the patient's nutritional balance, while minimizing the quantity of dietary fluids and endogenous secretions in the gastrointestinal tract. A period of 4 to 6 weeks' TPN therapy is warranted to allow for spontaneous closure of a low-output, distal fistula.

173. The answer is B (1, 3). *(Schwartz, 6/e, pp 981–982.)* Traumatic arterial injuries can be handled with several techniques. The basic principles of debridement of injured tissue and reestablishment of flow should be observed. Primary end-to-end anastomosis is preferable if this can be accomplished without tension. When 2 cm of artery has been destroyed it is often not possible to perform a tension-free primary anastomosis. In this case a reversed saphenous vein graft is the repair of choice. Ligation of the artery is to be avoided in order to prevent gangrene and limb loss. The use of prosthetic material (Goretex) in a potentially infected field is also to be avoided as infection at the suture line often leads to delayed hemorrhage.

174. The answer is C (2, 4). *(Cameron, 4/e, pp 657–659.)* Traumatic injuries to the diaphragm are associated with both blunt and penetrating trauma. Missed injuries lead to problems with herniation and bowel strangulation with sufficient frequency that repair should not be delayed. All such injuries require repair once the diagnosis is made and the patient has been stabilized. Most acute defects in the diaphragm can be repaired via an abdominal approach, which allows exploration for coexisting injuries.

175–177. The answers are 175-B, 176-C, 177-A. *(Davis, pp 2789–2790. Walters, Surg Gynecol Obstet 165:496–502, 1988.)* Peritoneal lavage is a diagnostic technique used to identify occult intraperitoneal injury in patients with abdominal trauma. An abnormal lavage is obtained when the lavage effluent exceeds allowable levels of blood, bile, or amylase; the presence of vegetable matter also constitutes an abnormal result. Lavage has been used most widely in the triage of hemodynamically stable victims of abdominal trauma who are suspected of having significant injuries but who manifest equivocal physical findings. Further indications for lavage are the suspicion of abdominal injury in patients with altered sensoria, with unexplained blood loss, and who require general anesthesia to treat other injuries. The technique is exquisitely sensitive to intraabdominal bleeding and will detect as little as 20 mL of free blood in the peritoneal cavity. Because stable retroperitoneal hematomas and minor lacerations of the liver and spleen often shed sufficient blood to produce a positive lavage, some authors have advocated abdominal CT as the preferred method of identifying occult operable injuries of the abdomen. Also, CT with oral and intravenous contrast can provide accurate images of the injured retroperitoneum and the solid intraabdominal viscera (as lavage cannot). Neither CT nor lavage has been a reliable indicator of small intestinal and diaphragmatic injuries; and neither has been useful in obtaining hemostasis nonoperatively. Angiography, however, may be employed to demonstrate visceral or pelvic arterial extravasation and to control hemorrhage by selective embolization.

178–180. The answers are 178-C, 179-C, 180-C. *(Feliciano, Ann Surg 211:569–582, 1990. Mizrahi, Arch Surg 124:863–865, 1989.)* Loss of splenic immunological function in the adult trauma patient may lead, in a small percentage of cases, to overwhelming postsplenectomy sepsis. In situ splenic salvage by debridement and splenorrhaphy has been performed with minimal morbidity in approximately 40 percent of patients in large combined series, although data on perioperative transfusion requirements are not reported in most studies published in the last 10 years. When splenectomy for hemostasis is deemed inevitable because of extensive splenic parenchymal or hilar injury, autotransplantation of thin slices of spleen tissue into the greater omentum has been successfully accomplished in stable patients without adverse sequelae. Postoperative radionuclide scanning has demonstrated viability of salvaged splenic tissue after both in situ splenorrhaphy and autotransplantation in the omentum. Both salvage techniques appear to restore some part of the spleen's immunological function, as suggested by normalization of serum IgM levels and absence of Howell-Jolly bodies on peripheral blood smear. Despite this evidence, however, reimplantation remains an unproven modality for protection against sepsis, as questions persist regarding the quantity both of reimplanted tissue and of blood flow needed to confer antistreptococcal immunity. Similarly, if splenorrhaphy entails ligation of the splenic artery or debridement of more than two-thirds of the spleen, the result may be marginal splenic trapping function and probable vulnerability to overwhelming sepsis.

181–185. The answers are 181-B, 182-E, 183-A, 184-D, 185-C *(Schwartz, 6/e, pp 672–684.)* Flail chest describes the paradoxical motion of the chest wall that occurs when consecutive ribs are broken in more than one place, usually following blunt trauma to the thorax. Respiratory distress may ensue when the noncompliant flail segment interferes with generation of adequate positive and negative intrathoracic pressure needed to move air through the trachea. In addition, a blow sufficiently violent to cause a flail chest may also contuse the underlying pulmonary parenchyma, which compounds the respiratory distress. Treatment consists of stabilizing the chest wall. Although some temporary benefit may be gained by external buttressing of the chest (e.g., with sandbags, or by turning the patient onto the affected side), endotracheal intubation provides rapid and safe control of the airway, as well as stabilization of the chest internally by positive pressure ventilation.

Airway obstruction denotes partial or complete occlusion of the tracheobronchial tree by foreign bodies, secretions, or crush injuries of the upper respiratory tract. Patients may present with symptoms ranging from cough and mild dyspnea to stridor and hypoxic cardiac arrest. An initial effort should be made to digitally clear the airway and to suction visible secretions; in selected, stable patients, fiberoptic endoscopy may be employed to determine the cause of obstruction and to retrieve foreign objects. Unstable patients whose airways cannot be quickly reestablished by clearing the oropharynx must be intubated. An endotracheal intubation may be attempted, but cricothyroidotomy is indicated in the presence of proximal obstruction or severe maxillofacial trauma.

Blunt or penetrating trauma to the pericardium and heart will result in pericardial tamponade when fluid pressure in the pericardial space exceeds central venous pressure and thus prevents venous return to the heart. The result is shock, despite adequate volume and myocardial function. The treatment is pericardial decompression. A subxiphoid, supradiaphragmatic incision and creation of a pericardial "window," ideally performed in the operating room, provides a rapid, safe means of confirming the diagnosis of tamponade and of relieving venous obstruction. If heavy bleeding is encountered on opening the pericardial window, a sternotomy may be performed.

Tension pneumothorax occurs when a laceration of the visceral pulmonary pleura acts as a one-way valve that allows air to enter the pleural space from an underlying parenchymal injury but not to escape. Increasing intrapleural pressure causes collapse of the ipsilateral lung, compression of the contralateral lung due to mediastinal shift toward the opposite hemithorax, and diminished venous return. Treatment consists of relieving the pneumothorax. This is best accomplished by tube thoracostomy.

Open pneumothorax occurs when a traumatic defect in the chest wall permits free communication of the pleural space with atmospheric pressure. If the defect is larger than two-thirds of the tracheal diameter, respiratory efforts will move air in and out through the defect in the chest wall rather than through the trachea. The immediate treatment is placement of an occlusive dressing over the defect; subsequent interventions include placement of a thoracostomy tube (preferably through a separate incision), formal closure of the chest wall, and ventilatory assistance if needed.

Transplants, Immunology, and Oncology

DIRECTIONS: Each question below contains five suggested responses. Select the **one best** response to each question.

186. Tumor necrosis factor (TNF) is among the monokines that appear in the tissues following injury or infection. Its origin is primarily from

(A) the damaged connective-tissue stroma cells
(B) the damaged vascular endothelial cells
(C) monocytes/macrophages
(D) the activated T lymphocytes
(E) the activated killer lymphocytes

187. A 28-year-old mountain guide has had a nonseminomatous testicular cancer treated. In following this patient for possible recurrent tumor, the most useful serum marker would be

(A) carcinoembryonic antigen (CEA)
(B) alpha fetoprotein (AFP)
(C) prostatic specific antigen (PSA)
(D) CA125
(E) p53 oncogene

188. In order to activate T-helper/inducer (CD4 +) lymphocytes, macrophages release

(A) interleukin 1
(B) interleukin 2
(C) interleukin 3
(D) interleukin 4
(E) interferon

189. Prior to performing an open biopsy of an enlarged cervical lymph node, all the following tests should be done EXCEPT

(A) sinus x-ray
(B) CT scan of the head and neck
(C) bone marrow biopsy
(D) nasopharyngoscopy
(E) indirect laryngoscopy

190. Each of the following statements regarding interferons are true EXCEPT

(A) they are maturation factors for interleukin 6
(B) they are effective in the treatment of hairy cell leukemia
(C) they are produced by leukocytes, lymphocytes, and fibroblasts
(D) they are the result of recombinant DNA technology
(E) they may cause severe congestive cardiomyopathy

191. Following intravenous administration of systemic chemotherapy,

(A) subcutaneous extravasation of carmustine (BCNU) or 5-fluorouracil (5-FU) usually causes ulceration
(B) doxorubicin extravasation rarely causes serious ulceration because the agent binds quickly to tissue nucleic acid
(C) serious and progressive ulceration can be expected following extravasation of vincristine or vinblastine
(D) problems of wound healing should be anticipated if systemic 5-FU therapy is begun less than 2 weeks postoperatively
(E) administration of folinic acid prevents most of the toxicity of methotrexate, but does not help to normalize wound healing

192. Which of the following immunological cells kills tumor cells in an immunologically specific manner?

(A) Macrophage
(B) Cytotoxic T lymphocyte
(C) Natural killer cell
(D) Polymorphonuclear leukocyte
(E) Helper T lymphocyte

193. For which of the following malignancies does histological grade best correlate with prognosis?

(A) Prostate cancer
(B) Melanoma
(C) Colonic adenocarcinoma
(D) Hepatocellular carcinoma
(E) Soft-tissue sarcoma

194. All the following statements regarding malignant parotid tumors are correct EXCEPT

(A) mucoepidermoid carcinoma accounts for nearly one-half of all malignant tumors of the parotid gland
(B) 20 to 35 percent of parotid neoplasms are malignant
(C) therapeutic regional node dissection is indicated for clinically positive neck nodes
(D) focal postoperative radiation allows preservation of facial nerve invaded by tumor
(E) carcinoma in mixed tumors may arise from previously benign tumors

Questions 195–199

A 27-year-old diabetic, hypertensive woman who has been receiving hemodialysis for 2 years is admitted to the hospital for cadaveric renal transplantation. She is blood type B and has had four transfusions of packed cells over the preceding 6 months.

195. Which of the following factors would preclude transplantation?

(A) Positive crossmatch
(B) Donor blood type O
(C) Two-antigen HLA match with donor
(D) Blood pressure of 180/100 mmHg
(E) Hemoglobin level of 8.2 g/dL

196. On the 14th posttransplant day, the recipient's temperature rises to 38.5°C (101°F). The serum creatinine level, previously 1.0 mg/dL, is 1.6 mg/dL. Renal scan shows good perfusion with delayed excretion. Ultrasound reveals a mildly enlarged transplant kidney with a small fluid collection near the upper pole. The white blood cell count is 3800/mm³ and the platelet count is 65,000/mm³. Appropriate management at this time might include all the following EXCEPT

(A) increased administration of prednisone
(B) administration of azathioprine
(C) administration of antilymphocyte globulin (ALG)
(D) administration of OKT3
(E) percutaneous needle biopsy of the graft

197. On the second postoperative day, the patient remains oliguric, but there is good perfusion on the renal scan and no hydronephrosis. The most commonly used immunosuppressive therapy at this time would be administration of

(A) cyclosporine A alone
(B) cyclosporine A and steroids
(C) cyclosporine A, steroids, and azathioprine
(D) OKT3 and steroids
(E) cyclophosphamide and steroids

198. On the 40th postoperative day, the patient feels well but is somewhat hypertensive. She had been started on ketoconazole for oral candidiasis. The serum creatinine level is 2.0 mg/dL and the serum cyclosporine level is 275 ng/mL. There are no fluid collections found on ultrasound. Appropriate initial management at this time would be to

(A) perform an immediate biopsy with management dependent on frozen section results
(B) discontinue immunosuppression with a diagnosis of systemic candidal infection
(C) decrease the cyclosporine and increase the prednisone
(D) start OKT3
(E) administer a bolus with intravenous steroids and plan biopsy in 3 days if there is no improvement

199. On the 21st posttransplant day, the patient is being maintained on cyclosporine A, azathioprine, and prednisone. The serum creatinine level is 1.2 mg/dL, temperature is 38.5°C (101°F), and ultrasound shows a normal-size kidney with a somewhat enlarged fluid collection at the upper pole. The renal scan is normal, white blood cell count is 13,500/mm³, and platelet count is 160,000/mm³. There is a hazy infiltrate on the left lower lobe on chest x-ray. The appropriate immediate therapeutic maneuvers would be

(A) withhold azathioprine, maintain cyclosporine, decrease prednisone dosage, aspirate the fluid collection, and perform bronchoscopy
(B) withhold azathioprine and cyclosporine, decrease prednisone dosage, and perform transplant nephrectomy with drainage of the fluid collection
(C) continue azathioprine and cyclosporine, decrease prednisone dosage, aspirate the fluid collection, and monitor serial antiviral antibody titers
(D) maintain immunosuppressive drugs, perform plasmapheresis with infusion of granulocytes, and begin antibiotics
(E) maintain immunosuppressive drugs, perform a bone marrow biopsy, and begin antibiotics

Questions 200–201

A 24-year-old woman presents with lethargy, anorexia, tachypnea, and weakness. Laboratory studies reveal a BUN of 150 mg/dL, serum creatinine of 16 mg/dL, and a potassium of 6.2 meq/L. Chest x-ray shows increased pulmonary vascularity and a dilated heart.

200. Management of this patient would include all the following EXCEPT

(A) peritoneal dialysis
(B) creation of a forearm arteriovenous fistula
(C) sodium polystyrene sulfonate (Kayexalate) enemas
(D) a 100-g protein diet
(E) renal biopsy

201. In the course of 3 months' treatment, the patient's congestive heart failure resolves, the lethargy and weakness diminish markedly, and she is able to return to work part-time. Family immune profile studies reveal that her mother and her father each are haplotype identical with regard to HLA antigens and that her sister is a six-antigen match. The patient at this time should be urged to

(A) continue hemodialysis three times a week
(B) undergo cadaveric renal transplantation
(C) accept a kidney transplant from her sister
(D) accept a kidney transplant from her father
(E) accept a kidney transplant from her mother

202. In centers with experienced personnel, 1-year liver transplant survival is now approximately

(A) 95 percent
(B) 80 percent
(C) 65 percent
(D) 50 percent
(E) 35 percent

203. The primary mechanism of action of cyclosporine A is inhibition of

(A) macrophage function
(B) antibody production
(C) interleukin 1 production
(D) interleukin 2 production
(E) cytotoxic T-cell effectiveness

204. A mother notices an abdominal mass in her 3-year-old son while giving him a bath. There is no history of any symptoms, but his blood pressure is elevated at 105/85 mmHg. Metastatic workup is negative and the patient is explored. The mass below is found within the left kidney. Which of the following statements concerning this disease is correct?

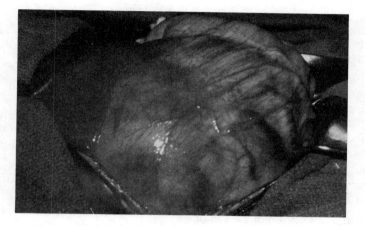

(A) This tumor is associated with aniridia, hemihypertrophy, and cryptorchidism

(B) The majority of patients present with an asymptomatic abdominal mass and hematuria

(C) Treatment with surgical excision, radiation, and chemotherapy results in survival of less than 60 percent even in histologically low-grade tumors

(D) Surgical excision is curative and no further treatment is ordinarily advised

(E) This tumor is the most common malignancy in childhood

Questions 205–206

A 30-year-old primigravida complains of headaches, restlessness, sweating, and tachycardia. She is 8 months pregnant and her blood pressure is 200/120 mmHg.

205. Appropriate workup might include all the following EXCEPT

(A) urine for epinephrine
(B) urine for norepinephrine
(C) chest x-ray
(D) abdominal CT scan
(E) abdominal ultrasonogram

206. Appropriate treatment might consist of all the following EXCEPT

(A) urgent excision of the tumor
(B) urgent excision of the tumor and a therapeutic abortion
(C) phenoxybenzamine and propranolol followed by a caesarean section and an elective excision of the tumor after delivery
(D) phenoxybenzamine and propranolol followed by a combined caesarean section and excision of the tumor
(E) metyrosine (Demser) blockade followed by a combined caesarean section and excision of the tumor

207. An 11-year-old girl presents to your office because of a family history of medullary carcinoma of the thyroid. Physical examination is normal. You would perform all the following tests EXCEPT

(A) urine vanillylmandelic acid (VMA)
(B) serum calcitonin
(C) serum gastrin
(D) serum calcium
(E) pentagastrin stimulation

208. Of the surgical procedures listed below, all are useful in the management of non-Hodgkin's lymphomas EXCEPT

(A) exploratory celiotomy for staging
(B) splenectomy for localized splenic involvement
(C) resection of small intestinal lesions
(D) excisional lymph node biopsy
(E) total gastrectomy for lesions localized to the stomach

209. All the following statements about hepatic resectional management of metastatic colorectal cancers are true EXCEPT that

(A) a small, solitary metastasis recognized at the time of colectomy should be removed by local excision or wedge resection

(B) patients with solitary metastases are those most likely to be cured

(C) mortality of lobectomy for resection of metastatic foci is less than 10 percent

(D) patient survival after surgery for metachronous metastases is significantly higher than with surgery for synchronous metastases

(E) 5-year survival rates of 20 to 40 percent can be expected when resection is possible

DIRECTIONS: Each question below contains four suggested responses of which **one or more** is correct. Select

A	if	**1, 2, and 3**	are correct
B	if	**1 and 3**	are correct
C	if	**2 and 4**	are correct
D	if	**4**	is correct
E	if	**1, 2, 3, and 4**	are correct

210. True statements regarding autoimmune hemolytic anemia include

(1) a relapse following successful splenectomy indicates possible presence of an accessory spleen
(2) splenectomy is first-line therapy for patients with severe hemolysis and symptomatic anemia
(3) patients with red cells coated by immunoglobulin G (IgG) respond better to splenectomy than those with IgM-coated cells
(4) splenectomy leads to complete remission in virtually all patients with secondary auto-immune hemolysis

211. Testicular carcinomas that require retroperitoneal lymph node dissection include

(1) embryonal carcinoma
(2) seminoma
(3) teratocarcinoma
(4) choriocarcinoma

212. Correct statements concerning human bone marrow transplants include which of the following?

(1) Marrow is highly immunogenic and easily rejected by the nonimmunosuppressed host
(2) Experimental techniques have shown promise for the induction of tolerance to organ allografts
(3) The major impediment to successful marrow grafting is the graft-versus-host response
(4) Marrow transplant must be performed with low-level immunosuppression to enhance the degree of chimerism

213. Correct statements concerning cancer and nutrition include which of the following?

(1) Levels of nitrates in food and drinking water are positively correlated with the incidence of gastric cancer
(2) Regular ingestion of vitamin C from childhood probably inhibits formation of gastric carcinogens
(3) Consumption of excessive amounts of animal dietary fats is associated with increased incidences of pancreatic, breast, and prostatic cancers
(4) Nutritional support of cancer patients improves response of the tumor to chemotherapy

214. Five-year survival rates in excess of 20 percent may be expected following resection of pulmonary metastases if

(1) no other organ metastases are present
(2) lung lesions are solitary
(3) the patient's condition and tumor location are favorable
(4) the tumor doubling time is less than 20 days

215. Graft-versus-host disease has occurred with the transplantation of which of the following?

(1) Kidney
(2) Liver
(3) Heart
(4) Bone marrow

216. Advantages of renal transplantation over dialysis include

(1) less expensive if the transplanted kidney survives 2 years
(2) increased number of pregnancies in female recipients
(3) less anemia
(4) increased 1-year survival of patient

217. Successful whole-organ pancreas transplantation in type I diabetes has been shown to

(1) maintain normal serum glucose levels
(2) prevent the recurrence of diabetic nephropathy in transplanted kidneys
(3) maintain normal oral glucose tolerance tests
(4) reverse the changes of diabetic retinopathy

218. Interferons are correctly characterized by which of the following statements?

(1) They are produced by virus-infected cells
(2) They inhibit viral replication
(3) They cause remission in hairy cell leukemia
(4) They cause malignant clonogenic cells to differentiate

219. Complications that are more common in patients receiving systemic chemotherapy include

(1) gastrointestinal bleeding
(2) perirectal abscesses
(3) pancreatitis
(4) sclerosing cholangitis

220. True statements about transmission of AIDS in a health care setting and recommendations to reduce the risk of transmission include

(1) a freshly prepared solution of dilute chlorine bleach adequately decontaminates clothing
(2) all needles should be capped immediately after use
(3) endoscopes should be cleaned and gas sterilized after use on an HIV seropositive patient
(4) double gloving is highly recommended

221. Characterization of T- and B-cell subpopulations by monoclonal anti-bodies is important for diagnosing

(1) acquired immune deficiency syndrome (AIDS)
(2) non-Hodgkin's lymphoma
(3) leukemia
(4) Hodgkin's lymphoma

222. Correct statements concerning the effects of radiation include which of the following?

(1) The excess risk of radiogenic cancer from diagnostic radiologic studies is estimated to be one case per million procedures per year
(2) Cellular hypoxia increases sensitivity to radiation
(3) The condition of the cell nucleus in relation to its mitotic cycle determines cell sensitivity to radiation
(4) In addition to natural background radiation, the safe limit for an average person is 0.5 rad per year (15 r/30 yr)

223. Correct statements concerning the behavior of tumor cells include which of the following?

(1) About 25 percent of the tumor cells invading the central circulation remain viable beyond 24 h
(2) It takes 1 billion cells for a tumor to become clinically detectable (1 cc)
(3) Most cells cloned from the same tumors have similar metastatic potential
(4) Local invasion is related to lytic enzymes produced by the tumor cells

224. True statements concerning the process involving the rejection of the kidney shown below include that

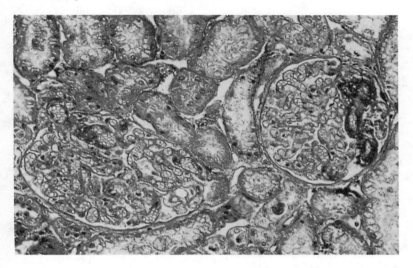

(1)   it is mediated by antibodies against donor HLA antigens
(2)   it can be avoided by performing cytotoxicity testing by incubating the recipient's serum with the donor lymphocytes
(3)   it is manifest grossly by a swollen, pale kidney at the time of transplant surgery
(4)   this form of rejection is associated with disseminated intravascular coagulation (DIC)

SUMMARY OF DIRECTIONS

A	B	C	D	E
1,2,3	1,3	2,4	4	All are
only	only	only	only	correct

225. Cardiac transplants differ from renal transplants in that

(1) negative lymphocyte cross-match is not necessary in heart transplantation
(2) cadaveric graft survival is significantly lower with heart transplants
(3) cadaveric kidneys can be preserved for substantially longer periods than hearts
(4) simple hypothermic preservation is inadequate for kidneys but satisfactory for hearts

226. Regarding cancer therapy with interleukin 2 (IL-2) and lymphokine-activated killer (LAK) cells,

(1) there is a marked increase in the peripheral lymphocyte count
(2) response rates of greater than 20 percent have been shown in melanoma, renal cell carcinoma, and non-Hodgkin's lymphoma
(3) examination of responsive tumors after such treatment shows infiltration of large, activated T cells
(4) LAK cell infusion without in vivo IL-2 is nearly as effective as the combination

DIRECTIONS: Each group of questions below consists of four lettered headings followed by a set of numbered items. For each numbered item select

A	if the item is associated with	(A) **only**
B	if the item is associated with	(B) **only**
C	if the item is associated with	**both** (A) and (B)
D	if the item is associated with	**neither** (A) nor (B)

Each lettered heading may be used **once, more than once, or not at all.**

Questions 227–230

(A) Fluid from which human immunodeficiency virus (HIV) has been isolated
(B) Fluid implicated in the transmission of HIV
(C) Both
(D) Neither

227. Human milk

228. Urine

229. Vaginal secretions

230. Sweat

Questions 231–233

(A) Tobacco smoking
(B) Alcohol ingestion
(C) Both
(D) Neither

231. Associated with esophageal carcinoma

232. Associated with bladder carcinoma

233. Associated with hepatocellular carcinoma

Questions 234–236

(A) Major histocompatibility complex (MHC) class I proteins
(B) MHC class II proteins
(C) Both
(D) Neither

234. Expressed on all nucleated cells

235. Expressed on B cells

236. Target of cytotoxic T cells

DIRECTIONS: The group of questions below consists of lettered headings followed by a set of numbered items. For each numbered item select the **one** lettered heading with which it is **most** closely associated. Each lettered heading may be used **once, more than once, or not at all.**

Questions 237–240

All the immunosuppressants currently used to prevent or treat allograft rejection have significant deleterious side effects. For each of the complications below, match the agent.

    (A) Azathioprine
    (B) Corticosteroids
    (C) Antilymphocyte serum
    (D) Cyclophosphamide
    (E) Cyclosporine

237. Nephrotoxicity

238. Hepatotoxicity

239. Testicular atrophy

240. Anaphylactoid reaction

Transplants, Immunology, and Oncology

Answers

186. The answer is C. *(Hall, pp 624–626.)* Tumor necrosis factor (TNF) is a peptide hormone produced by endotoxin-activated mono-cytes/macrophages and has been postulated to be the principal cytokine mediator in gram-negative shock and sepsis-related organ damage. Biological actions that have been attributed to TNF (cachectin) include polymorphonuclear neutrophil (PMN) activation and degranulation; increased nonspecific host resistance; increased vascular permeability in the gut; lymphopenia; promotion of interleukins 1, 2, and 6; capillary leak syndrome; microvascular thrombosis; anorexia and cachexia; and numerous other protective and adverse effects in sepsis. Its role in sepsis is providing a fertile field for research in critical care.

187. The answer is B. *(Way, 9/e, pp 936–937.)* In following patients with nonseminomatous testicular tumors, elevated serum levels of the beta subunit of human chorionic gonadotropin (hCG), alpha fetoprotein, and lactic dehydrogenase have been found to be useful indicators of tumor activity or recurrence. The discovery of prostate specific antigen has recently been touted as a major breakthrough in screening for prostate cancer, though some clinicians feel that early diagnosis may have no impact on survival in this disease. CA125 has been used to follow ovarian cancers; it is fairly nonspecific but can alert the physician to the need for a more aggressive search for persistent disease when relative increases are noted in a patient after therapy. The p53 oncogenes have been found in soft tissue sarcomas, osteogenic sarcomas, and colon cancers. Their significance is unknown.

188. The answer is A. *(Schwartz, 6/e, p 367.)* Interleukin 1 (Il-1) is a thymocyte mitogen produced by activated macrophages as well as many other types of cells (e.g., monocytes, dendritic cells, Langerhans cells, neutrophils, microglial cells). Il-1 induces interleukin 2 production by the T-helper cell, which initiates a cascade of immunoregulatory and inflammatory functions.

189. The answer is C. *(Schwartz, 6/e, pp 337–338, 607.)* Isolated enlarged cervical lymph nodes present a diagnostic problem. They may be involved with neoplasms that originate in the hypopharynx, piriform sinus, larynx, or thyroid or they may contain a lymphoma. It is important to ascertain the location of the primary neoplasm prior to excision, because curative surgery may involve a radical neck dissection, which would be complicated by a previous biopsy. There is also fear of tumor spread in an open biopsy. Bone marrow biopsy is not indicated prior to lymph node biopsy. It is done as part of the staging procedure, after a diagnosis of lymphoma has been made. Needle aspiration cytology is now being used more widely. It can often diagnose carcinomas, but is rarely useful for the diagnosis of lymphoma.

190. The answer is A. *(Schwartz, 6/e, pp 367, 379, 387.)* Interferons were discovered about 35 years ago as antiviral agents. Some early work encouraged many to believe a major new anticancer agent had appeared. Unfortunately, the early enthusiasm has dissipated after a sequence of disappointing clinical studies. Hairy cell leukemia and the Kaposi's sarcoma in AIDS patients seem to be the two neoplastic conditions in which interferon therapy has an established role. There are over a dozen physicochemically related interferons now identified; most are available through recombinant DNA technology. For the present, the interferons seem to be a solution searching for a problem.

191. The answer is D. *(Wilson, 12/e, pp 1587–1599.)* Since chemotherapy is generally most effective in killing rapidly dividing cells, the rapidly dividing cells of a fresh surgical wound should be in jeopardy when chemotherapy is given in the early postoperative period. Each of the phases of normal wound healing is theoretically at risk from one or another class of chemotherapeutic agents. Immediately following wounding, inflammation and vascular permeability lead to fibrin deposition and polymorphonuclear neutrophil (PMN), monocyte, and platelet influx. Macrophages are attracted by the activated complement system. By the fourth day, the proliferative phase begins and for the next 20 days fibroblasts produce mucopolysaccharides and collagen. Cross-linking of the collagen fibers then continues for several months in the maturation phase. It seems logical to delay antineoplastic agents for 10 to 14 days unless there are compelling clinical indications (e.g., superior vena cava syndrome) for more urgent treatment. Administration of folinic acid simultaneously with methotrexate normalizes wound healing. Extravasation of chemotherapeutic agents during intravenous administration may result in severe ulceration and sloughing. The nature of the injury is largely related to the nucleic acid–binding characteristics of the agent. Those agents that do not bind to tissue nucleic acid (vincristine, vinblastine, nitrogen mustard, BCNU, 5-FU) generally cause only local damage from the immediate injury. These substances are quickly metabolized or inactivated, and usual patterns of wound healing can be expected. On the other hand, agents that bind the nucleic acid (doxorubicin, dactinomycin, mitomycin C, mithramycin, and daunorubicin) cause not only immediate toxic reaction in the tissues but, unless excised, continuing and progressive tissue damage. Though some authors have reported success with elevation and ice packs, most recommend surgical excision if there is severe pain, any sign of early necrosis, or significant blistering.

192. The answer is B. *(Schwartz, 6/e, pp 385–387.)* Unlike the granulocyte line, T lymphocytes express the T-cell receptor. This receptor imports antigen specificity to T cells. The helper T cell, when stimulated by interleukin 1 and antigens, produces various lymphokines that ultimately produce effector cells. One of these effector cells is the cytotoxic T cell, which will kill cells that express specific antigens including viral tumor and nonbiologic antigens. Macrophages and natural killer cells have some tumoricidal activity; however, this is not specific for tumors.

193. The answer is E. *(Way, 9/e, pp 645, 1216, 1221.)* The management of malignant tumors may be guided by knowledge obtained by grading and staging the tumors. Histological *grading* reflects the degree of anaplasia of tumor cells. Tumors in which histological grading seems to have prognostic value include soft-tissue sarcoma, transitional cell cancers of the bladder, astrocytoma, and chondrosarcoma. Grading has been of little predictive value in melanoma, hepatocellular carcinoma, or osteosarcoma. *Staging* is based on the extent of spread rather than histological appearance and is more relevant in predicting the course of prostate and colorectal cancers.

194. The answer is D. *(Schwartz, 6/e, p 654.)* Acinar, adenoid cystic, and low grades of mucoepidermoid carcinomas exhibit moderately malignant behavior. Undifferentiated, squamous, and high grades of mucoepidermoid carcinomas are considered highly malignant tumors. Regional node dissection is indicated for malignant tumors because of the high (up to 50 percent) incidence of occult regional metastases. Facial nerve preservation should be attempted when the margins are adequate and the tumor is well localized. The minimal appropriate procedure is a superficial parotidectomy with nerve preservation. The nerve must be partially or totally sacrificed if the tumor directly involves the nerve trunk or its branches.

195–199. The answers are 195-A, 196-B, 197-D, 198-C, 199-A *(Schwartz, 6/e, pp 437–448.)* A positive crossmatch means that the recipient has circulating antibodies that are cytotoxic to donor strain lymphocytes. This incompatibility, which almost always leads to an acute humoral rejection of the graft, precludes transplantation. Blood type matching prior to organ allograft is similar to cross-matching prior to transfusion; O is the universal donor and AB the universal recipient. Minor blood group factors do not appear to act as histocompatibility antigens. Matching of HLA antigens in cadaveric renal transplants may improve graft survival, but the impact is relatively minor. While attempts are made to pair recipient and donor by tissue typing, a two-antigen match is perfectly acceptable and even zero-antigen matches can be transplanted with good results. Neither hypertension nor anemia is a contraindication to transplantation; indeed, hypertension may be cured or ameliorated following successful transplantation. Patients with end-stage renal failure generally are anemic and can be transfused, if necessary, intra- or postoperatively. Anemia generally also improves following transplantation because of increased erythropoietin production by the graft.

The differential diagnosis of the oliguric patient in the early post-transplant period includes technical error with the vascular or ureteral anastomosis, accelerated rejection, or acute tubular necrosis (ATN). Good perfusion on the renal scan eliminates the arterial anastomosis as the problem and makes antibody-mediated rejection very unlikely. The lack of hydronephrosis eliminates ureteral obstruction as the source of oliguria. ATN is the diagnosis by exclusion. Most transplant centers will withhold cyclosporine in the setting of ATN because of the known potentiation of cyclosporine nephrotoxicity in this setting. Although some transplant centers will treat with azathioprine and steroids in this setting, most are now using an antilymphocyte preparation such as OKT3 or antilymphocyte globulin (ALG) until the ATN resolves. At that time, cyclosporine therapy is initiated.

The findings on the 14th day suggest that the patient has suffered a rejection episode. Because of the depressed white blood cell and platelet counts, azathioprine must be withheld to avoid further bone marrow suppression. Rejection treatment in this setting generally includes increased steroid administration. Definitive diagnosis by biopsy is indicated, inasmuch as infection and rejection can be confused or may co-exist. With infection present, immunosuppressants must be withheld or decreased, regardless of the effect on the graft survival. If rejection is confirmed by biopsy and there is no response to steroids, then an anti-lymphocyte preparation is usually started. ALG and OKT3 are both very effective agents. ALG will frequently cause thrombocytopenia and therefore OKT3 is currently being used more often.

Temperature elevation, chest film findings, and lack of evidence for rejection suggest the presence of pneumonitis. The first priority is the patient's survival, not allograft salvage. The current mortality level in transplant patients is approximately 5 to 10 percent, with infection the major cause of death. Immunosuppressed patients are at high risk for viral, fungal, and protozoal infections, all of which are difficult to di-agnose. Aggressive measures, including bronchoscopy, aspiration, and biopsy, are imperative for appropriate diagnosis and treatment. Immu-nosuppressant dosages must be reduced. Cyclosporine is the most spe-cific of the agents this patient is being treated with. It decreases anti-bacterial defense mechanisms less than do steroids or azathioprine and can sometimes be maintained throughout the course of a controlled in-fection. Percutaneous drainage of perirenal fluid collections for culture may reveal an infected lymphocele as a coexisting or primary infectious locus. Transplant nephrectomy is not necessary at this stage since the graft may survive the period of infection despite withdrawal of immu-nosuppressants.

Cyclosporine nephrotoxicity must be suspected whenever there is an asymptomatic rise in serum creatinine. Many drugs, one of which is ketoconazole, influence the hepatic metabolism of cyclosporine and can produce elevated serum levels (therapeutic range is 100 to 200 ng/mL) without dosage changes. In the setting described on the 40th postoper-ative day, the cyclosporine dose should be decreased. Many transplant surgeons would simultaneously increase other immunosuppressive agents to guard against rejection. If there is no improvement in serum creatinine after this step, then renal biopsy is indicated.

200–201. The answers are 200-D, 201-C. (*Wilson, 12/e, pp 1151, 1158–1159.*) Hemodialysis, rather than management by dietary manipulation alone, should be instituted in patients with end-stage renal failure whose serum creatinine is over 15 mg/dL or whose creatinine clearance is less than 3 mL/min. It is important that hemodialysis be initiated prior to the onset of uremic complications. These complications include hyper-kalemia, congestive heart failure, peripheral neuropathy, severe hypertension, pericarditis, bleeding, and severe anemia. The uremic hyperkalemic patient in congestive heart failure may require emergency dialysis in addition to the standard conservative measures, which include (1) limitation of protein intake to less than 60 g/day and restriction of fluid intake; and (2) reduction of elevated serum potassium levels by insulin-glucose or sodium polystyrene sulfonate (Kayexalate) enema treatment. Arteriovenous fistulas require about 2 weeks to develop adequate size and flow. While awaiting maturation, temporary dialysis can be satisfactorily performed using either an external arteriovenous shunt or the peritoneal cavity. Renal biopsy would be performed in an attempt to obtain a diagnosis of the underlying renal disease.

Patients who are acceptable candidates for kidney transplantation usually should undergo this form of treatment rather than chronic hemodialysis, the mortality for which is now higher than for transplantation. Despite adequate dialysis, problems of neuropathy, bone disease, anemia, and hypertension remain difficult to manage. Compared with chronic dialysis, transplantation restores more patients to happier and more productive lives. It has been conjectured that, all other issues being equal, sex matching was important in the graft survival and that a mother-daughter graft was preferred to a father-daughter. Review of the current data does not support such a conclusion. The best graft survival rates for living related transplants—over 90 percent at 5 years—are obtained when all six histocompatibility loci are identical. All family members of potential transplant recipients should be tissue typed and the donor selected on the basis of closest match, if psychological and medical evaluation makes this feasible. With the development of cyclosporine-based immunosuppression, cadaveric kidney graft survival has approached that of living-related transplantation. There are some transplanters who believe that the slight improvement with living-related kidneys does not justify the risk to the donor and that these transplantations should no longer be performed.

202. The answer is B. *(Schwartz, 6/e, pp 414–419.)* With the introduction of cyclosporine in the early 1980s and the rapidly accumulated experience with liver transplantation, graft and patient survivals have improved markedly. In the azathioprine and steroid era, 1-year graft survival was in the range of 25 percent. More recently, most centers are experiencing 1-year graft survival rates of approximately 80 percent.

203. The answer is D. *(Schwartz, 6/e, pp 398–399.)* Cyclosporine is a highly effective immunosuppressive agent produced by fungi. It is more specific than the anti-inflammatory agents such as steroids or the anti-proliferative agents such as azathioprine. The effectiveness of cyclosporine in preventing allograft rejection is related to its ability to inhibit interleukin 2 production. Without interleukin 2 from helper T cells, there is no clonal expansion of alloantigen-directed cytotoxic T cells and no stimulation of antibody production by B cells.

204. The answer is A. (*Way, 9/e, pp 1203–1204.*) This is a nephroblastoma (Wilms' tumor) adherent to the left kidney. These tumors are associated with aniridia (rarely) and with hemihypertrophy, cryptorchidism, or hypospadias in about 10 percent of cases. Most patients present with an asymptomatic mass found by a parent. Less than one-third of patients experience hematuria. As would be expected in over half such cases, this child is hypertensive, probably due to compression of the renal artery by the mass. Treatment with excision, radiation, vincristine, and actinomycin D results in survival of over 90 percent in stage I and II tumors. While computed tomography (CT) or magnetic resonance imaging (MRI) evaluates metastatic disease, intravenous pyelography (IVP) is better at differentiating this tumor from polycystic kidney or neuroblastoma. Wilms' tumor is the most common abdominal malignancy of childhood, but represents only about 10 percent of childhood malignant tumors.

205–206. The answers are 205-D, 206-B. (*Schwartz, 6/e, pp 1586–1593.*) This young pregnant woman presents with the symptoms of a pheochromocytoma. These tumors can become initially symptomatic during pregnancy. A noninvasive workup should be performed. Ultrasonography of the abdomen is frequently sufficient to localize the tumor to the right or left adrenal; an abdominal CT scan with its large dose of radiation should be avoided in pregnancy. The treatment can be early excision of the pheochromocytoma, and in three cases in pregnant women this was done with survival of two of the three infants. A therapeutic abortion, especially at 8 months, is not indicated. The more current approach is α- and β-adrenergic blockade followed by vaginal delivery or caesarean section with excision of the tumor at the same time as delivery or electively after delivery. Metyrosine (Demser) inhibits tyrosine hydroxylase and results in a decrease in endogenous levels of catecholamines. This form of treatment is also acceptable.

207. The answer is C. (*Schwartz, 6/e, pp 1638–1639.*) Medullary carcinomas occur in families as part of syndromes called multiple endocrine neoplasia (MEN), type IIA and type IIB. MEN-IIA consists of multicentric medullary thyroid cancer, pheochromocytomas or adrenal medullary hyperplasia, and hyperparathyroidism. MEN-IIB consists of medullary cancer, pheochromocytoma and mucosal neuromas, gangliomas, and a Marfan-like habitus. These patients may develop medullary carcinoma at a very young age, and any patient with MEN-IIB should be assumed to have medullary cancer until proved otherwise. Patients are followed carefully for pheochromocytoma with urine VMA, for hyperparathyroidism with serum calcium, and for medullary carcinoma with serum calcitonin. However, as some patients have a normal basal calcitonin, a pentagastrin or calcium infusion test should be performed in these high-risk patients. Gastrin levels should be obtained in patients thought to have MEN-I syndrome (pituitary, parathyroid, and pancreatic tumors) or Zollinger-Ellison syndrome.

208. The answer is E. (*Copeland, pp 640–641, 644–646.*) Although somewhat controversial, staging laparotomy is generally recommended for many patients with non-Hodgkin's lymphoma whose disease is localized to a single lymph node region. Since most patients with non-Hodgkin's lymphoma (over 90 percent) have anatomically disseminated disease at time of presentation, however, this issue is not often germane. Treatment usually consists of combination chemotherapy and radiation, but surgery is important in establishing the diagnosis and in resection of extranodal lymphomas. These may arise in the gastrointestinal tract, bone, soft tissue, skin, and nasopharynx. Lymphomas constitute 3 percent of all malignant gastric tumors. Ninety percent of these lymphomas are non-Hodgkin's. For early lesions, resections can achieve a 30 percent 5-year survival rate. If a total gastrectomy is necessary to remove the lesion, resection should not be performed and chemoradiotherapy should be employed.

209. The answer is D. (*Copeland, pp 618–620.*) Ten percent of patients with colorectal cancer have liver metastases at time of initial presentation. Thirty to forty percent of patients with recurrent disease have liver metastases. Patients with metastatic disease localized to resectable portions of the liver who are suitable candidates for surgery should undergo appropriate local excision or lobectomy since 5-year survival rates of 20 to 40 percent can be anticipated. Patients with solitary metastases have the most favorable prognosis, but cures after lobectomy for multiple metastases are also reported. Operative mortality of less than 10 percent should be expected after lobectomy and less than 5 percent for local or wedge resections. Data from the Liver Tumor Study on colorectal hepatic metastases have shown no survival benefit to patients with synchronous as opposed to metachronous disease.

210. The answer is B (1, 3). *Collins, Semin Hematol 29:64–74, 1992.)* Autoimmune hemolytic anemia results from acute red blood cell destruction secondary to complement fixation of antibodies bound to the surface of the erythrocytes. Medications that induce antibody synthesis, viral infections, malignancies, and other inflammatory processes can trigger autoimmune hemolytic anemia. Therapy with corticosteroids results in an 80 percent response even in cases of severe hemolysis. Red cell transfusions may be needed in the acute phase if the patient has symptomatic anemia. With the hemolysis thus under control, the underlying problem is addressed (e.g., withdrawing a drug, awaiting resolution of a viral illness, treatment of a malignancy). Generally, the steroid dose can be tapered so that a small maintenance dose will control the disease well. A positive direct Coombs test confirms the diagnosis of autoimmune hemolytic anemia. This bioassay results in hemolysis when complement is added to a sample of the patient's red blood cells. The anemia is associated with either cold (IgM) or warm (IgG) antibodies. Warm antibodies are more common, and since the IgG-erythrocyte complex is destroyed in the spleen, splenectomy may benefit these patients. Splenectomy or other immunosuppressive drugs (azathioprine or cyclophosphamide) should be tried if the response to steroids is poor or if steroid-associated complications develop. Patients with cold-induced (IgM) hemolysis are rarely helped by splenectomy alone since the IgM-erythrocyte complex is primarily destroyed in the liver. These patients may be helped by avoiding the cold or by using heated gloves and socks. Occasionally plasmapheresis is required to decrease the cold agglutinin titer during an acute phase of hemolysis.

211. The answer is B (1, 3). *(Schwartz, 6/e, pp 1731, 1764–1765.)* After radical orchiectomy, lymph node dissection is indicated in embryonal carcinoma, teratocarcinoma, and adult teratoma if there is no supradiaphragmatic spread. This dissection increases the 5-year survival and helps in staging. Seminoma is extremely radiosensitive and lymph node dissection is unnecessary. Choriocarcinoma is associated with pulmonary metastases in 81 percent of cases and is treated with chemotherapy.

212. The answer is A (1, 2, 3). *(Schwartz, 6/e, pp 410–411.)* Bone marrow cells are highly immunogenic. Successful engraftment requires the use of immunosuppressants that permit the transplanted cells not only to survive but also to mount a graft-versus-host response against recipient tissues. The graft-versus-host response is the major impediment to more widespread clinical use of this technique. Despite these barriers, human bone marrow transplantation has had important clinical application in the treatment of aplastic anemias and congenital immunodeficiency diseases and several hematologic malignancies. In experimental models, work with bone marrow transplantation for the induction of tolerance to organ allografts has proved highly promising. This may provide a key for the development of treatment protocols in organ transplant recipients that would avoid or reduce the need for toxic systemic immunosuppressants.

213. The answer is A (1, 2, 3). *(Heys, Br J Surg 79:614–623, 1992.)* Malignant tumors require energy substrates to grow and ordinarily claim these substrates from the host. In animal studies, withholding dietary proteins diminishes the rate of tumor growth. There is no evidence in the human to suggest acceleration of tumor growth when nutritional support is provided. There is also no evidence that nutritional therapy improves the response of the tumor to therapy. For nearly a century, the association of stomach cancer and diet has been recognized. Among the wide variety of substances incriminated are nitrates and nitrosamides in food and drinking water. There is evidence that regular ingestion of vitamin C from childhood may reduce the formation of carcinogens, though reduction in the incidence of cancer has not been demonstrated. Excess amounts of dietary fat and deficiency of fiber have been clearly associated with colon cancer. Animal fats have also been associated with cancer of the exocrine pancreas, the breast, the prostate, and the endometrium.

214. The answer is A (1, 2, 3). *(Schwartz, 6/e, pp 370, 752–753.)* Resection of metastases of lung, liver, and brain can result in occasional 5-year cures. In general, surgery should be undertaken only when the primary tumor is controlled, diffuse metastatic disease has been ruled out, and the affected patient's condition and the location of the metastasis permit safe resection. Five-year survivals as high as 18 percent have been reported for selected patients with liver metastases from colorectal primaries. However, the best results have come from resection of pulmonary metastases, in which 5-year survival rates exceed those of resection for primary bronchogenic carcinoma. Autopsy reviews have demonstrated that many patients with pulmonary metastases have no other evidence of tumor, which suggests that resectional treatment may be justified even when the lung foci are not solitary. Selection of patients for pulmonary resections may be aided by measurement of tumor doubling times; patients with doubling times greater than 40 days appear to benefit most, while those with doubling times less than 20 days are not significantly helped.

215. The answer is C (2, 4). *(Cerilli, pp 413–418.)* Donor-type lymphoid cells transplanted within a graft may recognize the host's tissue as foreign and mount an immune response against the host. This response, termed graft-versus-host disease (GVHD), is common in bone marrow transplantation and is an important source of morbidity and mortality. Treatment requires more aggressive immunosuppression. Current clinical practice includes depletion of lymphocytes from the marrow graft in order to prevent the development of GVHD. GVHD has been documented following liver transplantation—presumably because of the large amount of lymphoid tissue in the donor liver. GVHD has not been described following heart or kidney transplantation.

216. The answer is A (1, 2, 3). *(Cerilli, pp 361–377.)* Renal transplantation is less expensive than dialysis if the graft functions for more than 2 years. Recipients with functioning grafts are less anemic because of erythropoietin production by the graft. As more dialysis patients are treated with recombinant erythropoietin, this advantage may disappear. Females have more normal menses and an increased number of successful pregnancies. The patient survival in the two groups is comparable at 1 year.

217. The answer is A (1, 2, 3). *(von Schilfgaarde, pp 86–106.)* Whole-organ pancreas transplantation is the only therapy for type I insulin-dependent diabetes that maintains normal serum glucose levels and normal glucose tolerance tests. When the pancreas is transplanted along with a kidney, the tight glucose control generally prevents the recurrence of diabetic nephropathy. No series has shown the reversal of diabetic retinopathy after pancreas transplantation.

218. The answer is E (all). *(Schwartz, 6/e, pp 366, 379, 387.)* The interferons are a group of glycoproteins first found as products of virus-infected cells that inhibited viral replication. Subsequently, they have been shown to have a variety of effects on both cells of the immune system and malignant cells. Interferons cause Burkitt's lymphoma cell lines to differentiate and lose the capacity to divide. Hematological malignancies are very responsive to the interferons; up to 100 percent of hairy cell leukemias show some degree of remission.

219. The answer is E (all). *(Schwartz, 6/e, pp 353–362.)* A surgeon frequently is asked to evaluate patients who are receiving chemotherapy. Most complications do not require surgical therapy. Gastrointestinal bleeding occurs secondary to mucosal irritation and thrombocytopenia. Perirectal abscesses are more common in these immunosuppressed patients. Pancreatitis is uncommon, but is associated with L-asparaginase use. Up to 20 percent of patients treated with floxuridine by continuous hepatic artery infusion develop some degree of inflammation and obstruction of the bile duct.

220. The answer is B (1, 3). *(Rhame, Postgrad Med 91:141–152, 1992. Wilson, Postgrad Med 88:193–201, 1990.)* The risk of contracting AIDS is much less than the risk of contracting hepatitis B from a patient. Although the risk of transmission of AIDS in the health care setting is very low, there are reported cases of seroconversion after parenteral exposure. Particular precautions should be taken in operating upon patients who are known to be seropositive for HIV or who have known risk factors. Recommendations include elimination of inexperienced personnel or personnel with open lesions on body surfaces from the operating room. Disposable gowns, drapes, masks, and eye shields should be used. Clothing should be soaked in a dilute solution (1:10) of chlorine bleach prior to washing and personnel should shower after the procedure. Double gloving does not reduce the major intraoperative risk of needle puncture, which is the primary source of risk to the operating team. Needles should never be capped; an uncapped needle is less dangerous than are the maneuvers to recap needles.

221. The answer is E (all). *(Schwartz, 6/e, pp 364, 366, 1263–1265.)* Acquired immune deficiency syndrome (AIDS) is characterized by a reversal in the normal T-lymphocyte helper-to-suppressor ratio. Monoclonal antibodies are helpful in detecting this reversal in peripheral blood samples and in lymph node biopsies, especially when lymphocyte numbers and lymph node architecture appear normal. They are also important in the diagnosis of lymphomas, both non-Hodgkin's and Hodgkin's, and of leukemias. Monoclonal antibodies have been made to "TdT," a marker on immature B and T lymphocytes. This is especially helpful in differentiating lymphocytes from myelocytes in bone marrow biopsies, which is necessary in distinguishing acute myelocytic leukemia (AML) from acute lymphocytic leukemia (ALL). Monoclonal antibodies are also used for checking the clonal nature of B cells. If this is present, a lymphoma can be diagnosed even in the presence of a node that appears normal. A Hodgkin's lymphoma can be differentiated from a high-grade T lymphoma by the polyclonal nature of the cells in the former. Monoclonal antibodies to Reed-Sternberg cells have been made and are being used experimentally.

222. The answer is B (1, 3). (*Hall, Cancer 55:2051–2057, 1985. Kohn, N Engl J Med 310:504–511, 1984. Wilkening, Med Clin North Am 74:489–507, 1990.*) Among the basic principles of radiation biology are the observations that the sensitivity of mammalian cells to radiation varies with their position in the cell-division (mitotic) cycle. The percentage of cells killed by a given dose of x-rays or gamma rays is greatly increased by molecular oxygen; cells deficient in oxygen are resistant to radiation. Only about 30 percent of the biologic damage from x-rays is due to the direct effects on the target molecule. The remainder is due to an indirect action mediated by free radicals and can be modified by free radical scavengers such as sulfhydryl. Workers at the Oak Ridge National Laboratory have identified the safe radiation limit for an average person as 0.17 rad per year, with a 30-year maximum of 5 rad. This is superimposed on the 12 rad the average U.S. citizen will accumulate from natural sources by age 65. It is difficult to estimate cancer risk from radiation up to 10 rad above background since there is variation in risk per rad depending on dose, dose-rates, and the linear energy transfer (LET) of the radiation source. Low-LET radiation (e.g., gamma rays, x-rays, and beta rays) becomes less damaging to tissue per rad as the dose falls; high-LET radiation (e.g., neutrons and alpha particles) does not. The exposures from radiological examinations are low-LET exposures in low-dose, low-dose-rate ranges, and the risk associated with them is difficult to estimate. That risk has been estimated to be about one case of radiogenic cancer per million procedures per year.

223. The answer is C (2, 4). (*Fidler, Cancer Bull 39:126–131, 1987.*) Tumor metastases occur as a result of a complex process of tumor cell factors and host responses. At the lower limit of clinical detectability (1 cc), there are already 1 billion aggregated tumor cells. Experimental work confirms that cells or cell aggregates cultured from metastases are both biologically and immunologically heterogeneous, despite their similar histological appearance; they also have markedly variable potential for establishing viable metastases. In experimental models, 99 percent of radiolabeled tumor cells introduced into the circulation are dead by the end of the first 24 h and less than 0.1 percent survive to produce metastases. Most injected tumor cells are destroyed by the mechanical stress of blood turbulence. Local invasion seems to be the consequence of several interrelated factors: the forcing of cords of cells along lower resistance paths as a result of mechanical pressure from the proliferating tumor mass; tumor cell motility; and, more clearly, specific tissue destruction and destabilization caused by destructive lytic enzymes produced by the neoplastic cells.

224. The answer is E (all). *(Schwartz, 6/e, pp 446–447.)* Hyperacute rejection is mediated by cytotoxic antibodies with subsequent triggering of the complement, coagulation, and kinin systems. It can occur during surgery after the clamps are released from the vascular anastomosis and the recipient's antibodies are exposed to the donor's passenger lymphocytes and kidney tissue. It is the cause of immediate and early oliguria and biopsies should be performed intraoperatively or early postoperatively. Hyperacute rejection is characterized pathologically by fibrin and platelet thrombosis and necrosis of the glomerular tufts, renal arterioles, and small arteries. Massive polymorphonuclear infiltrate with tubular necrosis occurs 24 to 36 h after transplantation. The intravascular coagulation can rarely result in a systemic coagulopathy. Careful crossmatching can test for cytotoxic antibodies.

225. The answer is B (1, 3). *(Schwartz, 6/e, pp 419–426.)* Cardiac transplantation has become an acceptable clinical treatment modality for selected patients with end-stage cardiac failure. Allograft survivals are now comparable to those of cadaveric renal transplants—approximately 70 percent at 1 year and 50 percent at 5 years as reported by the Stanford group. Although kidneys can be safely preserved by either hypothermic storage or hypothermic perfusion for periods up to 48 h, donor hearts, protected by simple hypothermia, should be transplanted within 4 h. For this reason the usual tissue-typing procedures used in kidney transplantation are impractical in cardiac transplantation. The role of prospective tissue-typing is not clear in cardiac transplantation and it is frequently not performed. In pairing donor and recipient for heart transplants there must be at least ABO blood group compatibility. Cyclosporine has improved results in both cardiac and renal transplantation despite its major drawback of dose-related nephrotoxicity.

226. The answer is A (1, 2, 3). *(Schwartz, 6/e, pp 366–367, 619.)* With the availability of recombinant IL-2, multiple trials of cancer therapy with this lymphokine have been undertaken. The most successful trials include the reinfusion of in vivo IL-2. Rosenberg's group has documented complete or partial responses in 33, 23, and 100 percent of renal cell, melanoma, and non-Hodgkin's lymphoma patients, respectively. Infusion of either LAK cells or IL-2 alone was not nearly as effective. The therapy is not innocuous: there were 4 deaths among 106 patients treated. All patients exhibit a marked lymphocytosis, eosinophilia, fluid retention, fever, and decrease in peripheral vascular resistance.

227–230. The answers are 227-C, 228-A, 229-C, 230-D *(Recommendations for prevention of HIV transmission in health care settings. NY State J Med 88:25–31, 1988. Rhame, Postgrad Med 91:141–144, 1992.)* Human immunodeficiency virus (HIV) has been isolated from blood, semen, vaginal secretions, saliva, tears, breast milk, cerebrospinal fluid, amniotic fluid, and urine. It is an extremely fastidious virus that ordinarily is transmitted only after repeated admixture of body fluids. Blood and semen are by far the major transmission fluids, though vaginal secretions have been weakly implicated in the transmission of HIV by epidemiological evidence. Breast milk is probably another mode of transmission.

231–233. The answers are 231-C, 232-A, 233-B. *(Schwartz, 6/e, pp 309–311, 1087–1098, 1337, 1761.)* Both alcohol ingestion and tobacco smoking appear to carry an increased risk of carcinoma. Both have been implicated in esophageal carcinoma, while smoking alone is associated with bladder carcinoma. Alcoholic cirrhosis as well as cirrhosis from other causes is associated with hepatocellular carcinoma.

234–236. The answers are 234-A, 235-C, 236-C. *(Cirelli, pp 37–66.)* Major histocompatibility complex (MHC) proteins are polymorphic cell surface molecules that are important in lymphocyte-lymphocyte and lymphocyte-target interactions. All nucleated cells express MHC class I proteins. B lymphocytes, macrophages, and activated T lymphocytes express both MHC class I and class II. The specificity of killing by cytotoxic T cells occurs via recognition of specific MHC class I molecules on target cells. The initiation of the immune response, however, requires presentation of antigen on cells that express MHC class II molecules.

237–240. The answers are 237-E, 238-A, 239-D, 240-C. *(Schwartz, 6/e, pp 395–406.)* Despite recent advances in tissue typing and immune modifications of graft and host, the major obstacle to successful transplantation remains rejection. Immunosuppressive regimens are required in virtually all patients. The major complications resulting from these agents are infection and bone marrow suppression.

The most recent addition to the available agents is cyclosporine A. This fungal derivative has proved, in numerous animal and human studies, to be a highly effective immunosuppressant with minimal side effects of infection. Its major clinical drawback is dose-related nephrotoxicity, which makes its use in renal transplantation difficult though still efficacious.

Azathioprine and cyclophosphamide both inhibit cell division and cause bone marrow suppression. Cyclophosphamide can cause testicular atrophy and sterility but is often substituted for azathioprine when hepatocellular damage occurs.

Antilymphocyte serum is used both prophylactically to prevent rejection and to treat acute cellular rejection. Anaphylactoid reactions occur but are generally manageable and rarely either preclude use of the serum or lead to lethal sequelae. Thrombocytopenia is a common side effect.

Corticosteroids are used as adjuncts to all the other immunosuppressive agents listed for long-term graft maintenance and for treatment of rejection episodes. The attendant complications are well known and include, most importantly, predisposition to infection, gastrointestinal ulceration, aseptic necrosis of bone, and impaired wound healing. The recent trend toward use of substantially lower doses has led to a decrease in complications with no apparent increase in rejection rates.

Endocrine Problems and Breast

DIRECTIONS: Each question below contains five suggested responses. Select the **one best** response to each question.

241. Regarding adrenal cortical insufficiency all the following are true EXCEPT that

(A) adrenal insufficiency may be precipitated by anticoagulation with either warfarin (Coumadin) or heparin

(B) it is characteristically seen as a consequence of metastasis to the adrenal glands, especially from lung or breast

(C) adrenal insufficiency in the postoperative patient may have an insidious onset with gradually progressive hypoglycemia, hyponatremia, and hyperkalemia

(D) the most common underlying cause is poor administration of exogenous steroids

(E) the electrolyte changes of adrenal insufficiency secondary to prior chronic exogenous steroids may not occur until late in the postoperative course

242. The thyroid scan shown below exhibits a pattern that is more consistent with which of the following disorders?

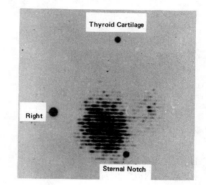

(A) Hypersecreting adenoma
(B) Graves' disease
(C) Lateral aberrant thyroid
(D) Papillary carcinoma of thyroid
(E) Medullary carcinoma of thyroid

243. A 17-year-old girl presents with an anterior neck mass. Her thyroid scan, shown below, is most consistent with which of the following disorders?

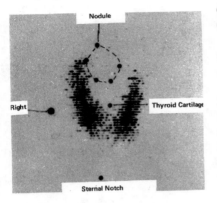

(A) Hypersecreting adenoma
(B) Parathyroid adenoma
(C) Thyroglossal duct cyst
(D) Graves' disease
(E) Carcinoma

244. The radiographic (mammographic and xeroradiographic) findings that require breast biopsy include all the following EXCEPT

(A) breast calcifications larger than 2 mm in diameter
(B) five or more clustered breast microcalcifications per square centimeter
(C) stellate-shaped breast mass
(D) breast mass with ill-defined borders
(E) dominant, well-circumscribed smooth breast mass

245. Estrogen receptor activity is clinically useful to predict

(A) presence of ovarian cancer
(B) presence of metastatic disease
(C) response to chemotherapy
(D) response to hormonal manipulation
(E) likelihood of development of osteoporosis

246. When galactorrhea occurs in a high school student, a diagnostic associated finding would be

(A) gonadal atrophy
(B) bitemporal hemianopia
(C) exophthalmos and lid lag
(D) episodic hypertension
(E) a "buffalo hump"

247. The diagnosis of primary hyperparathyroidism is most strongly suggested by

(A) serum acid phosphatase above 120 IU/L
(B) serum alkaline phosphatase above 120 IU/L
(C) serum calcium above 11 mg/dL
(D) urinary calcium below 100 mg/day
(E) parathyroid hormone levels below 5 pmoles/L

248. Somatostatin contributes to the regulation of each of the following EXCEPT

(A) adrenocortical cells
(B) pancreatic alpha cells
(C) antral gastrin cells
(D) secretin-producing cells in the duodenum
(E) GI motility

249. All the following statements concerning Cushing's syndrome secondary to adrenal adenoma are true EXCEPT that

(A) the tumors are only rarely malignant
(B) biochemical and x-ray procedures generally make preoperative isolation of the tumors possible
(C) exploration of both adrenal glands is frequently indicated
(D) for uncomplicated tumors an abdominothoracic incision is usually employed
(E) postoperative corticoid therapy is required to prevent hypoadrenalism

250. A 40-year-old woman is found to have a 1- to 2-cm, slightly tender cystic mass in her breast; she has no perceptible axillary adenopathy. What course would you follow?

(A) Reassurance and reexamination in the immediate postmenstrual period
(B) Immediate excisional biopsy
(C) Aspiration of the mass with cytological analysis
(D) Fluoroscopically guided needle localization biopsy
(E) Mammography and reevaluation of options with new information

251. Which statement concerning radiation-induced thyroid cancer is true?

(A) It usually follows high-dose radiation to the head and neck
(B) A patient with a history of radiation is safe if no cancer has been found 20 years after exposure
(C) Approximately 25 percent of patients with a history of head and neck irradiation develop thyroid cancer
(D) Most radiation-induced thyroid cancers are follicular
(E) The treatment of choice is a near-total (or total) thyroidectomy

252. The course of papillary carcinoma of the thyroid is best described by which of the following statements?

(A) Metastases are rare; local growth is rapid; erosion into the trachea and large blood vessels is frequent

(B) Local invasion and metastases almost never occur, which makes the term "carcinoma" misleading

(C) Bony metastases are frequent and produce an osteolytic pattern particularly in vertebrae

(D) Metastases frequently occur to cervical lymph nodes; distant metastases and local invasion are rare

(E) Rapid, widespread metastatic involvement of the liver, lungs, and bone marrow results in a 5-year survival rate of approximately 10 percent

253. Fibrocystic disease of the breast has been associated with elevated blood levels of

(A) testosterone
(B) progesterone
(C) estrogen
(D) luteinizing hormone
(E) aldosterone

254. A 14-year-old black girl had her right breast removed because of a large mass. The tumor weighed 1400 g and was found to have a bulging, very firm, lobulated surface with a whorl-like pattern, as illustrated below. This neoplasm is most likely

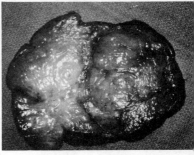

(A) cystosarcoma phylloides
(B) intraductal carcinoma
(C) malignant lymphoma
(D) fibroadenoma
(E) juvenile hypertrophy

255. As an incidental finding during an upper abdominal CT scan, a 2 × 2 cm mass in the adrenal gland is noted. The appropriate next step in analysis and management of this finding would be

(A) observation
(B) CT-guided needle biopsy
(C) excision of the mass
(D) measurement of urine catecholamine excretion
(E) cortisol provocation test

Questions 256–257

A 53-year-old woman presents with complaints of weakness, anorexia, malaise, constipation, and back pain. While being evaluated, she becomes somewhat lethargic. Laboratory studies include a normal chest x-ray, serum albumin of 3.2 mg/dL, serum calcium of 14 mg/dL, serum phosphorus of 2.6 mg/dL, serum chloride of 108 mg/dL, BUN of 32 mg/dL, and creatinine of 2.0 mg/dL.

256. Appropriate initial management would include

(A) intravenous normal saline infusion
(B) administration of thiazide diuretics
(C) administration of intravenous phosphorus
(D) use of mithramycin
(E) neck exploration and parathyroidectomy

257. After appropriate immediate management, the patient's symptoms resolve. Appropriate diagnostic tests to perform at this point would include all the following EXCEPT

(A) abdominal and chest CT scans
(B) measurement of serum parathyroid hormone levels
(C) a Kveim test
(D) serum and urine protein electrophoresis
(E) mammography and breast examination

258. All the following statements concerning fat necrosis of the breast are true EXCEPT that

(A) it usually is associated with a history of trauma
(B) it usually occurs in large, pendulous breasts
(C) it predisposes patients to the development of breast cancer
(D) liquefaction of fat may produce cystic spaces
(E) the treatment of choice is local excision

Questions 259–260

259. The most likely diagnosis in a patient with hypertension, hypokalemia, and a 7-cm suprarenal mass is

(A) hypernephroma
(B) Cushing's disease
(C) adrenocortical carcinoma
(D) pheochromocytoma
(E) carcinoid syndrome

260. Appropriate treatment of this condition would include all the following EXCEPT

(A) surgical resection
(B) ketoconazole
(C) mitotane
(D) hydrocortisone
(E) phenoxybenzamine

Questions 261–262

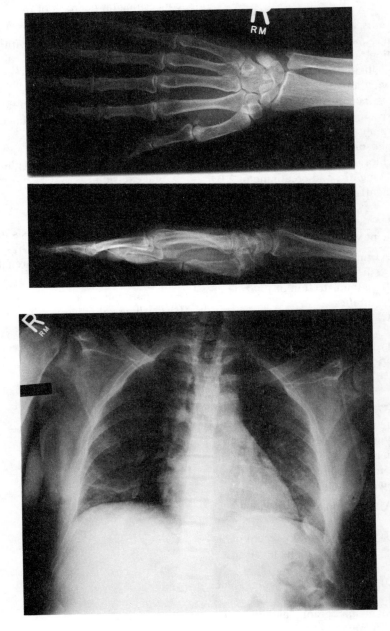

261. This 30-year-old woman presented with weakness, bone pain, an elevated parathormone level, and a serum calcium level of 15.2 mg/dL. Skeletal survey films were taken including the hand films and chest x-ray shown. The most likely cause of these findings is

(A) sarcoidosis
(B) vitamin D intoxication
(C) Paget's disease
(D) metastatic carcinoma
(E) primary hyperparathyroidism

262. Following correction of her hypercalcemia with hydration and gentle diuresis with furosemide, the most likely therapeutic approach would be

(A) administration of maintenance doses of steroids
(B) radiation treatment for bony metastases
(C) neck exploration and resection of three out of four parathyroid glands
(D) neck exploration and resection of a parathyroid adenoma
(E) avoidance of sunlight, vitamin D, and calcium-containing dairy products

DIRECTIONS: Each question below contains four suggested responses of which **one or more** is correct. Select

A	if	**1, 2, and 3**	are correct
B	if	**1 and 3**	are correct
C	if	**2 and 4**	are correct
D	if	**4**	is correct
E	if	**1, 2, 3, and 4**	are correct

263. Correct statements regarding management of pregnant patients who have breast cancer include

(1) modified radical mastectomy is the accepted standard of therapy for stage I or II carcinoma during pregnancy

(2) carcinoma of the breast behaves more aggressively in pregnant women owing to hormonal stimulation

(3) administration of adjuvant chemotherapy is safe for the fetus during the second and third trimesters

(4) termination of a first-term pregnancy will decrease hormonal stimulation of the tumor and improve long-term survival of the patient

264. True statements regarding Paget's disease of the breast include

(1) Paget's disease of bone usually precedes development of Paget's disease of the breast

(2) most patients present with nipple-areolar eczematous changes

(3) involvement of axillary lymph nodes is uncommon, which makes node dissection unnecessary

(4) less than 1 in 25 patients with breast cancer has Paget's disease of breast

265. A 40-year-old man who has a long history of peptic ulcer disease that has not responded to medical therapy is admitted to the hospital. His serum gastrin levels are markedly elevated; at celiotomy, a small firm mass is palpated in the tail of the pancreas. Correct statements concerning this patient's condition include which of the following?

(1) Histamine or a protein meal will markedly increase basal acid secretion
(2) Secretin administration will suppress acid secretion
(3) The pancreatic mass will probably be benign
(4) Distal pancreatectomy is the treatment of choice

266. Complications of surgical extirpation of the thyroid or parathyroid glands include

(1) injury to the recurrent laryngeal nerve
(2) injury to the superior laryngeal nerve
(3) symptomatic hypocalcemia
(4) postoperative hemorrhage and wound hematoma

267. A 25-year-old woman is found to have an anterior neck mass. Her thyroid scan, shown below, exhibits findings that are consistent with which of the following disorders?

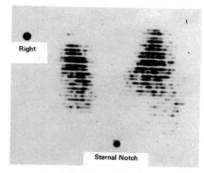

(1) Carcinoma
(2) Hyperfunctioning adenoma
(3) Follicular adenoma
(4) Graves' disease

268. Incisional biopsy of a breast mass in a 35-year-old woman demonstrates a hypercellular fibroadenoma (cystosarcoma phylloides) at the time of frozen section. Appropriate management of this lesion could include

(1) wide local excision with a rim of normal tissue
(2) lumpectomy and axillary lymphadenectomy
(3) simple mastectomy for very large lesions
(4) excision and postoperative radiotherapy

SUMMARY OF DIRECTIONS

A	B	C	D	E
1,2,3 only	1,3 only	2,4 only	4 only	All are correct

269. A 36-year-old woman, 20 weeks pregnant, presents with a 1.5-cm right thyroid mass. Fine-needle aspiration is consistent with a papillary neoplasm. The mass is "cold" by scan and solid by ultrasound. Acceptable management of this lesion would include

(1) right thyroid lobectomy
(2) total thyroidectomy
(3) subtotal thyroidectomy
(4) ^{131}I radioactive ablation of the thyroid gland

270. True statements about discharges from the nipple include

(1) intermittent thin or milky discharge can be physiological
(2) expressible nipple discharge is an indication for open biopsy
(3) bloody discharge may indicate Paget's disease of the nipple
(4) bloody discharge usually indicates an underlying malignancy

271. A 28-year-old man presents with a 2.5-cm mass in the anterior triangle of the left neck. The mass moves with swallowing and has slowly enlarged over the past 1 to 2 years. His past medical history is notable for high-dose irradiation to the chest and abdomen for Hodgkin's lymphoma 8 years prior to presentation. Thyroid scan shows a "cool" lesion. Fine-needle aspiration cytology is "suspicious." Core-needle biopsy shows features suggestive of a follicular neoplasm. Appropriate management for this patient would include

(1) left thyroid lobectomy
(2) ^{131}I radioactive ablation of the thyroid
(3) total thyroidectomy
(4) TSH suppression with thyroid hormone (Synthroid)

272. Correct statements concerning Hürthle-cell carcinoma of the thyroid include which of the following?

(1) It is a form of follicular cancer
(2) It metastasizes via the blood to bone, lung, and liver
(3) Treatment consists of a near-total (or total) thyroidectomy
(4) Microscopically it consists of clusters of cells separated by areas of collagen and amyloid

273. True statements regarding Cushing's disease and syndrome include which of the following?

(1) Adrenocortical hyperplasia is the most common cause of Cushing's syndrome

(2) Overproduction of ACTH is pathognomonic of Cushing's disease

(3) The pituitary may be suppressed in the syndrome

(4) Chromophobe pituitary tumors are a cause of Cushing's disease

274. A 34-year-old woman has recurrent fainting spells induced by fasting. Her serum insulin levels during these episodes are markedly elevated. Correct statements regarding this patient's condition include which of the following?

(1) The underlying lesion is probably an alpha-cell tumor of the pancreas

(2) She should be screened for a pheochromocytoma

(3) These lesions are usually malignant

(4) Serum calcium levels may be elevated

275. The incidence of breast cancer

(1) increases with increasing age

(2) has declined since the 1940s

(3) is twice as high for women 80 to 85 compared with women 60 to 65

(4) is greater among black women than white women

DIRECTIONS: Each group of questions below consists of four lettered headings followed by a set of numbered items. For each numbered item select

A	if the item is associated with	(A) **only**
B	if the item is associated with	(B) **only**
C	if the item is associated with	**both** (A) and (B)
D	if the item is associated with	**neither** (A) nor (B)

Each lettered heading may be used **once, more than once, or not at all.**

Questions 276–278

(A) Propylthiouracil (PTU)
(B) Methimazole (Tapazole)
(C) Both
(D) Neither

276. Will decrease peripheral tissue conversion of T_4 to T_3

277. Will decrease uptake of iodine by the thyroid

278. Will alter the iodination and coupling of tyrosine moieties in thyroglobulin

Questions 279–281

(A) Hormone (estrogen and progesterone) receptor proteins
(B) Lymph node metastasis
(C) Both
(D) Neither

279. Adversely prognostic in breast cancer

280. Relevant to operability in breast cancer

281. Relevant to choice of adjuvant therapy in breast cancer

DIRECTIONS: The group of questions below consists of lettered headings followed by a set of numbered items. For each numbered item select the **one** lettered heading with which it is **most** closely associated. Each lettered heading may be used **once, more than once, or not at all.**

Questions 282–286

For each clinical description select the appropriate stage of breast cancer

(A) Stage I
(B) Stage II
(C) Stage III
(D) Stage IV
(E) Inflammatory carcinoma

282. Tumor not palpable, clinically positive lymph nodes fixed to one another, no evidence of metastases

283. Tumor 5.0 cm; clinically positive, movable ipsilateral lymph nodes; no evidence of metastases

284. Tumor 2.1 cm, clinically negative lymph nodes, no evidence of metastases

285. Tumor not palpable but breast diffusely enlarged and erythematous, clinically positive supraclavicular nodes, and evidence of metastases

286. Tumor 0.5 cm, clinically negative lymph nodes, pathological rib fracture

Questions 287–290

A 43-year-old man presents with signs and symptoms of peritonitis in the right lower quadrant. The clinical impression and supportive data suggest acute appendicitis. At exploration, however, a tumor is found; frozen section suggests carcinoid features. For each tumor described, choose the most appropriate surgical procedure.

(A) Appendectomy
(B) Segmental ileal resection
(C) Cecectomy
(D) Right hemicolectomy
(E) Hepatic wedge resection and appropriate bowel resection

287. A 2.5-cm tumor at the base of the appendix

288. A 1.0-cm tumor at the tip of the appendix

289. A 0.5-cm tumor with serosal umbilication in the ileum

290. A 1.0-cm tumor of the midappendix; 1-cm firm, pale lesion at the periphery of the right lobe of the liver

Endocrine Problems and Breast

Answers

241. The answer is B. *(Hardy, 2/e, pp 434–436.)* Failure to recognize adrenal cortical insufficiency particularly in the postoperative patient may be a fatal error. This error is especially regrettable because therapy (exogenous steroid) is effective and relatively easy to apply. Adrenal insufficiency may occur in a host of settings including tuberculosis (formerly the most common cause), autoimmune states, severe infections (classically, meningococcal septicemia), pituitary insufficiency, after burns, during anticoagulant therapy, and after chronic administration of exogenous steroids. Although the adrenal gland is a fairly common site for metastases, it is rare for there to be enough destruction of the glands to produce clinical adrenal deficiency. Chronic adrenal insufficiency (classic Addison's disease) should be recognizable preoperatively by the constellation of skin pigmentation, weakness, weight loss, hypotension, nausea, vomiting, abdominal pain, hypoglycemia, hyponatremia, and hyperkalemia. Death may occur within hours of surgery if a patient with Addison's disease is operated on without recognition of the adrenal insufficiency. An acute adrenal crisis involving fever, shock, and depressed mental status may occur as a response to surgery or other trauma. Patients who have adrenal insufficiency as a result of exogenous steroid therapy may not develop the classic electrolyte abnormalities until the preterminal period. Adrenal insufficiency may also develop insidiously in the postoperative period progressing over a course of several days. This insidious type tends to occur when the actual adrenal defect itself occurs in the perioperative period as would be the case with adrenal damage from hemorrhage into the gland. Measurement of blood corticosteroid levels, urinary corticosteroid secretion, urinary sodium levels, and the response to exogenous steroids is helpful in establishing the diagnosis of adrenal insufficiency.

242. The answer is A. *(Schwartz, 6/e, pp 1629–1633.)* The thyroid scan illustrated in the question shows a single focus of increased isotope uptake, often referred to as a "hot" nodule; the remainder of the thyroid gland has not taken up radioactive iodine. Hyperfunctioning adenomas become independent of thyroid stimulating hormone (TSH) control and secrete thyroid hormone autonomously, which results in clinical hyperthyroidism. The elevated thyroid hormone levels ultimately diminish TSH levels severely and thus depress function of the remaining normal thyroid gland. An isolated focus of increased uptake on a thyroid scan is virtually diagnostic of a hyperfunctioning adenoma. Carcinomas usually display diminished uptake and are called "cold" nodules. Graves' disease would probably manifest as a diffusely hyperactive gland without nodularity. Multinodular goiter would display many nodules with varying activity.

243. The answer is C. *(Schwartz, 6/e, pp 1629–1633, 1683–1684.)* The thyroid gland originates embryologically from the foramen cecum at the base of the tongue. Normally, the thyroglossal duct becomes obliterated and resorbed, but portions may remain patent and become filled with serous fluid, which produces a midline cervical mass. Observe that in the scan of the patient described in the question, the mass is central and appears not to be part of the gland itself.

244. The answer is A. *(Schwartz, 6/e, pp 540–544.)* Breast biopsies have traditionally been performed to identify clinically suspicious palpable masses; also, in settings where multicentric or bilateral breast disease is likely to be encountered (e.g., lobular carcinoma), random or "blind" biopsies have been advocated by some to detect occult lesions. In more recent years the advent of screening mammography and xeroradiography has led to the discovery of nonpalpable but radiographically suspicious breast lesions that have a strong correlation with breast cancer. These clinically occult, mammographically detected lesions are (1) breast calcifications that are (a) smaller than 2 mm, (b) punctate, microlinear, or branching, (c) clustered along ducts, or (d) concentrated in clusters greater than five calcifications per square centimeter; (2) stellate-shaped lesions; (3) masses with ill-defined borders or nodular contours; (4) dominant, well-circumscribed, smooth masses that are significantly larger than any other mass in either breast; and (5) areas of increased tissue density or distorted breast architecture.

245. The answer is D. *(Schwartz, 6/e, pp 582–583.)* The likelihood of response of a breast cancer to hormonal therapy is dependent on the presence of hormone receptors in the cytoplasm of the breast cancer cells. Receptors for corticosteroids, progesterone, prolactin, and estrogen have been identified. Eighty percent of patients with tumors that exhibit receptors to both estrogen and progesterone will respond favorably to hormonal manipulation. Estrogen receptor activity has no predictive value in diagnosing ovarian cancer or metastatic disease, forecasting the development of osteoporosis, or determining the likelihood of a beneficial response to chemotherapy.

246. The answer is B. *(Schwartz, 6/e, pp 1553–1554.)* Prolactin-secreting tumors in the pituitary gland (previously called *chromophobe adenomas*) may grow to large size and cause bitemporal hemianopia because of proximity to the optic chiasm. They typically are associated with amenorrhea and galactorrhea (the "A/G syndrome") in women. In both sexes lack of libido and impotence or infertility may be noted. Sexual vigor is usually restored after removal of the adenomas. These tumors are not life-threatening; if their physical size is not an issue or the relative sexual dysfunction is not a problem, benign neglect is sometimes recommended.

247. The answer is C. *(Norton, Ann Surg 215:297–299, 1992. Potts, Ann Intern Med 114:593–597, 1991.)* Primary hyperparathyroidism is a common disease with over 100,000 new cases diagnosed each year in the U.S., usually in women. Essential to the diagnosis of hyperparathyroidism is the finding of hypercalcemia. Though there are many causes of hypercalcemia, hyperparathyroidism is by far the most prevalent. With rare exceptions operations for primary hyperparathyroidism should not be performed unless the patient is hypercalcemic. Parathyroid hormone (PTH) is not invariably elevated, but it should be elevated relative to the serum calcium level. Ordinarily, high serum calcium levels suppress parathyroid secretion. Therefore, in the presence of hypercalcemia, normal levels of PTH are "abnormal." Patients with primary hyperparathyroidism have either normal or elevated urinary calcium. As the name suggests, patients with familial hypocalciuric hypercalcemia (FHH) have hypercalcemia. They also usually have elevated PTH, but surgery is not indicated in this relatively rare setting of hypercalcemia.

248. The answer is A. *(Polk, 4/e, pp 204–205.)* Somatostatin is produced by D cells in the pancreatic islets and in a variety of other tissue sites in the central nervous system, gut, and elsewhere. It is a potent regulator of intestinal hormones and motility. Because it was originally found in the hypothalamus, somatostatin earned its name because it was believed to be a major inhibitor of secretion of growth hormone. It has now been shown to inhibit the secretion of most GI hormones, particularly insulin and glucagon, as well as thyroid-stimulating hormone (TSH), renin, and calcitonin. It is occasionally of value in controlling bowel fistulas by sharply reducing the amount of drainage. It has no known effect on adrenocortical cells.

249. The answer is D. *(Hardy, 2/e, pp 425–436.)* A hyperfunctioning adrenal adenoma can often be palpated or visualized on x-ray. In 10 to 15 percent of cases, adenomas are bilateral, and they are occasionally malignant. To rule out multiple adenomas and to exclude malignancy it is advisable to explore both glands. The bilateral posterolateral approach avoids invasion of the peritoneal cavity and is generally less traumatic than the anterior approach, which should be reserved for complicated cases such as large or obviously malignant lesions. After tumor excision, corticosteroid therapy to correct postoperative hypoadrenalism is necessary and adrenocorticotropic hormone (ACTH), inhibited by the corticosteroid output of the autonomous tumor, returns to normal levels.

250. The answer is C. *(Polk, 4/e, pp 386–388.)* Most clinicians would recommend aspiration and cytological examination of the cyst fluid in this situation. Cysts are common lesions in the breasts of women in their thirties and forties; malignancies are relatively rare. All such lesions justify attention, however, and physicians must not underestimate the fear associated with the discovery of a mass in the breast, even in low-risk situations. If the lesion does not completely disappear after aspiration, excision is advised. In young women the breast parenchyma is dense, which limits the diagnostic value of mammography. The American Cancer Society (ACS) does not suggest a baseline mammographic examination until age 35 unless a suspicious lesion exists.

251. The answer is E. *(Hardy, 2/e, pp 395–404.)* Radiation-induced thyroid cancer was first recognized in 1950 by Duffy and Fitzgerald. It usually follows *low*-dose external radiation. Most cancers occur after exposure to 1500 rads or less to the neck, but an increase in thyroid cancer has been noted after as little as 6 rads. Salivary gland tumors and possibly parathyroid adenomas are also associated with radiation. The latent period for these tumors is 30 years or longer. Of all patients who have low-dose radiation, about 9 percent have been found to have thyroid cancer, usually of the papillary type. Treatment consists of a near-total thyroidectomy because there is a high incidence of bilaterality and because there is a greater incidence of complications if a second operation is necessary.

252. The answer is D. *(Hardy, 2/e, pp 395–404.)* Papillary carcinoma of the thyroid frequently metastasizes to cervical lymph nodes, but distant metastasis is uncommon. The nonaggressive nature of this tumor locally and the infrequency of distant metastases combine to produce an 80 to 95 percent 5-year survival rate. A contributing factor to the success of thyroid surgery for papillary carcinoma is the easy accessibility of cervical nodes for examination and dissection. Slow growth and a predilection for local extension are characteristics of this tumor that contribute to a high survival rate in affected persons. This is true even of patients who have limited surgery, which has led to considerable controversy regarding the extent of the indicated surgical procedure.

253. The answer is C. *(Way, 9/e, pp 302–303.)* Fibrocystic disease (chronic cystic mastitis) is a common disorder of the adult female breast. It is rare after cessation of ovarian function, either natural or induced. Its association with estrogens is inferential. In postmenopausal women it only occurs when replacement estrogen therapy is in use. Its main clinical significance relates to the need to differentiate irregular breast tissue from cancer. Patients afflicted with this disorder are often frustrated by the repeated biopsies that may be recommended.

254. The answer is D. *(Schwartz, 6/e, pp 550–551.)* Fibroadenomas occur infrequently before puberty but are the most common breast tumors between puberty and the early thirties. They usually are well demarcated and firm. Although most fibroadenomas are no larger than 3 cm in diameter, giant or juvenile fibroadenomas frequently are very large. The bigger fibroadenomas (greater than 5 cm) occur predominantly in adolescent black girls. The average age at onset of juvenile mammary hypertrophy is 16 years. This disorder involves a diffuse change in the entire breast and does not usually manifest clinically as a discrete mass; it may be unilateral or bilateral and can cause an enormous and incapacitating increase in breast size. Regression may be spontaneous and sometimes coincides with puberty or pregnancy. Cystosarcoma phylloides may also cause a large lesion. Together with intraductal carcinoma, it characteristically occurs in older women. Lymphomas are less firm than fibroadenomas and do not have a whorl-like pattern. They display a characteristic fish-flesh texture.

255. The answer is A. *(Gajraj, Br J Surg 80:422–426, 1993. Way, 9/e, pp 724–725.)* With the increasing use of CT and MRI scans for other purposes, small "incidentalomas" of the adrenal gland are becoming a frequent finding. In the absence of any clinical signs or symptoms of endocrine dysfunction, most experts now recommend observation and a search for evidence of endocrine dysfunction for lesions less than 5 cm in diameter. Lesions below that size are common and are usually asymptomatic, nonfunctional adenomas or adrenal cysts. Functional neoplasms secrete an excess of hormones, which produce clinical signs and symptoms. All functional tumors and solid tumors greater than 5.0 cm in diameter should be removed. Cystic masses greater than 5 cm may be aspirated with a fine needle. Clear fluid suggests a benign lesion; if the fluid is bloody or aspiration produces solid tissue, then the lesion should be resected.

Cystic tumors ranging from 3.5 to 5.0 cm may also be aspirated. If bloody fluid is obtained or if the lesion is solid, then resection should be considered in a patient who is otherwise a healthy surgical candidate. Both solid and cystic masses less than 3.5 cm may be followed and can be considered benign if they do not increase in size or become functional.

256. The answer is A. *(Schwartz, 6/e, pp 1648–1658.)* The patient described is exhibiting classic signs and symptoms of hyperparathyroidism. In addition, if a history is obtainable, frequently the patient will relate a history of renal calculi and bone pain—the syndrome characterized as "groans, stones, and bones." The acute management of the hypercalcemic state includes vigorous hydration to restore intravascular volume, which is invariably diminished. This will establish renal perfusion and thus promote urinary calcium excretion. Thiazide diuretics are contraindicated, as they frequently will cause patients to become hypercalcemic. Instead, diuresis should be promoted with the use of "loop" diuretics such as furosemide (Lasix). The use of intravenous phosphorus infusion is no longer recommended, as precipitation in the lungs, heart, or kidney can lead to serious morbidity. Mithramycin is an antineoplastic agent that in low doses inhibits bone resorption and thus diminishes serum calcium levels; it is used only when other maneuvers fail to decrease the calcium level. Calcitonin is useful at times. Bisphosphonates are newer agents particularly useful for lowering calcium levels in resistant cases, such as those associated with humoral malignancy. Finally, "emergency" neck exploration is seldom warranted. In unprepared patients, the morbidity is unacceptably high.

257. The answer is C. (*Schwartz, 6/e, pp 1650–1655.*) The mechanism of hypercalcemia of malignancy is thought to be due to either elaboration of a "PTH-like" humoral factor or, many times, direct bone destruction by metastatic disease. Breast, prostatic, pulmonary, and hematologic malignancy all may give rise to hypercalcemia. Sarcoidosis also may produce hypercalcemia, but the presence of the normal chest x-ray essentially rules out this possibility. Thus, a Kveim test is not indicated.

258. The answer is C. (*Schwartz, 6/e, pp 540–545.*) Injury to breast tissue may cause necrosis of mammary adipose tissue and lead to the formation of a tender, localized, firm mass. A history of trauma is often elicited from affected patients, but less apparent factors, such as prolonged pressure, may also produce fat necrosis; half the patients in whom the diagnosis is made do not recall a history of trauma. The pathophysiology of this lesion seems to involve early development of liquefaction of mammary fat with the formation of a cystic mass. Through a process of fibrosis, this lesion evolves into a firm, sometimes calcified lump that may be difficult to distinguish from carcinoma. Excisional biopsy is usually required for definitive diagnosis; if the diagnosis of fat necrosis is confirmed, simple excision is curative.

259–260. The answers are 259-C, 260-E. (*Friesen, pp 405–433.*) The constellation of symptoms in this patient is typical of a functional adrenocortical tumor. Masculinization in females is also a common finding. Elevated urine 17-ketosteroids will be found in this patient. Any adrenocortical tumor larger than 6 cm should be considered a carcinoma rather than an adenoma. Treatment should include resection of as much tumor as possible. This would include invaded adjacent organs such as the kidney or the tail of the pancreas. Symptoms related to hormone production can be minimized by complete resection despite the inability to cure advanced disease. The most effective adjuvant therapy is mitotane, which is toxic for functional adrenocortical cells. When mitotane is used, therefore, glucocorticoids must be administered. Ketoconazole has been found to inhibit the production of various steroid hormones and may be useful in the treatment of hormone-related symptoms. The overall 5-year survival of patients with adrenocortical carcinoma treated with resection and mitotane is 20 percent.

261–262. The answers are 261-E, 262-D. (*Cameron, 4/e, pp 461–462.*) This patient's presentation and films are consistent with primary hyperparathyroidism. The elevated parathormone level (PTH) confirms the diagnosis. Her chest film demonstrates marked osteopenia and the hand films are classic for this disease with severe demineralization and periosteal bone resorption most prominent in the middle phalanges. The films show no evidence of malignant lesions or mediastinal adenopathy consistent with sarcoidosis, and an elevated PTH level is not found in Paget's disease or vitamin D intoxication.

Treatment for primary hyperparathyroidism in this setting is resection of the diseased parathyroid glands after initial correction of the severe hypercalcemia. A neck exploration would yield a single parathyroid adenoma in about 85 percent of cases. Two adenomata are found less often (approximately 5 percent) and hyperplasia of all four glands occurs in about 10 to 15 percent of patients. If hyperplasia is found, treatment would include resection of three and one-half glands. The remnant of the fourth gland can be identified with a metal clip in case reexploration becomes necessary. Alternatively, all four glands can be removed with autotransplantation of a small piece of parathyroid tissue into the forearm or sternocleidomastoid muscle. Subsequent hyperfunction, should it develop, can then be treated by removal of this tissue. A patient with osteopenia this severe will need calcium supplementation postoperatively. Vitamin D supplementation may also be necessary if hypocalcemia develops and persists despite treatment with oral calcium.

263. The answer is B (1, 3). *(Barnavon, Surg Gynecol Obstet 171:347–352, 1990.)* Approximately 2 percent of American women who develop carcinoma of the breast will be pregnant at the time of diagnosis. The therapeutic approach to these patients has changed considerably in recent years. Though changes in the breast that occur during pregnancy often lead to a delay in diagnosis of breast carcinoma, there is no convincing evidence that breast carcinoma in pregnant women behaves differently or is histologically different from that in nonpregnant women. Furthermore, when patients are matched for age and stage of disease, no significant differences in survival rates are found. The majority of breast cancers in these patients, as with most premenopausal patients, is estrogen-receptor negative and not hormonally sensitive. Therefore, elective termination of pregnancy is generally no longer indicated to decrease estrogen stimulation of the tumor. Since radiation exposure endangers the fetus and there is no evidence that general anesthesia and nonabdominal surgery increase premature labor, modified radical mastectomy is recommended for stage I or II carcinoma (tumor less than 4 cm in diameter). Patients in later stages of pregnancy, however, can start radiation therapy shortly after delivery, and some of them may be candidates for breast-conserving surgery and adjuvant radiotherapy.

Chemotherapy does not appear to increase the risk of congenital malformation when given in the second or third trimester of pregnancy. Patients who require adjuvant chemotherapy during the first trimester may opt for a therapeutic abortion, however, since there is a slightly increased risk of fetal malformation in that circumstance.

264. The answer is C (2, 4). *(Osther, Acta Chir Scand 156:343–352, 1990.)* Paget's disease of the breast is unrelated to Paget's bone disease. It represents a small percentage (1 to 4 percent) of all breast cancers and is thought to originate in the retroareolar lactiferous ducts. It progresses toward the nipple-areola complex in most patients, where it causes the typical clinical finding of nipple eczema and erosion. Up to 20 percent of patients with Paget's disease have an associated breast mass, and these patients are more likely to have involvement of axillary nodes. Nipple-areolar disease alone usually represents in situ cancer; these patients have a 10-year survival rate of over 80 percent. In contrast, if Paget's disease presents with a mass, it behaves like an infiltrating ductal carcinoma. The generally recommended surgical procedure for Paget's disease is currently a modified radical mastectomy. The validity of breast-saving surgery and adjuvant radiation therapy for patients without an associated mass is underinvestigated.

265. The answer is D (4). *(Davis, pp 1444–1445, 1466–1467.)* The syndrome of a gastrin-secreting non-beta-cell pancreatic tumor is a rare entity first described by Zollinger and Ellison. They originally described a triad of (1) fulminant, complicated peptic ulceration; (2) extreme gastric hypersecretion; and (3) a non-beta-cell tumor of pancreatic islets. Over 50 percent of the tumors are malignant, and 40 percent of them have metastases at the time of surgery. Until recently, total gastrectomy had been the primary operation for this tumor; however, it is now believed that operative exploration of the patient with resection of the tumor should be done if possible. H-receptor antagonists have also proved very promising in the management of these patients. Patients with Zollinger-Ellison tumors have very high basal gastric acid (greater than 35 meq/h) and serum gastrin levels (usually greater than 200 pg/mL). A protein meal or histamine usually does *not* increase acid and gastrin levels as it would in conventional duodenal ulcer patients. A paradoxical *rise* in serum gastrin after intravenous secretin is diagnostic of Zollinger-Ellison syndrome.

266. The answer is E (all). (*Schwartz, 6/e, pp 1642–1644.*) The incidence of complications with thyroidectomy or parathyroidectomy is relatively low in most series. The likelihood of serious complications increases with the extent of resection ("total thyroidectomy" versus "subtotal thyroidectomy") and with the number of neck explorations (initial exploration versus reexploration). Injury to the recurrent laryngeal nerve can compromise the airway, as can hemorrhage into the wound. Superior laryngeal nerve injury causes annoying voice "fatigue," but rarely is of significant consequence. Hypocalcemia is usually transient, but can at times necessitate permanent calcium supplementation. Perforation of hollow neck structures very seldom occurs, and unless it is massive or not appreciated, usually causes no morbidity.

267. The answer is B (1, 3). (*Davis, p 2553.*) The thyroid scan of the patient discussed in the question shows a discrete area of decreased radioactive iodine uptake with the remainder of the gland accepting iodine normally. This means the tissue that composes the nodule is not endocrinologically active for thyroid hormone. The two major mass lesions of the thyroid that can produce this pattern are a nonfunctioning follicular adenoma and a carcinoma. Carcinomas seldom produce thyroid hormone. Adenomas may be very active and suppress the remaining gland, but hyperactive adenomas are uncommon. Most thyroid adenomas are not hormone-producing and appear as "cold" nodules on a thyroid scan. Graves' disease produces a diffusely hyperactive gland without nodularity. A large parathyroid adenoma could conceivably displace the thyroid gland and produce a pattern similar to the one shown, but it would be unusual. A localized infectious process also could produce such a pattern. The essential point is that a "cold" thyroid nodule may represent a carcinoma, and needle biopsy or surgical excision is indicated to rule out this possibility.

268. The answer is B (1, 3). (*Schwartz, 6/e, pp 550–551.*) Cystosarcoma phylloides is a tumor most often seen in younger women. It can grow to enormous size and at times ulcerate through the skin. Still, it is a lesion with low propensity toward metastasis. Local recurrence does occur, especially if the initial resection was inadequate. Simple reexcision with adequate margins is curative. Very large lesions may necessitate simple mastectomy to achieve clear margins. Axillary lymphadenectomy, however, seldom is indicated without biopsy-positive demonstration of tumor in the nodes. The low incidence of metastatic disease suggests that adjunctive therapy is indicated only for known metastatic disease, even when the tumors are quite large and ulcerated.

269. The answer is A (1, 2, 3). *(Schwartz, 6/e, pp 1633–1636.)* This patient has cytological evidence of a papillary lesion, possibly papillary carcinoma. Papillary carcinoma is a relatively nonaggressive lesion with long-term survival (>20 years) of more than 90 percent. The lesion is frequently multicentric, which argues for more complete resection. Metastases, when they occur, are usually responsive to surgical resection or radioablation therapy. Removal of the involved lobe, and possibly the entire thyroid gland, is appropriate. Papillary carcinoma is frequently multifocal. Bilateral disease mandates total thyroidectomy. The use of radioactive ^{131}I, however, is contraindicated in pregnancy and should be used with caution in women of childbearing age.

270. The answer is B (1, 3). *(Schwartz, 6/e, pp 532–536.)* Expression of discharge from the nipple, even if bloody, is rarely an indication for biopsy. The presence of spontaneous nipple discharge in the presence of a breast mass is an indication for open biopsy. Most lesions (more than 80 percent) are proved benign upon histological examination. Friable, blood-encrusted nipples would raise suspicion of Paget's disease of the breast and biopsy is indicated. Clear or milky discharge from the nipple is usually elicited and is a physiological response to nipple stimulation.

271. The answer is B (1, 3). *(Schwartz, 6/e, pp 1629–1633.)* Thyroid nodules are somewhat less common in men and always should suggest malignancy. The history of irradiation to the chest and the findings on biopsy mandate resection of the lesion in this patient. The optimum management of thyroid carcinoma remains controversial. Thyroid lobectomy, subtotal thyroidectomy, and total thyroidectomy are all acceptable techniques for treatment. Removal of the gland permits more accurate histological diagnosis, particularly with regard to the relatively radioresistant Hürthle-cell follicular variant. Removal of the gland also makes subsequent treatment of metastases with radioactive iodine more effective. Suppression with thyroid hormone (Synthroid) in the setting of abnormal cytology is not recommended.

272. The answer is A (1, 2, 3). *(Schwartz, 6/e, pp 1637–1638.)* Hürthle-cell cancer is a type of follicular cancer, but it tends to recur more often than other types. Follicular cancer spreads hematogenously to distant sites. This is unlike papillary cancer, which metastasizes via the lymphatics. Amyloid deposits in the stroma of a thyroid tumor are diagnostic of medullary carcinoma. The treatment of choice is a near-total thyroidectomy to facilitate later body scanning for metastases and treatment with ^{131}I.

273. The answer is B (1, 3). *(Hardy, 2/e, pp 425–430.)* Cushing's disease refers to the syndrome caused by a functional pituitary tumor. Harvey Cushing first described basophilic pituitary tumors that caused truncal obesity, hypertension, hirsuitism, and the other characteristics of the disease. Pathological anatomy in the adrenals is usually secondary adrenocortical hyperplasia. Primary steroid-producing adrenal or ovarian tumors may cause the syndrome, with suppression of the normal pituitary. Similar pituitary suppression may be caused by ACTH-secreting tumors elsewhere, such as oat cell lesions of the lung. Evaluation of patients has been simplified recently by availability of ACTH radioimmunoassay. Patients with both elevated 17-hydroxycorticosteroids and ACTH levels must have either a pituitary tumor (further confirmed by CT scan or MRI scan) or an occult ACTH-producing tumor in another site. Extrapituitary ACTH tumors generally are not suppressible by high-dose dexamethasone. Elevated steroid and undetectable ACTH levels eliminate the pituitary as the cause for Cushing's syndrome and place the disorder at the level of one or both adrenals, or occasionally in an ovary or testis (carcinoma, adenoma, or 1° hyperplasia).

274. The answer is D (4). *(Hardy, 2/e, pp 454–456. Schwartz, 6/e, pp 1426–1427.)* Insulin-secreting *beta*-cell tumors of the pancreas produce paroxysmal nervous system manifestations that may be a consequence of hypoglycemia, although the blood glucose level may bear little relation to the severity of the symptoms, even in the same patient from episode to episode. Most insulinomas are single discrete tumors. If a careful examination of the entire gland reveals one or more specific adenomata, these can be locally excised. Excision of these tumors may be difficult because the tumors often are small and, in 10 to 15 percent of cases, multiple. Subtotal pancreatectomy is sometimes indicated to increase the probability of complete tumor removal. Patients with insulinoma may have associated "APUD" tumors of the pituitary and parathyroid (MEN-I). Insulinomas are not associated with MEN-II, which comprises coexistent medullary thyroid cancer, parathyroid hyperplasia, and pheochromocytoma. About one in seven of these tumors is malignant. Streptozotocin, a potent antibiotic that selectively destroys islet cells, can be useful in controlling symptoms from unresectable malignant tumors of the islet cells but probably has little to offer in the definitive management of the typical benign islet cell insulinoma.

275. The answer is B (1, 3). *(Schwartz, 6/e, pp 554–557.)* Breast cancer is rarely seen before the age of 20, but thereafter its incidence increases inexorably. While the prevalence of breast cancer (the raw number of patients alive with disease) is greatest among perimenopausal women, the incidence of breast cancer (the number of new cases per 100,000 population) rises so sharply that it is twice as common among women between 80 and 85 years of age as among those 60 to 65. In addition, the age-adjusted incidence has increased steadily since the mid-1940s. Approximately one in fourteen black women will develop breast cancer; the incidence among white women is one in ten.

276–278. The answers are 276-A, 277-D, 278-C. *(Wilson, 12/e, p 1705.)* Propylthiouracil (PTU) and methimazole are the two most commonly prescribed antithyroid medications used in the U.S. for medical therapy of thyrotoxic states. Potassium iodide and potassium perchlorate also are used and are especially useful for preoperative preparation. Propranolol is useful in diminishing the physiological symptoms of thyrotoxicosis, but has no direct action upon the thyroid itself. Only PTU diminishes the peripheral conversion of T_4 to T_3. Both PTU and methimazole affect the iodination of tyrosine moieties of thyroglobulin within the thyroid gland. Subsequent coupling of monoiodotyrosine and diiodotyrosine to form T_4 and T_3 also is diminished. Neither medication decreases the uptake of iodine by the thyroid; this is achieved by the use of ionic inhibitors such as potassium perchlorate.

279–281. The answers are 279-B, 280-B, 281-C. *(Davis, pp 1275–1390. Hardy, 2/e, pp 339–364.)* Normal mammary glandular cells bind estrogen and progesterone to cytoplasmic membrane binding sites, or receptors. Breast cancers retain the ability to bind hormones to a variable degree. The older the patient and the better differentiated the tumor, the more likely the tumor is to contain a high concentration of hormone receptors. Tumors that are rich in estrogen or progesterone receptors tend to respond favorably to hormonal manipulation, usually in the form of an oral antiestrogen medication (tamoxifen). The likelihood that a tumor low or absent in hormone receptors will respond to hormonal therapy is small; these tumors have poorer prognosis than tumors that have equivalent stages in the TNM system but have high levels of receptor proteins. The status of a tumor's hormone receptors helps to guide the selection of appropriate adjuvant therapy, but does not determine a tumor's operability.

The presence of lymph node metastasis is the single most important prognostic factor in breast cancer. Tumor metastasis to even a single lymph node dramatically worsens the patient's probability of survival. Metastasis to axillary lymph nodes mandates adjuvant therapy (usually cytotoxic chemotherapy in premenopausal women, regardless of hormone receptor status, and hormonal manipulation with or without additional adjuvant therapy in postmenopausal women). Metastasis to supraclavicular or infraclavicular lymph nodes constitutes stage IV disease irrespective of the size of the tumor or the presence of distant metastasis and precludes the possibility of curative surgery.

282–286. The answers are 282-C, 283-B, 284-B, 285-E, 286-D *(Schwartz, 6/e, pp 557–559.)* The American Joint Committee on Cancer has defined a four-tiered staging system for breast cancer based on the clinical criteria of tumor size, involvement of lymph nodes, and metastatic disease. In one version of this system, a separate category is reserved for inflammatory breast cancer. While the grouping of breast cancers into stages provides a useful shorthand for expressing a patient's survival probability, it is noteworthy that considerable heterogeneity exists both with respect to tumor size and nodal characteristics among tumors that are classified within a given stage.

The TNM stage of breast cancer is assigned by measuring the greatest diameter of the tumor ("T"), assessing the axillary and clavicular lymph nodes for enlargement and fixation ("N"), and judging whether metastatic disease is present ("M"). In general, the worst of the three TNM parameters will determine the stage assignment.

Tumors that are not palpable are classified T0; tumors 2 cm or less, T1; tumors greater than 2 but not more than 5 cm, T2; tumors greater than 5 cm, T3; and tumors with extension into the chest wall or skin, T4.

Clinically negative lymph nodes are classified N0; positive, movable ipsilateral axillary nodes, N1; fixed ipsilateral axillary nodes, N2; and clavicular nodes, N3.

Absence of evidence of metastatic disease is classified M0; distant metastatic disease, M1.

The patient in question 282 has a T0, N2, M0 lesion. This is stage III (fixed or matted nodes are a poor prognostic sign).

The patient in question 283 has a T2, N1, M0 lesion. This is stage II.

The patient in question 284 has a T2, N0, M0 lesion. Though smaller than the tumor in question 283 and without clinically involved nodes, this tumor is also stage II.

The patient in question 285 has findings compatible with inflammatory breast cancer. A biopsy of the involved skin and a mammogram would confirm the diagnosis.

The patient in question 286 has a T1, N0, M1 lesion. This is stage IV (stage IV is any T, any N, M1).

287–290. The answers are 287-D, 288-A, 289-B, 290-E. *(Schwartz, 6/e, pp 1175–1177, 1316.)* Carcinoid tumors are most commonly found in the appendix and small bowel, where they may be multiple. They have a tendency to metastasize, which varies with the size of the tumor. Tumors < 1 cm uncommonly metastasize. Tumors >2.0 cm are more often found to be metastatic. Metastasis to the liver and beyond may give rise to the carcinoid syndrome. The tumors cause an intense desmoplastic reaction. Spread into the serosal lymphatics does not imply metastatic disease; local resection is potentially curative. When metastatic lesions are found in the liver, they should be resected when technically feasible to limit the symptoms of the carcinoid syndrome.

Gastrointestinal Tract, Liver, and Pancreas

DIRECTIONS: Each question below contains five suggested responses. Select the **one best** response to each question.

291. An 18-year-old woman presents with abdominal pain, fever, and leukocytosis. With the presumptive diagnosis of appendicitis, a right lower quadrant (McBurney) incision is made and the lesion pictured below is delivered. The process is 50 cm proximal to the ileocecal valve. This lesion

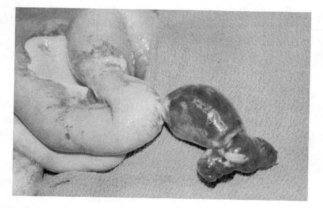

(A) can best be diagnosed by preoperative angiogram, which should be done whenever the diagnosis is suspected
(B) should routinely be removed when incidentally discovered during celiotomy
(C) is embryologically derived from a persistent vitelline duct (omphalomesenteric duct)
(D) often contains gastric mucosa or pancreatic tissue
(E) is frequently associated with cutaneous flushing and episodic tachycardia

292. Omeprazole has been added to the H_2-antagonists as a therapeutic approach to the management of acute gastric and duodenal ulcers. It acts by

(A) blocking breakdown of mucosal-damaging metabolites of NSAIDS
(B) providing direct cytoprotective effect
(C) buffering gastric acids
(D) inhibiting parietal cell hydrogen-potassium-ATPase
(E) inhibiting gastrin release and parietal cell acid production

293. Evidence that a splenectomy might benefit a patient with immune (idiopathic) thrombocytopenic purpura (ITP) includes

(A) a significant enlargement of the spleen
(B) a high reticulocyte count
(C) megakaryocytic elements in the bone marrow
(D) an increase in the platelet count on cortisone therapy
(E) patient's age less than 5

294. A 36-year-old former intravenous drug abuser with a prior history of *Pneumocystis carinii* pneumonia is seen for a complaint of diffuse abdominal pain and peritonitis. An abdominal x-ray reveals free intraperitoneal air. The most likely etiology for pneumoperitoneum in this patient is

(A) cytomegalovirus colitis with perforation
(B) diverticulitis
(C) necrotic bowel in a hernia
(D) perforated peptic ulcer
(E) perforated cecal carcinoma

295. The following statements concerning imperforate anus are true EXCEPT that

(A) imperforate anus affects males and females with equal frequency
(B) the rectum has descended to below the level of the levator ani muscle complex in most females
(C) the rectum usually ends in a fistulous communication
(D) the chance for eventual continence is greater when the rectum has descended to below the levator ani muscles
(E) immediate definitive repair of the anatomical defect is required to maximize the chance of eventual continence

Questions 296–297

A previously healthy 80-year-old woman presented with early satiety and abdominal fullness. The CT scan shown below was obtained.

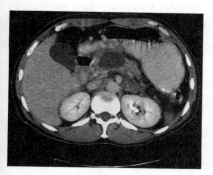

296. The lesion is most likely a

(A) pancreatic pseudocyst
(B) pancreatic adenocarcinoma
(C) pancreatic cystadenocarcinoma
(D) retroperitoneal lymphoma
(E) pancreatic serous cystadenoma

297. All the following statements about this lesion are correct EXCEPT

(A) neither clinical nor laboratory findings establish a preoperative diagnosis
(B) significant weight loss and back pain is the typical presentation
(C) the lesion may be multilocular or calcified
(D) it may be cured by resection even if large
(E) it is not associated with a history of pancreatitis

298. A patient with a history of familial polyposis undergoes a diagnostic polypectomy. Which of the following types of polyps is most likely to be found?

(A) Villous adenoma
(B) Hyperplastic polyp
(C) Adenomatous polyp
(D) Retention polyp
(E) Pseudopolyp

299. What is the most common serious complication of an end colostomy?

(A) Bleeding
(B) Skin breakdown
(C) Parastomal hernia
(D) Colonic perforation during irrigation
(E) Stomal prolapse

300. All the following statements regarding pancreatic carcinoma are true EXCEPT

(A) the majority of cases present with jaundice alone
(B) the overall rate of resectability for potential cure is 5 to 10 percent
(C) if a patient is jaundiced, the resectability rate is 10 to 25 percent
(D) 99 percent of patients with pancreatic cancer have metastatic disease at the time of diagnosis
(E) the 5-year survival rate after a Whipple procedure (pancreaticoduodenectomy) performed for cure is 5 to 20 percent

Questions 301–302

A 45-year-old woman is explored for a perforated duodenal ulcer 6 h after onset of symptoms. She has a history of chronic peptic ulcer disease treated medically with minimal symptoms.

301. The procedure of choice is

(A) simple closure with omental patch
(B) truncal vagotomy and pyloroplasty
(C) antrectomy and truncal vagotomy
(D) highly selective vagotomy
(E) hemigastrectomy

302. Six weeks after surgery, the patient returns complaining of postprandial weakness, sweating, light-headedness, crampy abdominal pain, and diarrhea. The best management would be

(A) antispasmodic medications (e.g., Lomotil)
(B) dietary advice and counseling that symptoms will probably abate within 3 months of surgery
(C) dietary advice and counseling that symptoms will probably not abate but are not dangerous
(D) workup for neuroendocrine tumor (e.g., carcinoid)
(E) preparation for revision to Roux-en-Y gastrojejunostomy

Questions 303–304

A 60-year-old male alcoholic is admitted to the hospital with hematemesis. His blood pressure is 100/60 mmHg, the physical examination reveals splenomegaly and ascites, and the initial hematocrit is 25 percent. Nasogastric suction yields 300 mL of fresh blood.

303. After initial resuscitation, this man should undergo

(A) esophageal balloon tamponade
(B) barium swallow
(C) selective angiography
(D) esophagogastroscopy
(E) exploratory celiotomy

304. A diagnosis of bleeding esophageal varices is made in this patient. Appropriate initial therapy would be

(A) intravenous vasopressin
(B) endoscopic sclerotherapy
(C) emergency portacaval shunt
(D) emergency esophageal transection
(E) esophageal balloon tamponade

305. During an operation for carcinoma of the hepatic flexure of the colon, an unexpected discontinuous 2 × 2 cm metastasis is discovered in the edge of the right lobe of the liver. The surgeon should

(A) terminate the operation, screen the patient for evidence of other metastases, and plan further therapy after the reevaluation

(B) perform a right hemicolectomy and a right hepatic lobectomy

(C) perform a right hemicolectomy and a wedge resection of the metastasis

(D) perform a cecostomy and schedule reoperation after a course of systemic chemotherapy

(E) perform local resection of the primary colon cancer and plan radiation therapy for the lesion on the liver

306. A 55-year-old man complains of chronic intermittent epigastric pain, and gastroscopy demonstrates a 2-cm ulcer of the distal lesser curvature. Endoscopic biopsy yields no malignant tissue. After a 6-week trial of H_2-blockade and antacid therapy, the ulcer is unchanged. Proper therapy at this point is

(A) repeat trial of medical therapy

(B) local excision of the ulcer

(C) Billroth I partial gastrectomy

(D) Billroth I partial gastrectomy with vagotomy

(E) vagotomy and pyloroplasty

307. Regarding regional enteritis, all the following are true statements EXCEPT that

(A) regional enteritis may involve any segment of the GI tract

(B) the most frequent site of involvement is the terminal ileum

(C) massive hemorrhage per rectum is common

(D) adenocarcinoma of the small bowel associated with the disease has a poor prognosis

(E) the actual cause of the disease is unknown

308. Which of the following hernias follows the path of the spermatic cord within the cremaster muscle?

(A) Femoral
(B) Direct inguinal
(C) Indirect inguinal
(D) Spigelian
(E) Interparietal

309. A spry octogenarian who has never before been hospitalized is admitted with signs and symptoms typical of a small bowel obstruction. Which of the following clinical findings would give most help in ascertaining the diagnosis?

(A) Coffee-grounds aspirate from the stomach
(B) Aerobilia
(C) A leukocyte count of 40,000/ mm³
(D) A pH of 7.5 P_{CO_2} 50 torr, and paradoxically acid urine
(E) A palpable mass in the pelvis

310. All the following disorders are thought to involve precancerous lesions of the colon EXCEPT

(A) ulcerative colitis
(B) villous adenomas
(C) familial polyposis
(D) Peutz-Jeghers syndrome
(E) Crohn's colitis

311. A 70-year-old woman has nausea, vomiting, abdominal distention, and episodic, crampy midabdominal pain. She has no history of previous surgery but has a long history of cholelithiasis for which she has refused surgery. Her abdominal radiograph reveals spherical density in the right lower quadrant. Correct treatment should consist of

(A) ileocolectomy
(B) cholecystectomy
(C) ileotomy and extraction
(D) nasogastric tube decompression
(E) intravenous antibiotics

312. Which of the following statements concerning Hirschsprung's disease is true?

(A) It is initially treated by colostomy
(B) It is best diagnosed in the newborn period by barium enema
(C) It is characterized by absence of ganglion cells in the transverse colon
(D) It is associated with high incidence of genitourinary tract anomalies
(E) It is the congenital disease that most commonly leads to subsequent fecal incontinence

313. A 36-hour-old infant presents with bilious vomiting and an increasingly distended abdomen. At exploration the segment below is found as the point of obstruction. Which of the following statements regarding this finding is true?

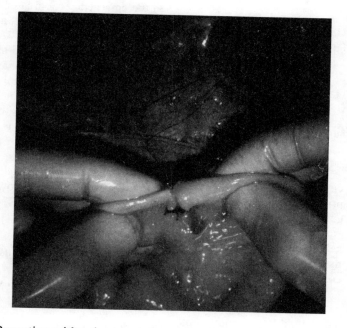

(A) Resection with primary anastomosis should not be performed
(B) Gentle, persistent traction on the specimen usually corrects the defect and removes the need for a resection
(C) The lesion is much more common in the jejunum than in the ileum in this age group
(D) This problem is probably related to mesenteric vascular insufficiency
(E) A properly monitored barium enema might have corrected this defect and removed the need for an operation

314. Spontaneous closure of which of the following congenital abnormalities of the abdominal wall generally occurs by the age of 4?

(A) Umbilical hernia
(B) Patent urachus
(C) Patent omphalomesenteric duct
(D) Omphalocele
(E) Gastroschisis

315. Laparoscopic cholecystectomy is relatively contraindicated in each of the following EXCEPT

(A) cirrhosis
(B) prior upper abdominal surgery
(C) suspected carcinoma of the gallbladder
(D) morbid obesity
(E) coagulopathy

316. Infants with anorectal anomalies tend to have other congenital anomalies. Associated abnormalities include all the following EXCEPT

(A) fistulas to the perineum or vagina
(B) fistulas to the urinary tract
(C) esophageal atresia
(D) heart disease
(E) corneal opacities

317. A 48-year-old woman develops pain of the right lower quadrant while playing tennis. The pain progresses and she presents to the emergency room later that day with a low-grade fever, a white blood count of 13,000, and complaints of anorexia and nausea as well as persistent, sharp pain of the right lower quadrant. On examination she is tender in the right lower quadrant with muscular spasm and there is a suggestion of a mass effect. An ultrasound is ordered and shows an apparent mass in the abdominal wall. Which of the following is the most likely diagnosis?

(A) Acute appendicitis
(B) Cecal carcinoma
(C) Hematoma of the rectus sheath
(D) Torsion of an ovarian cyst
(E) Cholecystitis

318. In determining the proper treatment for a sliding hiatal hernia, the most useful step would be

(A) barium swallow with cinefluoroscopy during Valsalva maneuver
(B) flexible endoscopy
(C) 24-h monitoring of esophageal pH
(D) measuring the size of the hernia
(E) assessing the patient's smoking and drinking history

319. All the following statements regarding the etiology of obstructive jaundice are true EXCEPT

(A) a markedly elevated alkaline phosphatase is usually associated with obstructive jaundice

(B) when extrahepatic biliary obstruction is suspected, the first test should be endoscopic retrograde cholangiopancreatography (ERCP)

(C) a Klatskin tumor will result in intrahepatic ductal dilation only

(D) a liver-spleen scan will add little to the diagnostic workup for obstructive jaundice

(E) carcinoma of the head of the pancreas can cause deep epigastric or back pain in as many as 30 percent of patients

320. A previously healthy 9-year-old child comes to the emergency room because of fulminant upper gastrointestinal bleeding. The hemorrhage is most likely to be the result of

(A) esophageal varices
(B) the Mallory-Weiss syndrome
(C) gastritis
(D) a gastric ulcer
(E) a duodenal ulcer

321. Intragastric pressure remains steady near 2 to 5 mmHg during slow gastric filling, but rises rapidly to high levels after reaching a volume of

(A) 400 to 600 mL
(B) 700 to 900 mL
(C) 1000 to 1200 mL
(D) 1300 to 1500 mL
(E) 1600 to 1800 mL

322. Regarding the effects of colon resection, all the following statements are true EXCEPT

(A) net absorption of water by the rectum has not been demonstrated in humans

(B) patients who undergo partial colon resections suffer little change in their bowel habits following operation

(C) patients may experience more frequent episodes of acute small-bowel–induced diarrhea following partial colectomy

(D) the right colon is better adapted for water and electrolyte absorption than the left colon

(E) the role of the ileocecal valve in normal colon function is not established

323. Operative planning and preoperative counseling for a patient with a rectal carcinoma can be best provided if the patient is staged before surgery by

(A) rigid proctoscopy
(B) barium enema
(C) MRI of the pelvis
(D) CT scanning of the pelvis
(E) rectal endosonography

324. True statements regarding absorption by the small intestine include all the following EXCEPT

(A) all but the fat in milk is digested and absorbed in normal humans by the end of the duodenum
(B) complete absorption of carbohydrates in a meal occurs in the first 200 cm of jejunum
(C) in short gut syndrome, much of the dietary carbohydrate appears in the stool
(D) aldosterone markedly increases sodium transport across the gut mucosa
(E) enzymes of the brush border of the small intestine can digest and absorb over 95 percent of an average protein meal in the complete absence of the pancreas

325. Local stimuli that cause the release of gastrin from the gastric mucosa include all the following EXCEPT

(A) small proteins
(B) 20-proof alcohol
(C) caffeine
(D) acidic antral contents
(E) antral distention

326. True statements regarding fat absorption include all the following EXCEPT

(A) half of neutral fat can be absorbed in the complete absence of bile and pancreatic lipase
(B) 10 to 15 percent of the total bile salt pool is lost in the stool and replaced daily by synthesis in the liver
(C) glycerol, short-chain fatty acids, and medium-chain triglycerides exit the mucosal cell in chylomicrons
(D) conjugated bile salts are actively resorbed in the distal ileum and returned to the liver via the portal vein
(E) conjugated bile salts from the gallbladder mix with emulsified lipids in the duodenum to produce water-soluble micelles

327. For a symptomatic partial duodenal obstruction secondary to an annular pancreas, the operative treatment of choice is

(A) a Whipple procedure
(B) gastrojejunostomy
(C) vagotomy and gastrojejunostomy
(D) partial resection of the annular pancreas
(E) duodenojejunostomy

328. After complete removal of a sessile polyp of 2 × 1.5 cm found one finger-length above the anal mucocutaneous margin, the pathologist reports it to have been a villous adenoma that contained carcinoma in situ. You would recommend that this patient undergo

(A) reexcision of biopsy site with wider margins
(B) abdominoperineal rectosigmoid resection
(C) anterior resection of rectum
(D) external radiation therapy to rectum
(E) no further therapy

329. A previously healthy 15-year-old boy is brought to the emergency room with complaints of about 12 h of progressive anorexia, nausea, and pain of the right lower quadrant. On physical examination, he is found to have a rectal temperature of 38.1° (100.5°F) and has direct and rebound abdominal tenderness localizing to McBurney's point as well as involuntary guarding in the right lower quadrant. At operation through a McBurney-type incision, his appendix and cecum are found to be normal, but the surgeon is impressed with the marked edema of the terminal ileum, which also has an overlying fibrinopurulent exudate. The correct procedure is to

(A) close the abdomen after culturing the exudate
(B) perform a standard appendectomy
(C) resect the involved terminal ileum
(D) perform the ileocolic resection
(E) perform an ileocolostomy to bypass the involved terminal ileum

330. A 32-year-old woman undergoes a cholecystectomy for acute cholecystitis and is discharged home on the sixth postoperative day. She returns to the clinic 8 months after the operation for a routine visit and is noted by the surgeon to be jaundiced. Laboratory values on readmission show total bilirubin 5.6 mg/dL, direct bilirubin 4.8 mg/dL, alkaline phosphatase 250 IU (normal 21 to 91 IU), SGOT 52 KU (normal 10 to 40 KU), and SGPT 51 KU (normal 10 to 40 KU). An ultrasonogram shows dilated intrahepatic ducts. She undergoes the transhepatic cholangiogram seen below. Appropriate management is

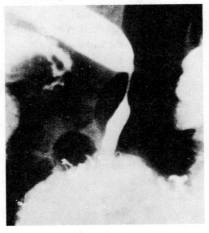

(A) choledochoplasty with insertion of a T tube
(B) end-to-end choledochocholedochal anastomosis
(C) Roux-en-Y choledochojejunostomy
(D) percutaneous transhepatic dilatation
(E) choledochoduodenostomy

331. A 55-year-old woman with cancer of the cervix undergoes hysterectomy and is found to have pelvic lymph nodes involved with cancer. She then receives a course of external beam radiation (4500 rads). When the physician counsels her prior to her radiation treatment, she should be told of all the possible complications of radiation enteritis. These include all the following EXCEPT

(A) malabsorption
(B) intussusception
(C) ulceration
(D) fistulization
(E) perforation

332. Which of the following would be expected to stimulate intestinal motility?

(A) Fear
(B) Gastrin
(C) Secretin
(D) Acetylcholine
(E) Cholecystokinin

333. All the following statements concerning carcinoma of the esophagus are true EXCEPT that

(A) alcohol has been implicated as a precipitating factor
(B) adenocarcinoma is the most common type at the cardioesophageal junction
(C) it has a higher incidence in males
(D) it occurs more commonly in patients with corrosive esophagitis
(E) surgical excision is the only effective treatment

Questions 334–335

334. A 30-year-old man with a duodenal ulcer is being considered for surgery because of intractable pain and a previous bleeding episode. Serum gastrin levels are found to be over 1000 pg/mL (normal 40 to 150) on three separate determinations. The patient should be told that the operation of choice is

(A) vagotomy and pyloroplasty
(B) highly selective vagotomy and tumor resection
(C) subtotal gastrectomy
(D) total gastrectomy
(E) partial pancreatectomy

335. Another 30-year-old man with the identical clinical situation presented in the previous question is being considered for surgery. His serum gastrin level, however, is 150 ± 10 pg/mL on three determinations. The surgeon should perform

(A) an arteriogram
(B) a secretin stimulation test
(C) a total gastrectomy
(D) a subtotal gastrectomy
(E) a highly selective vagotomy

336. The most common clinical presentation of idiopathic retroperitoneal fibrosis is

(A) ureteral obstruction
(B) leg edema
(C) calf claudication
(D) jaundice
(E) intestinal obstruction

337. A 55-year-old man who is extremely obese reports weakness, sweating, tachycardia, confusion, and headache whenever he fasts for more than a few hours. He has prompt relief of symptoms when he eats. These symptoms are most suggestive of which of the following disorders?

(A) Diabetes mellitus
(B) Insulinoma
(C) Zollinger-Ellison syndrome
(D) Carcinoid syndrome
(E) Multiple endocrine neoplasia, type II

338. In planning the management of a 2.8-cm epidermoid carcinoma of the anus, the first therapeutic approach should be

(A) abdominoperineal resection
(B) wide local resection with bilateral inguinal node dissection
(C) local radiation therapy
(D) systemic chemotherapy
(E) combined radiation therapy and chemotherapy

339. An 80-year-old man is admitted to the hospital complaining of nausea, abdominal pain, distention, and diarrhea. A cautiously performed transanal contrast study reveals an "apple-core" configuration in the rectosigmoid. Appropriate management at this time would include

(A) colonoscopic decompression and rectal tube placement
(B) saline enemas and digital disimpaction of fecal matter from the rectum
(C) colon resection and sigmoid colostomy
(D) oral administration of metronidazole and checking a *Clostridium difficile* titer
(E) evaluation of an electrocardiogram and obtaining an angiogram to evaluate for colonic mesenteric ischemia

340. Indications for operation in Crohn's disease include all the following EXCEPT

(A) intestinal obstruction
(B) enterovesical fistula
(C) ileum-ascending colon fistula
(D) enterovaginal fistula
(E) free perforation

341. A 50-year-old man presents to the emergency room with a 6-h history of excruciating abdominal pain and distention. The abdominal film shown below is obtained. The next diagnostic maneuver should be

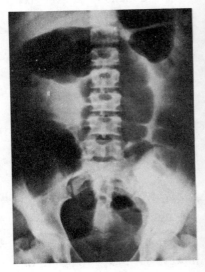

(A) emergency celiotomy
(B) upper gastrointestinal series with small bowel follow-through
(C) CT scan of the abdomen
(D) barium enema
(E) sigmoidoscopy

342. In the management of echinococcal liver cysts

(A) a large cyst should be treated by percutaneous aspiration of its contents

(B) medical treatment with albendazole usually preempts the need for surgical drainage

(C) negative serological tests suggest that the cyst is chronic and inactive and that no treatment is indicated

(D) leakage of cyst fluid puts the patient at risk for anaphylactic reaction

(E) coexistent extrahepatic cysts are uncommon

343. Each of the following statements regarding appendicitis during pregnancy is correct EXCEPT

(A) appendicitis is the most prevalent extrauterine indication for celiotomy during pregnancy

(B) appendicitis occurs in pregnant and nonpregnant women of comparable age with equal frequency

(C) suspected appendicitis in a pregnant woman necessitates prompt surgical intervention

(D) noncomplicated appendicitis results in 20 percent fetal mortality and 10 percent premature labor rate

(E) general anesthesia for appendectomy causes no increase in fetal damage or loss

344. Which of the following organisms is most closely associated with gastric and duodenal ulcer disease?

(A) *Campylobacter*

(B) Cytomegalovirus

(C) *Helicobacter*

(D) *Mycobacterium avium-intracellulare*

(E) *Yersinia enterocolitica*

345. On Monday morning, a septuagenarian man has a moderate-sized abdominal aneurysm resected. On Friday, he is noted to be markedly distended with an abdominal radiograph on which the cecum is measured as 12 cm across. Proper management at this time would be

(A) decompression of the large bowel via colonoscopy

(B) replacement of the nasogastric tube and administration of low-dose cholinergic drugs

(C) continued nothing-by-mouth orders, administration of a gentle saline enema, and encouragement of ambulation

(D) immediate return to the operating room for operative decompression by transverse colostomy

(E) right hemicolectomy

346. Which of the following is most likely to require surgical correction?

(A) Large sliding esophageal hiatal hernia
(B) Paraesophageal hiatal hernia
(C) Traction diverticulum of esophagus
(D) Schatzki's ring of distal esophagus
(E) Esophageal web

347. A 65-year-old man who is hospitalized with pancreatic carcinoma develops abdominal distention and obstipation. The following abdominal radiograph is obtained. Appropriate management would now include

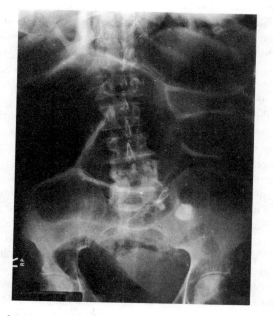

(1) urgent colostomy or cecostomy
(2) discontinuation of anticholinergic medications and narcotics and correction of metabolic disorders
(3) digital disimpaction of fecal mass in rectum
(4) diagnostic and therapeutic colonoscopy

SUMMARY OF DIRECTIONS

A	B	C	D	E
1,2,3	1,3	2,4	4	All are
only	only	only	only	correct

---

348. True statements regarding the Zenker's diverticulum include

(1) aspiration pneumonitis is likely
(2) it is an acquired abnormality
(3) the most common symptom is a sensation of high obstruction on swallowing
(4) it is a pulsion-type diverticulum

349. True statements regarding hemobilia include which of the following?

(1) The classic presentation includes biliary colic, jaundice, and gastrointestinal bleeding
(2) Iatrogenic injury has become the major cause
(3) Angiographic embolization is preferred treatment in cases of significant intrahepatic bleeding
(4) Surgery is advocated for extrahepatic hemobilia

350. The routine treatment of acute pancreatitis usually includes

(1) nothing by mouth
(2) administration of parenteral fluids
(3) administration of parenteral analgesics
(4) administration of steroids

351. True statements regarding the management of patients with asymptomatic, ultrasonographically documented gallstones include which of the following?

(1) Prophylactic cholecystectomy should be considered for diabetics with asymptomatic gallstones
(2) Most patients with asymptomatic gallstones can be managed by observation alone
(3) Gallstones detected incidentally at laparotomy are more likely to become symptomatic and cause complications if left untreated than gallstones detected by ultrasonography
(4) Cholecystectomy for asymptomatic gallstones is justified to prevent development of gallbladder carcinoma

352. An upper GI series is performed on a 71-year-old woman who presented with several months of chest pain that occurred when she was eating. The film below was obtained. Investigation revealed a microcytic anemia and erosive gastritis on upper endoscopy. True statements about her condition include

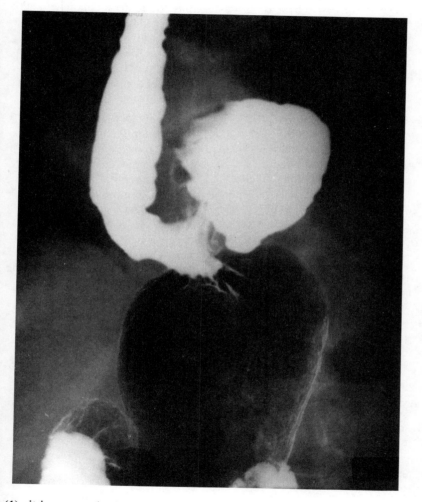

(1) it is an acquired condition
(2) the gastroesophageal junction is above the diaphragm
(3) ulceration, gastritis, or anemia is common
(4) it usually is controlled by contemporary medical therapy

SUMMARY OF DIRECTIONS

A	B	C	D	E
1,2,3 only	1,3 only	2,4 only	4 only	All are correct

353. True statements regarding adenocarcinoma of the pancreas include that it

(1) occurs most frequently in the body of the gland
(2) carries a 1 to 2 percent 5-year survival rate
(3) is nonresectable if it presents as painless jaundice
(4) is associated with diabetes mellitus

354. Correct statements concerning intussusception in infants include which of the following?

(1) Recurrence rates following treatment are high
(2) It is frequently preceded by a gastrointestinal viral illness
(3) A 1- to 2-week period of parenteral alimentation should precede surgical reduction when surgery is required
(4) Hydrostatic reduction without surgery usually provides successful treatment

355. A 32-year-old woman presents to the hospital with a 24-h history of abdominal pain of the right lower quadrant. She undergoes an uncomplicated appendectomy for acute appendicitis and is discharged home on the fourth postoperative day. The pathologist notes the presence of a carcinoid tumor (1.2 cm) in the tip of the appendix. Correct statements include that

(1) the patient should be advised to undergo ileocolectomy
(2) the most common location of carcinoids is in the appendix
(3) the carcinoid syndrome occurs in more than half the patients with carcinoid tumors
(4) the tumor is an apudoma

356. Correct statements regarding direct inguinal hernias include that

(1) they are the most common inguinal hernias in women
(2) they protrude medial to the inferior epigastric vessels
(3) they should be opened and ligated at the internal ring
(4) Cooper's ligament repair is recommended

357. A 35-year-old woman presented with pancreatitis. Subsequent endoscopic retrograde cholangiopancreatography (ERCP) revealed the congenital cystic anomaly of her biliary system illustrated in the film below. True statements regarding this problem include

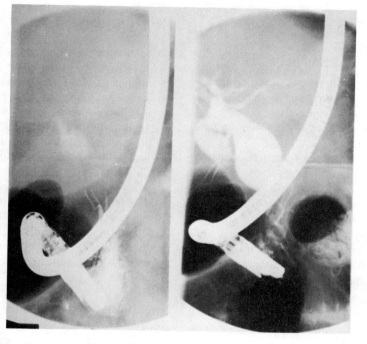

(1) treatment consists of internal drainage via choledochoduodenostomy
(2) malignant changes may occur within this structure
(3) most patients present with the classic triad of epigastric pain, an abdominal mass, and jaundice
(4) cystic dilatation of the intrahepatic biliary tree may coexist

SUMMARY OF DIRECTIONS

A	B	C	D	E
1,2,3 only	1,3 only	2,4 only	4 only	All are correct

358. True statements regarding stress ulceration include

(1) it is true ulceration, extending into and through the muscularis mucosa
(2) it classically involves the antrum
(3) increased secretion of gastric acid has been shown to play a causative role
(4) it frequently involves multiple sites

359. Correct statements concerning cholangitis include which of the following?

(1) The most common infecting organism is *E. coli*
(2) The diagnosis is suggested by Charcot's triad
(3) The disease occurs primarily in elderly patients
(4) Cholecystostomy is the procedure of choice in affected patients

360. Correct statements regarding colorectal carcinoma include which of the following?

(1) The 5-year survival rate in patients with carcinomas limited to the bowel wall is 80 percent
(2) Chemotherapeutic agents have been of little benefit for palliation of metastatic disease, but dramatic improvement of survival rates has been noted when the agents are used as adjuvant therapy following curative resection
(3) The survival rate for patients with carcinomas of the colon has remained essentially the same for the last 30 years
(4) Radiotherapy is quite helpful in treating recurrent disease that is confined to the bowel wall

361. Dieulafoy's lesion of the stomach is characterized by

(1) a large mucosal defect with underlying, friable vascular plexus
(2) frequent rebleeding after endoscopic treatment
(3) massive bleeding that requires subtotal gastrectomy
(4) location in the proximal stomach

362. A 45-year-old alcoholic man presents to the hospital after a weekend drinking binge with abdominal pain, nausea, and vomiting. On physical examination he is afebrile and is noted to have a palpable tender mass in the epigastrium. Laboratory tests reveal an amylase of 250 U/dL (normal < 180). A CT scan done on the second hospital day is pictured below. Appropriate statements concerning this patient's condition include

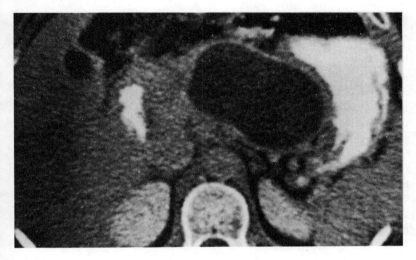

(1) the mass may result in gastric outlet or extrahepatic biliary obstruction
(2) spontaneous resolution commonly occurs
(3) the mass may be seen with acute and chronic pancreatitis
(4) the mass has an epithelial lining

---

363. Pancreatitis usually warrants surgical intervention in the presence of

(1) acute peritonitis
(2) severe cramping pain
(3) severe hypocalcemia
(4) common duct stones

364. A patient who has a total pancreatectomy might be expected to develop which of the following complications?

(1) Diabetes mellitus
(2) Iron deficiency
(3) Malabsorption
(4) Hypophosphatemia

365. A 28-year-old previously healthy woman arrives in the emergency room complaining of 24 h of anorexia and nausea and lower abdominal pain that is more intense in the right lower quadrant than elsewhere. On examination she has peritoneal signs of the right lower quadrant and a rectal temperature of 38.3°C (101°F). At exploration through incision of the right lower quadrant, she is found to have a small, contained perforation of a cecal diverticulum. True statements regarding this situation include which of the following?

(1) Cecal diverticula are acquired disorders
(2) Cecal diverticula are often solitary
(3) Cecal diverticula are mucosal herniations through the muscularis propria
(4) Diverticulectomy, closure of the cecal defect, and appendectomy are indicated

366. True statements regarding cavernous hemangiomata of the liver in adults include

(1) the majority are asymptomatic
(2) they may undergo malignant transformation
(3) they enlarge under hormonal stimulation
(4) they should be resected to avoid spontaneous rupture and life-threatening hemorrhage

367. Indications for surgical removal of polypoid lesions of the gallbladder include

(1) size greater than 1.0 cm
(2) presence of clinical symptoms
(3) patients over 50 years of age
(4) presence of multiple small lesions

368. Correct statements regarding rectal carcinoid tumors include

(1) endoscopic resection is sufficient for tumors smaller than 2 cm
(2) patients frequently present with the carcinoid syndrome
(3) they are rapidly growing tumors
(4) local recurrence is rare with complete resection of the primary lesion

369. Correct statements regarding carcinoembryonic antigen (CEA) and colorectal tumors include which of the following?

(1) Elevated CEA is indicative of a tumor of gastrointestinal origin

(2) A low CEA level after resection of a colon tumor is a good marker of disease control

(3) Ninety percent of colorectal tumors produce CEA

(4) There is a high likelihood of liver involvement if the CEA level is high (greater than 100 ng/mL)

DIRECTIONS: The group of questions below consists of four lettered headings followed by a set of numbered items. For each numbered item select

A	if the item is associated with	(A) **only**
B	if the item is associated with	(B) **only**
C	if the item is associated with	**both** (A) and (B)
D	if the item is associated with	**neither** (A) nor (B)

Each lettered heading may be used **once, more than once, or not at all.**

Questions 370–373

 (A) Ulcerative colitis
 (B) Crohn's disease (Crohn's colitis)
 (C) Both
 (D) Neither

370. Risk factor for colon cancer

371. Megacolon

372. Perianal fistulas

373. Transmural disease

DIRECTIONS: Each group of questions below consists of lettered headings followed by a set of numbered items. For each numbered item select the **one** lettered heading with which it is **most** closely associated. Each lettered heading may be used **once, more than once, or not at all.**

Questions 374–377

Match each sign below with the appropriate disorder.

(A) Acute cholecystitis
(B) Acute pancreatitis
(C) Acute cholangitis
(D) Splenic rupture
(E) Pancreatic cancer

374. Kehr's sign

375. Murphy's sign

376. Cullen's sign

377. Courvoisier's sign

Questions 378–380

Match the following.

(A) Rupture of the diaphragm
(B) Paraesophageal hiatal hernia
(C) Sliding hiatal hernia
(D) Foramen of Bochdalek hernia
(E) Foramen of Morgagni hernia

378. The most common congenital diaphragmatic hernia in infants

379. The hernia most likely to cause acute respiratory distress in infants

380. A congenital hernia that is most frequently discovered as an incidental finding in adults

Gastrointestinal Tract, Liver, and Pancreas

Answers

291. The answer is C. *(Schwartz, 6/e, pp 1179–1180.)* This is an in flamed Meckel's diverticulum. This common lesion is often clinically indistinguishable from acute appendicitis. It is the remnant of the vitel line duct. Meckel's diverticula are usually located 50 to 75 cm proxima to the ileocecal valve, are antimesenteric, and may contain either gastric and pancreatic or pancreatic tissue. Hemorrhage or obstruction is a more common presentation than inflammation. ^{99m}Tc pertechnetate ha affinity for gastric mucosa and a scan with this isotope can aid in the diagnosis of this anomaly as a cause of lower gastrointestinal hemor rhage in a child. Angiography is more useful when looking for arterio venous malformations. Since complications are relatively rare, most au thors do not recommend removing asymptomatic diverticula when they are incidentally discovered during abdominal procedures. Those diver ticula with a narrow neck, palpable heterotopic tissue, or nodularity are prone to obstruction and should be excised. In addition, patients ex plored for abdominal pain of unknown etiology should also undergo di verticulectomy, as should those operated on for appendicitis who are to be left with a scar of the right lower quadrant.

292. The answer is D. *(McQuaid, Surg Clin North Am 72:285–316 1992.)* Omeprazole (Prilosec) irreversibly inhibits the hydrogen-potas sium-ATPase (proton pump) in the secretory canaliculus of the gastric parietal cell. This blocks the last step in the acid-secretory process Omeprazole's duration of action exceeds 24 h and doses of 20 to 30 m per day inhibit more than 90 percent of 24-h acid secretion. Omeprazol provides excellent suppression of meal-stimulated and nocturnal aci secretion. It seems very safe for short-term therapy. However, its safet for long-term use is uncertain since it produces significant hypergastri nemia, hyperplasia of enterochromaffin-like cells, and carcinoid tumor in laboratory animals with prolonged administration.

293. The answer is D. *(Way, 9/e, pp 591–592.)* Patients with ITP who have mild symptoms need no therapy, but they are usually advised to avoid contact sports and elective surgery. When symptoms (e.g., easy bruising, menorrhagia, bleeding gums) are troublesome, the bleeding time will be prolonged, capillary fragility greatly increased, and clot retraction poor. Corticosteroid therapy will increase the platelet count in over 75 percent of cases and provides the best indication that splenectomy will be of lasting benefit. The platelet count can be expected to rise shortly after splenectomy and prolonged remissions are anticipated in 80 percent of cases. The size of the spleen and the state of function in the bone marrow have no predictive value in assessing the likelihood of response to splenectomy. In children, complete spontaneous remissions are common (80 percent of cases) and surgical intervention should be avoided.

294. The answer is A. (*Wilson, Ann Surg 210:428–434, 1989.*) Perforated peptic ulcer, perforated colon carcinoma, diverticulitis, and necrotic intestine from strangulated obstruction are common causes of pneumoperitoneum and peritonitis in the general population. This patient's history of prior drug use and opportunistic infection, however, suggests the presence of the acquired immunodeficiency syndrome and points to a second opportunistic infection, most commonly cytomegalovirus colitis, as the etiology of the current problem. The prognosis for these patients is poor. Over 50 percent in one series presenting with peritonitis did not survive.

295. The answer is E. (*Schwartz, 6/e, pp 1703–1704.*) Imperforate anus affects males and females with equal frequency, occurring in 1 of each 20,000 live births. It is due to failure of descent of the urorectal septum. Imperforate anus may be broadly classified into "high" or "low," depending on whether the rectum ends above or below the level of the levator ani complex. In 90 percent of females, but only 50 percent of males, the lesion is of the low variety. The rectal fistula may end in the prostatic urethra or vagina in the high cases, while the low cases terminate in a perineal fistula. For the low cases, only a perineal operation may be required and these children will be expected to be continent. A pull-through procedure will be required for the high imperforate anus and the chances for continence are less. If there is doubt about the level or location of the termination of the rectum, it is better to perform a colostomy than to compromise chances of continence by an injudicious perineal approach.

296–297. The answers are 296-C, 297-B. (*Cameron, 4/e, pp 449–450.*) This woman had a cystadenocarcinoma arising from the pancreatic body and tail, which was successfully resected. About 90 percent of primary malignant neoplasms of the exocrine pancreas are adenocarcinomas of duct cell origin. The remaining neoplasms include adenosquamous carcinoma, mucinous carcinomas, microadenocarcinoma, giant cell carcinoma, and cystadenocarcinoma of uncertain histogenesis. The clinical presentation is usually quite subtle with symptoms related primarily to the enlarging mass. There are no diagnostic laboratory findings and definitive preoperative diagnosis is rare. An elderly patient with no history of pancreatitis is unlikely to have a pseudocyst and a benign neoplasm is also less likely in this age group. These less common carcinomas are often several times the size of typical ductal cancers and often arise in the body or tail of the pancreas. They may become very large without invading adjacent viscera and do not generally cause significant pain or weight loss. Therefore, even large tumors may be cured by resection, and aggressive surgical management is indicated.

298. The answer is C. *(Schwartz, 6/e, pp 1266–1267.)* Varying types of colonic polyps can be distinguished on pathological examination. Adenomatous polyps are distributed throughout the entire large bowel, more commonly in the right and left colon than the rectum. They are often pedunculated and show an increased number of glands compared with normal mucosa. Although polyps that appear in familial polyposis are indistinguishable from single adenomatous polyps, they are manifested much earlier in life. Carcinomatous changes in patients who have familial polyposis occur approximately 20 years before carcinomatous changes of the bowel occur among patients in the general population.

299. The answer is C. *(Schwartz, 9/e, pp 1153–1154.)* According to the United Ostomy Association Data Registry, the most frequent serious complication of end colostomies is parastomal herniation, which commonly occurs when the stoma is placed lateral to, rather than through, the rectus muscle. Symptomatic herniation requires operative relocation of the stoma or mesh herniorrhaphy. Minor problems are frequently encountered with colostomies. They include irregularity of function, irritation of the skin due to leakage of enteric contents, or bleeding from the exposed mucosa following trauma. Prolapse occurs most frequently with transverse loop colostomies and is likely due to the use of the transverse loop to decompress distal colon obstructions. As the intestine decompresses, it retracts from the edge of the surrounding fascia, which allows prolapse or herniation of the mobile transverse colon. Optimal treatment of stomal prolapse is restoration of intestinal continuity or conversion to an end colostomy. Perforation of a stoma is usually due to careless instrumentation with an irrigation catheter. Perforations that cause minimal peritoneal contamination may be treated with observation and antibiotics, while more extensive leaks require operative closure.

300. The answer is A. *(Cameron, 4/e, pp 441–448.)* The prognosis for a patient with carcinoma of the pancreas is dismal. The majority of cases (46 percent) present as pain without jaundice, 34 percent present as pain with jaundice, and only 13 percent present with jaundice alone. Tumors over 1 to 2 cm may be seen by ultrasonography, computed tomography, or magnetic resonance imaging, but none of these methods can visualize smaller tumors. Endoscopic retrograde pancreaticocholangiography is helpful in distinguishing the more favorable tumors of the duodenum, ampulla, and common bile duct and lymphomas from cancer of the head of the pancreas. A combination of techniques including CT, angiography, and laparoscopy will accurately determine resectability in 97 percent of cases. Overall, the rate of resectability for cure is dismal: 5 to 10 percent of all patients and 10 to 25 percent of patients who present with jaundice alone. Ninety-nine percent of patients have metastatic disease at the time of diagnosis, and only 5 to 20 percent will be alive at 5 years following a pancreaticoduodenectomy.

301. The answer is C. *(Schwartz, 6/e, pp 1134–1142.)* Perforation of a duodenal ulcer is an indication for emergency celiotomy and closure of the perforation. In patients with no prior history of peptic ulcer disease, simple closure with an omental patch is recommended. Seventy-two percent of patients who are asymptomatic preoperatively will remain so postoperatively. Patients with long-standing ulcer disease require a definitive acid-reducing procedure, except in high-risk situations. The choice of procedure is made by weighing the risk of recurrence against the incidence of undesirable side effects of the procedure, and considerable controversy persists about this issue. Antrectomy and truncal vagotomy offers a recurrence rate of 1 percent, but carries a 15 to 25 percent incidence of sequelae such as diarrhea, dumping syndrome, bloating, and gastric stasis. Highly selective vagotomy, if technically feasible, offers a 1 to 5 percent incidence of side effects but carries a recurrence rate of 10 to 13 percent in some series, although results are better when gastric and prepyloric ulcers are excluded. In general, definitive acid-reducing procedures should be postponed if the perforation is more than 12 h old, or if there is extensive peritoneal soilage. Pyloroplasty and truncal vagotomy carries intermediate rates of recurrence and side effects, but has the advantage of speed in the setting of very ill patients with acute perforation.

302. The answer is B. (*Sawyers, Am J Surg 159:8–14, 1990.*) Though reminiscent of the carcinoid syndrome, this patient's complaints in the context of recent gastric surgery are highly suggestive of "the dumping syndrome," seen after gastroenteric bypass such as antrectomy and gastrojejunostomy. Dumping syndrome presents as vasomotor symptoms (weakness, sweating, syncope) and intestinal symptoms (bloating, cramping, diarrhea). The etiology of dumping has best been attributed to the rapid influx of fluid with a high osmotic gradient into the small intestine from the gastric remnant. Medical management consists of reassurance and frequent small meals that are low in carbohydrates (to limit the osmotic load). Antispasmodic medications are sometimes used if dietary adjustments are unsuccessful. The majority of cases will resolve within 3 months of operation on this regimen. Surgery for intractable dumping consists of creation of an antiperistaltic limb of jejunum distal to the gastrojejunostomy.

303–304. The answers are 303-D, 304-B. (*Schwartz, 6/e, pp 1346–1349.*) The diagnosis of bleeding esophageal varices is aided in the adult by stigmata of portal hypertension. Upper gastrointestinal hemorrhage in cirrhotics is due to esophageal varices in less than half of patients. Gastritis and peptic ulcer disease account for the majority of cases. Esophagoscopy is the single most reliable means of establishing the source of bleeding, though variations in transvariceal blood flow may result in nonvisualization of the varices. In addition, endoscopic sclerotherapy is reported to control acute variceal hemorrhage in 80 to 90 percent of cases and carries an acute mortality lower than other procedures. Barium swallow has a high false negative rate and offers no therapeutic advantage. Celiac angiography will rule out arterial hemorrhage and will demonstrate venous collateral circulation, but will not demonstrate variceal bleeding. Parenteral vasopressin controls variceal hemorrhage by constriction of the splanchnic arteriolar bed and a resultant drop in portal pressure. Intraarterial vasopressin offers no advantage over intravenous administration and requires a mesenteric catheter. The reported control rate is 50 to 70 percent. Esophageal balloon tamponade controls variceal hemorrhage in two-thirds of patients, but may also control bleeding ulcers and thereby obscure the diagnosis. Although balloon tamponade has reduced the mortality and morbidity from variceal hemorrhage in good-risk patients, an increased awareness of associated complications (aspiration, asphyxiation, and ulceration at the tamponade site), as well as a rebleeding rate of 40 percent, has reduced its use. It is indicated as a temporary measure when vasopressin and sclerotherapy fail. Emergency portacaval shunt is advised in good-risk cirrhotic patients whose bleeding is not controlled with vasopressin or sclerosis. The mortality for patients with bleeding varices not subjected to shunting is between 66 and 73 percent, whereas operative mortality of emergency shunts ranges from 20 to 50 percent. Esophageal transection with the autostapler carries the same mortality as shunt procedures and the rebleeding rate is estimated to be 50 percent at 1 year.

305. The answer is C. *(Schwartz, 6/e, pp 1272–1275.)* Since approximately 5 percent of colorectal cancers will be associated with resectable hepatic metastases, appropriate preoperative discussion should include obtaining permission for removal of synchronous peripheral hepatic lesions if they are found. If gross tumor is removed, a 25 percent "cure" rate can be anticipated. Adequate local resection, either by wedge or by limited partial hepatectomy, may be carried out whenever no extrahepatic disease is found and the hepatic lesion is technically removable. Any option that leaves the potentially obstructing primary cancer unremoved would be unacceptable. Radiation therapy has little to offer in colon cancer or its hepatic metastases. Local infusion of floxuridine (FUDR) via an implantable Infusaid pump for 14 days at 0.3 mg/kg/per day has been reported to provide some acceptable palliation in selected patients with unresectable hepatic lesions.

306. The answer is C. *(Cameron, 4/e, pp 53–56.)* Benign gastric ulcers have a peak incidence in the fifth decade, with male predominance. About 95 percent of gastric ulcers are located near the lesser curvature. It should be recognized that up to 16 percent of patients with gastric carcinoma pass a 12-week healing trial and that benign ulcers may enlarge during medical therapy. Therefore, the possibility of malignancy must be assessed by biopsy despite a 5 to 10 percent false negative rate. Six weeks of medical therapy will heal many gastric ulcers, but a recurrence rate as high as 63 percent and the serious consequence of complications in this older group of patients warrant surgery for recurrent or nonhealing ulcers. A distal gastrectomy with gastroduodenostomy is usually feasible in the absence of duodenal disease. Vagotomy, while advocated by some, is generally not included. Local excision with definitive distal resection or vagotomy and pyloroplasty is appropriate for a proximal ulcer that would otherwise require a subtotal gastrectomy.

307. The answer is C. *(Cameron, 4/e, pp 102–107.)* Regional enteritis may involve any segment of the GI tract from the esophagus to the rectum and often shows skip areas. The commonest area of involvement is the terminal ileum with minimal or no cecal involvement. The disease may also commonly involve both the small bowel and the right colon or present as jejunoileitis. The diarrhea in regional enteritis is of less frequency than that seen with ulcerative colitis and does not usually contain mucus, pus, or blood, although occult bleeding sufficient to produce anemia is a typical feature. Massive rectal bleeding is rare. The number of cases of adenocarcinoma of the small bowel associated with regional enteritis is small, but the association is probably significant. The 5-year survival is less than 10 percent. Although certain infectious agents such as enteroviruses, *Yersinia,* or *Campylobacter* have been linked to the acute variety of the disease, the cause of the typical chronic form is really not known. Viruses, immune deficiency, and genetic and toxic causes have all come under scrutiny as possible causes.

308. The answer is C. *(Cameron, 4/e, pp 526–543.)* An indirect inguinal hernia leaves the abdominal cavity by entering the dilated internal inguinal ring and passing along the anteromedial aspect of the spermatic cord. The internal inguinal ring is an opening in the transversalis fascia for the passage of the spermatic cord; an indirect inguinal hernia, therefore, lies within the fibers of the cremaster muscle. Repair consists of removing the hernia sac and tightening the internal inguinal ring. A femoral hernia passes directly beneath the inguinal ligament at a point medial to the femoral vessels, and a *direct* inguinal hernia passes through a weakness in the floor of the inguinal canal medial to the inferior epigastric artery. Each is dependent on defects in Hesselbach's triangle of transversalis fascia and neither lies within the cremaster muscle fibers. Repair consists of reconstructing the floor of the inguinal canal. Spigelian hernias, which are rare, protrude through an anatomic defect that can occur along the lateral border of the rectus muscle at its junction with the linea semilunaris. An interparietal hernia is one in which the hernia sac, instead of protruding in the usual fashion, makes its way between the fascial layers of the abdominal wall. These unusual hernias may be preperitoneal (between the peritoneum and transversalis fascia), interstitial (between muscle layers), or superficial (between the external oblique aponeurosis and the skin).

309. The answer is B. *(Schwartz, 6/e, p 1381.)* The finding of air in the biliary tract of a nonseptic patient is diagnostic of a biliary enteric fistula. When the clinical findings also include small bowel obstruction in an elderly patient without a history of prior abdominal surgery (a "virgin" abdomen), the diagnosis of gallstone ileus can be made with a high degree of certainty. In this condition, a large chronic gallstone mechanically erodes through the wall of the gallbladder into adjacent stomach or duodenum. As the stone moves down the small intestine, mild cramping symptoms are common. When the gallstone arrives in the distal ileum, the caliber of the bowel no longer allows passage and obstruction develops. Surgical removal of the gallstone is necessary. The diseases suggested by each of the other response items (bleeding ulcer, peritoneal infection, pyloric outlet obstruction, pelvic neoplasm) are common in elderly patients, but each of them would probably present with symptoms other than those of small bowel obstruction.

310. The answer is D. *(Schwartz, 6/e, pp 1259–1262.)* Cancer of the colon in patients with chronic ulcerative colitis is ten times more frequent than in the general population. Duration of disease is very important; the risk of developing cancer in the first 10 years is low but thereafter rises about 4 percent per year. The average age of cancer development in patients with chronic ulcerative colitis is 37 years; idiopathic carcinoma of the colon, however, develops at an average age of 65 years. Crohn's colitis is currently felt to be a precancerous condition as well. The chance of development of carcinoma of the colon in patients with familial polyposis is essentially 100 percent. Treatment of the patient with familial polyposis generally consists of subtotal colectomy with ileoproctostomy and regular proctoscopic examination of the rectal stump. Villous adenomas have been demonstrated to contain malignant portions in about one-third of affected persons and invasive malignancy in another one-third of removed specimens. Anterior resection is performed for large lesions or those containing invasive carcinomas when the lesion is above the peritoneal reflection. Abdominoperineal resection is indicated for low-lying rectal villous adenomas when they have demonstrated invasive carcinomas. Transrectal excision with regular follow-up examinations is sufficient for lesions without invasive carcinomas. Peutz-Jeghers syndrome is characterized by intestinal polyposis and melanin spots of the oral mucosa. Unlike the adenomatous polyps seen in familial polyposis, the lesions in this condition are hamartomas, which have no malignant potential.

311. The answer is C. *(Schwartz, 6/e, p 1381.)* Gallstone ileus is due to erosion of a stone from the gallbladder into the gastrointestinal tract (most commonly into the duodenum). The stone becomes lodged in the small bowel—usually in the terminal ileum—and causes small-bowel obstruction. Plain films of the abdomen that demonstrate small-bowel obstruction and air in the biliary tract are diagnostic of the condition. Treatment consists of ileotomy, removal of the stone, and cholecystectomy if it is technically safe. If there is significant inflammation of the right upper quadrant, ileotomy for stone extraction followed by an interval cholecystectomy is often a safer alternative.

312. The answer is A. (*Schwartz, 6/e, pp 1702–1703.*) Hirschsprung's disease, which is the congenital absence of ganglion cells in the rectum or rectosigmoid colon, is definitively diagnosed by rectal biopsy. The typical findings on barium enema, a distal narrow segment of bowel with markedly distended colon proximally, may not be seen early in life. Symptoms may go unrecognized in the newborn period with consequent development of malnutrition or enterocolitis. Initial treatment is colostomy decompression. Definitive repair is best delayed until nutritional status is adequate and the chronically distended bowel has returned to normal size. Unlike the situation with imperforate anus, which is associated with a high incidence of genitourinary tract anomalies and a 50 percent incidence of long-term fecal incontinence, in Hirschsprung's disease repair leads to satisfactory bowel function in most affected patients.

313. The answer is D. (*Way, 9/e, pp 1184–1185.*) This is an example of an ileal atresia. Whether the atresia is jejunal or ileal does not affect treatment and there is no predilection for one site over the other. Resection and primary anastomosis should be performed if possible, but the bowel should be exteriorized if there is a question of viability or there is a large size discrepancy between two segments. Plain films will reveal a small bowel obstruction with no gas beyond the lesion. A carefully administered meglumine diatrizoate (Gastrografin) enema can help in the differential diagnosis. Midgut volvulus and meconium ileus can be apparent on an enema, which is important as meconium ileus should be managed nonoperatively. The basis of jejunoileal atresia is probably a mesenteric vascular accident during intrauterine growth.

314. The answer is A. (*Schwartz, 6/e, pp 1706–1707.*) Omphalocele and gastroschisis result in evisceration of bowel and require emergency surgical treatment to effect immediate or staged reduction and abdominal wall closure. Patent urachal or omphalomesenteric ducts result from incomplete closure of embryonic connections from the bladder and ileum, respectively, to the abdominal wall. They are appropriately treated by excision of the tracts and closure of the bladder or ileum. In most children, umbilical hernias close spontaneously by the age of 4 and need not be repaired unless incarceration or marbled enlargement and distortion of the umbilicus occur.

315. The answer is D. *(Schirmer, Ann Surg 216:146–152, 1992.)* Laparoscopic cholecystectomy is now viewed as the treatment of choice for most patients with symptomatic gallstones. This procedure has frequently been performed in obese patients with the same efficiency, morbidity, and mortality rates and length of hospitalization as in the average-weight population. The other conditions listed represent currently accepted relative contraindications, but as experience increases and techniques and instruments improve, the safe indications for laparoscopic cholecystectomies are likely to expand and some presently contraindicated procedures may become laparoscopically approachable.

316. The answer is E. *(Schwartz, 6/e, pp 1703–1704.)* Congenital anorectal anomalies are frequently associated with other congenital anomalies including heart disease, esophageal atresia, abnormalities of the lumbosacral spine, double urinary collecting systems, hydronephrosis, and communication between the rectum and the urinary tract, vagina, or perineum. Congenital anorectal anomalies are not as common as congenital megacolon (Hirschsprung's disease), and their cause is unknown. They occur in approximately 1 in 2000 live births. Depending on the type of anomaly, a variety of surgical procedures has been devised to treat the problem. However, even when anatomical integrity is established, the prognosis for effective toilet training is poor. In 50 percent of cases continence is never achieved. Corneal opacities have no significant association with congenital anorectal anomalies.

317. The answer is C. *(Schwartz, 6/e, pp 1485–1487.)* Hematomas of the rectus sheath are more common in women and present most often in the fifth decade. A history of trauma, sudden muscular exertion, or anticoagulation can usually be elicited. The pain is of sudden onset and is sharp in nature. The hematoma is most common in the right lower quadrant and irritation of the peritoneum leads to fever, leukocytosis, anorexia, and nausea. Preoperatively the diagnosis can be established with an ultrasound or CT scan showing a mass within the rectus sheath. Management is conservative unless symptoms are severe and bleeding persists, in which case surgical evacuation of the hematoma and ligation of bleeding vessels is required.

318. The answer is B. *(Polk, 4/e, pp 296–297.)* Surgical treatment for sliding esophageal hernias should only be considered in symptomatic patients with objectively documented esophagitis or stenosis. The overwhelming majority of sliding hiatal hernias are totally asymptomatic—even many of those with demonstrable reflux. Even in the presence of reflux, esophageal inflammation rarely develops because the esophagus is so efficient at clearing the refluxed acid. Symptomatic hernias should be treated vigorously by the variety of medical measures that have been found helpful. Patients who do have symptoms of episodic reflux and who remain untreated can expect their disease to progress to intolerable esophagitis or fibrosis and stenosis. Neither the presence of the hernia nor its size is important in deciding on surgical therapy. Once esophagitis has been documented to persist under adequate medical therapy, manometric or pH studies may help determine the optimum surgical treatment.

319. The answer is B. *(Schwartz, 6/e, pp 1035–1038.)* While elevation of SGOT and SGPT are indicative of hepatocellular disease, elevated alkaline phosphatase is indicative of biliary obstruction. Based on safety and cost, ultrasonography is the initial diagnostic procedure. Once ductal dilation is identified, a percutaneous transhepatic cholangiogram or ERCP may be performed to localize and characterize the obstruction. If a distal common bile duct obstruction is noted, a CT scan is recommended to image the head of the pancreas. In most instances, a liver-spleen scan adds little to the diagnostic workup. This also applies to the upper gastrointestinal series.

320. The answer is A. *(Schwartz, 6/e, pp 1347–1348.)* Massive hematemesis in children is almost always due to variceal bleeding. The varices usually result from extrahepatic portal vein obstruction consequent to bacterial infection transmitted via a patent umbilical vein during infancy. In spite of this common cause, a history of neonatal omphalitis is infrequently obtainable. Bleeding can be massive but is usually self-limited and esophageal tamponade or vasopressin is usually not necessary. Elective portal-systemic decompression is recommended for recurrent bleeding episodes.

321. The answer is C. *(Davis, pp 236–237.)* The proximal stomach can distend or accommodate a large volume without any increase in intragastric pressure. This phenomenon permits solid food to settle along the greater curvature while liquids are propelled along the lesser curvature by slow tonic contractions of the upper stomach. In the normal state, once a volume of 1000 to 1200 mL is reached, intragastric pressure rises to high levels. While the stomach's ability to accommodate large volumes is necessary for normal gastric motor activity, a potentially deleterious effect is seen in patients with gastric atony. These patients may accumulate several liters of gastric juice in their stomach without sensing fullness, and this often leads to massive emesis and aspiration.

322. The answer is D. *(Davis, pp 251–260.)* Because the reserve capacity of the colon for water absorption greatly exceeds the normal requirements for maintaining stable bowel function, patients may undergo resection of a large fraction of their colon and suffer little change in bowel habits. Neither the right nor the left colon appears to be a site of preferential water and electrolyte absorption, nor does the ileocecal valve play a noticeable role in fluid homeostasis. However, in diseases characterized by increased fluid secretion of the small bowel, the colon is more likely to be overwhelmed by the absorptive demand following partial colectomy than in the intact state. The rectum does not appear to play a role in fluid absorption.

323. The answer is E. *(Cameron, 4/e, pp 191–200.)* Workup of a patient with a diagnosed rectal cancer should include CT scan of the upper abdomen in search of liver metastases and assessment of the depth of local invasion by transanal ultrasound. Sonographic staging of the rectal wall and pararectal lymph nodes has become crucial in planning the magnitude of the resection and choice of preoperative treatment. The survival advantages of neoadjuvant radiation therapy now seem clear. Administering radiation preoperatively to large or deeply invasive tumors often reduces the tumor mass and permits clean resection of previously bulky disease. In addition, the cytoreductive effect of preoperative radiation therapy now allows many patients to undergo sphincter-saving procedures and avoid the morbidity of proctectomy and colostomy.

324. The answer is C. *(Davis, pp 244–251.)* Digestion and absorption of dietary carbohydrate by the duodenum and small intestine are so avid that complete absorption has already occurred by the time ingested food has traversed 200 cm of jejunum. Simple fluids that require minimal digestion, such as milk, are entirely absorbed save for their fat content within the duodenum. Even in the short gut syndrome, virtually all di-

etary carbohydrate is absorbed within the residual jejunum. While pancreatic peptidases are important to protein digestion, redundant digestive enzymes are so widely distributed within the duodenal and jejuna
brush border that 95 percent of a protein meal can be absorbed in the
absence of the pancreas. Salt and water flux in the small intestine is
influenced by a variety of hormones; aldosterone markedly increases
sodium uptake, while prostaglandins stimulate fluid and electrolyte secretion.

325. The answer is D. *(Davis, pp 240–242.)* Gastrin, an aqueous ex
tract of the antral G cell, stimulates acid and pepsin secretion. A variet
of local stimuli cause the release of gastrin. The most potent of these
are small proteins, 20-proof alcohol, and caffeine. Acidic antral content
inhibit gastrin secretion; alkalinization of the antrum is stimulatory. Me
chanical distention of the antrum will also stimulate gastrin secretion.

326. The answer is C. *(Davis, pp 250–251.)* As it does with carbohy
drate digestion, the gastrointestinal tract exhibits remarkable redun
dancy and alternative pathways to facilitate fat uptake. In the norma
state, water-insoluble dietary lipid is rendered into soluble micelle
through mixing with pancreatic and intestinal lipase and with bile. How
ever, lipases of the stomach and small intestine permit absorption o
approximately half of neutral dietary fat in the absence of bile and pan
creatic secretion. Small breakdown products of complex fats—such a
glycerol, short-chain fatty acids, and medium-chain triglycerides—ca
be transported directly from the jejunal mucosal cell into the portal ve
nous system, whereas larger triglycerides, resynthesized by the mu
cosal cells from fatty acids, are deposited in chylomicrons and release
into the lymphatic system. Enterohepatic recirculation of bile with ac
tive resorption in the ileum and secretion into the portal venous system
yields an effective bile salt pool six to eight times its actual volume
Normal daily losses of bile into the stool represent 10 to 15 percent c
the total bile salt pool; these losses can usually be replaced by new
synthesis in the liver. Bile salt-wasting states, however, such as inflam
matory bowel disease or ileal resection, may exceed the liver's capacit
to maintain an adequate volume of bile.

327. The answer is E. *(Schwartz, 6/e, pp 1405–1406.)* A bypass proce
dure is the operation of choice for obstruction secondary to an annula

pancreas. A Whipple procedure is too radical a therapy for this benign disease, and a partial resection of the annular pancreas often is complicated by fistula. Duodenojejunostomy is much more physiologic than gastrojejunostomy and does not require a vagotomy to prevent marginal ulceration; it is therefore the procedure of choice.

328. The answer is E. *(Way, 9/e, pp 952–954.)* Many authorities now recommend abandonment of the phrase *carcinoma in situ* because it gives a misleading impression to patient and family regarding the true implications of severe dysplasia. Almost all agree that no further treatment is indicated when a polyp has been adequately removed and such changes are found. Only when malignant cells penetrate the muscularis mucosae is there any potential for metastases, and only when that depth of penetration is seen should the term *carcinoma* be used. Even then resection is probably not indicated if the gross and microscopic margins are clear, the tumor is well differentiated, and the stalk is not invaded.

329. The answer is B. *(Schwartz, 6/e, pp 1166–1167.)* Patients with regional enteritis usually have a chronic and slowly progressive course with intermittent symptom-free periods. The usual symptoms are anorexia, abdominal pain, diarrhea, fever, and weight loss. There are extraintestinal syndromes that may be seen with the disease such as ankylosing spondylitis, polyarthritis, erythema nodosum, pyoderma gangrenosum, gallstones, hepatic fatty infiltration, and fibrosis of the biliary tract, pancreas, and retroperitoneum. However, in about 10 percent of patients, especially those who are young, the onset of the disease is abrupt and may be mistaken for acute appendicitis. Appendectomy is indicated in such patients as long as the cecum at the base of the appendix is not involved, otherwise the risk of fecal fistula must be considered. Interestingly, about 90 percent of patients who present with the acute appendicitis-like form of regional enteritis will not progress to develop the full-blown chronic disease. Thus, resection or bypass of the involved areas is not indicated at this time.

330. The answer is C. *(Moosa, Arch Surg 125:1028–1031, 1990. Schwartz, 6/e, pp 1386–1387.)* The scenario in the question is a typical course of a patient with iatrogenic injury of the common bile duct. These injuries commonly occur in the proximal portion of the extrahepatic biliary system. The transhepatic cholangiogram documents a biliary stricture, which in this clinical setting is best dealt with surgically. Choledochoduodenostomy generally cannot be performed because of the proximal location of the stricture. The best results are achieved with end-to-side choledochojejunostomy (Roux-en-Y) performed over a stent. Percutaneous transhepatic dilation has been attempted in select cases, but follow-up is too short to make an adequate assessment of this technique. Primary repair of the common bile duct may result in recurrent stricture.

331. The answer is B. *(Cameron, 4/e, pp 181–185.)* The effects of radiation on the intestine depend on a variety of factors, which include the age of the patient, temperature, degree of oxygenation, and metabolic activity. Acute intestinal radiation injury is manifested in the bowel by the cessation of viable cell production and is seen clinically as diarrhea or gastrointestinal bleeding. Progressive vasculitis and fibrosis are seen in the latter stages of radiation injury and may result in malabsorption, ulceration, fistulization, or perforation. Intussusception is generally not associated with radiation injury.

332. The answer is D. *(Schwartz, 6/e, pp 1158–1160.)* Drugs, hormones, or emotional states (e.g., fear) that stimulate or simulate sympathetic activity will inhibit intestinal motility. Those factors that arouse parasympathetic activity (acetylcholine) will stimulate motility. Gastrin has specific delaying effects on gastric emptying. Secretin and cholecystokinin are potent regulators of intestinal and digestive activities but probably have no effect on motility per se.

333. The answer is E. *(Schwartz, 6/e, pp 1088–1089.)* Carcinoma of the esophagus occurs primarily in the sixth and seventh decades of life in a male:female ratio of 3:1. Although the cause is unknown, alcohol, tobacco, and dietary factors have been implicated as causative agents. A high incidence is reported in patients with corrosive esophagitis. The malignant tumors arising in the esophagus usually are squamous cell carcinomas except those involving the espohagogastric junction, which usually are adenocarcinomas. Even though squamous cell carcinomas are weakly radiosensitive, surgical extirpation affords reasonable, if short-term, palliation. Some authorities recommend radiotherapy for palliation alone or in combination with surgery to treat this lesion. Adenocarcinomas are not particularly radiosensitive and surgical treatment is generally employed. Following resection for esophageal carcinoma among the highly select group of patients whose tumors are still resectable when the diagnosis is made, survival is only about 14 percent at 5 years. The overall 5-year survival is under 5 percent.

334–335. The answers are 334-B, 335-B. *(Schwartz, 6/e, pp 1427–1428.)* Total gastrectomy was formerly the procedure of choice for patients with Zollinger-Ellison syndrome (ZES). However, with the knowledge that most patients will die of metastatic disease and that the symptoms can often be controlled with H_2-receptor antagonists, the role for surgery has changed. Initial surgical exploration is aimed at curative resection of the tumor. Unfortunately metastatic disease is often present or will develop at a later date despite tumor resection. Therefore, highly selective vagotomy is also added to the procedure to reduce the required dose of H_2-receptor antagonists.

The second patient has a gastrin level suggestive of but not diagnostic of ZES. A secretin stimulation test will cause a significant rise in serum gastrin levels in patients with ZES.

336. The answer is A. *(Schwartz, 6/e, pp 1509–1511.)* Idiopathic retroperitoneal fibrosis is a nonsuppurative inflammatory process of the retroperitoneum that causes problems by extrinsic compression of retroperitoneal structures. The ureters, aorta, and inferior vena cava are most at risk; however, the aorta is quite resistant to compression and the inferior vena cava has multiple collaterals so that ureteral obstruction is the most common presentation of this disease process. The common bile duct and duodenum may be compressed and obstructed, but this occurs much less frequently. Treatment of ureteral obstruction includes conservative therapy with steroids. Often surgical intervention is required and ureterolysis with intraperitoneal transplantation is the current procedure of choice. Biopsies must also be taken to exclude a malignant process as the cause of the fibrosis.

337. The answer is B. *(Schwartz, 6/e, pp 1426–1427.)* Tumors arising from the pancreatic beta cells give rise to hyperinsulinism. Seventy-five percent of these tumors are benign adenomas and in fifteen percent of affected patients the adenomas are multiple. Symptoms relate to a rapidly falling blood glucose level and are due to epinephrine release triggered by hypoglycemia (sweating, weakness, tachycardia). Cerebral symptoms of headache, confusion, visual disturbances, convulsions, and coma are due to glucose deprivation of the brain. Whipple's triad summarizes the clinical findings in patients with insulinomas: (1) attacks precipitated by fasting or exertion; (2) fasting blood glucose concentrations below 50 mg/dL; (3) symptoms relieved by oral or intravenous glucose administration. These tumors are treated surgically and simple excision of an adenoma is curative in the majority of cases.

338. The answer is E. *(Schwartz, 6/e, pp 1299–1300.)* Epidermoid cancers of the anal canal metastasize to inguinal nodes as well as to the perirectal and mesenteric nodes. The results of local radical surgery have been disappointing. Combined external radiation (dose range 3500 to 5000 cG) with synchronous chemotherapy (fluorouracil and mitomycin) is now recommended as the means for controlling the disease. Radical surgical approaches are now generally reserved for treatment failures and recurrences.

339. The answer is C. *(Schwartz, 6/e, pp 1274–1275.)* A markedly distended colon could have many causes in this 80-year-old man. The contrast study, however, reveals a classic "apple-core" lesion in the distal colon, which is diagnostic of colon cancer. No further diagnostic studies are appropriate prior to relief of this large bowel obstruction. After medical preparation (e.g., hydration, normalization of electrolytes), this patient should undergo prompt surgical management of his mechanical obstruction; conservative management by resection and proximal colostomy would generally be preferred in this elderly patient with an obstructed, unprepared bowel.

340. The answer is C. *(Schwartz, 6/e, pp 1249–1250.)* Surgical treatment of Crohn's disease is aimed at correcting complications that are causing symptoms. Intestinal obstruction is usually partial and secondary to a fixed stricture that is not responsive to anti-inflammatory agents. When the obstruction causes symptoms that compromise nutritional status, surgery is warranted. Fistula formation in itself is not an indication for surgery. Fistulas between the intestine and the bladder and the intestine and the vagina, however, generally cause significant symptoms and warrant surgical intervention, while an ileum-ascending colon fistula is very common yet rarely symptomatic. Perforation of bowel into the free abdominal cavity is obviously a surgical emergency.

341. The answer is E. *(Schwartz, 6/e, pp 1192–1193.)* The film shows a markedly distended colon. The differential diagnosis includes tumor, foreign body, and colitis, but far more likely is either cecal or sigmoid volvulus. Sigmoid volvulus may be ruled out quickly by proctosigmoidoscopy, which is preferable to barium enema, since sigmoid volvulus may be treated successfully by rectal tube decompression via the sigmoidoscope. If sigmoidoscopy is negative, the working diagnosis, based on this classic film, must be cecal volvulus; barium enema would clinch the diagnosis, but the colon might rupture in the intervening 1 to 2 h. Emergency celiotomy should be done.

342. The answer is D. *(Case records, N Engl J Med 317:1209–1218, 1987.)* Hydatid cysts secondary to echinococcal infection are most common in the liver in adults. Up to 25 percent of patients with hepatic cysts also have cysts in their lungs. In general, serological tests are more likely to be positive the longer the lesion has been present, but false negativity occurs with sufficient frequency that results should not influence the decision to treat hepatic hydatid cysts. Spontaneous rupture of the cyst or leakage of cyst fluid during diagnostic or therapeutic aspiration may cause anaphylactic reactions or peritoneal dissemination of the disease. Definitive treatment requires surgical resection, enucleation, or evacuation of the cysts. Agents such as 0.5% silver nitrate or hypertonic saline are introduced into the cyst at the time of surgery, and efforts are made to avoid spillage and contamination of the peritoneal cavity. Treatment of patients with liver cysts with mebendazole or albendazole has not been effective enough to replace the need for surgery.

343. The answer is D. *(Mahmoodian, South Med J 85:19–24, 1992.)* Appendicitis complicates approximately 1 in 1700 pregnancies at an incidence comparable with that in nonpregnant women matched for age. The duration of gestation does not influence the severity of the disease, but the diagnosis does become more difficult as the pregnancy progresses. By the twentieth week of gestation the appendix often lies at the level of the umbilicus and more lateral than usual. Pregnancy should not delay surgery if appendicitis is suspected; appendiceal perforation greatly increases the chance of premature labor and fetal mortality (approximately 20 percent for each). In contrast, negative laparotomy and nonperforated appendicitis are associated with very low risk to both the fetus and mother (less than 1 percent and 5 percent, respectively).

344. The answer is C. *(Graham, Gastroenterology 105:279–282, 1993.)* *Helicobacter pylori* is a spiral-shaped, gram-negative bacterium that is found in the viscous gastric mucus layer and has an affinity for epithelial cells. It was originally classified as a form of *Campylobacter,* but its genomic and phenotypic characteristics were subsequently found to be unique and it was given a new genus name. Urease and other peptides released by *H. pylori* may be toxic and cause direct gastroduodenal injury. Evidence is strong that *H. pylori* plays a role in the etiology of ulcer disease. There is an almost 100 percent association between gastric *H. pylori* infection and duodenal ulcer disease, and about 70 percent of patients with gastric ulcers are also infected with *H. py-*

lori. Furthermore, colonization with *H. pylori* increases the risk of developing a duodenal ulcer by up to twenty-fold. Eradication of *H. pylori* from the stomach markedly decreases the rate of ulcer recurrence. This generally requires "triple therapy" with colloidal bismuth (Pepto-Bismol), an antibiotic (amoxicillin or ampicillin), and a nitroimidazole such as metronidazole. Recent studies have also demonstrated a possible association between *H. pylori* infection and gastric carcinoma.

345. The answer is E. *(Schwartz, 6/e, pp 1202–1203.)* The history, x-ray, and clinical findings are typical of a postoperative cecal volvulus, a condition in which the cecum is twisted on its mesentery (often, after aneurysm resection, a neomesentery) and becomes acutely obstructed. At 12 cm, the cecum is in imminent danger of perforation. Particularly in the presence of a prosthetic graft, cecal perforation is a catastrophe. Urgent decompression is needed. To attempt colonoscopic decompression would necessitate insufflation of additional air and increase the stress on the already compromised cecal wall. A transverse colostomy "decompression" would not decompress the cecum nor would it provide detorsion of the cecal mesentery to allow restoration of adequate blood supply to the right colon. While untwisting the cecum and fixing it to the lateral abdominal wall (to inhibit recurrence) by a decompressing cecostomy might be advocated in some settings, the risk of contaminating the aortic graft would be excessive. Resection of the offending organ with ileotransverse colostomy would be the procedure of choice.

346. The answer is B. *(Schwartz, 6/e, pp 1111–1112.)* Normal respiration creates negative pressure in the thoracic cavity. As a result of the pressure gradient, blood enters the chest via the venae cavae and air via the trachea; both are life-sustaining results of this pressure gradient. The pathophysiological consequence of a hole in the diaphragm is that eventually abdominal viscera will be aspirated into the thorax. The sliding hernia, contained in the lower mediastinum by intact pleura, may rarely cause symptoms of reflux that would justify surgical attention, but such patients are in no danger of vascular compromise, nor of obstructive displacement of hollow viscera. The paraesophageal hernia, on the other hand, leaves the patient at substantial risk for both strangulation and obstruction. Either result would be a surgical catastrophe; with rare exceptions, paraesophageal hernias should be surgically repaired whenever diagnosed. A traction diverticulum is usually caused by inflammatory contraction around mediastinal nodes, is rarely of any symptomatic consequence, and need not be repaired. Neither the Schatzki ring nor the esophageal web justifies esophageal surgery. They can be ignored or dilated as symptoms demand.

347. The answer is D (4). *(Cameron, 4/e, pp 168–170.)* As classically described, Olgilvie's syndrome was associated with the rare occurrence of malignant infiltration of the colonic sympathetic nerve supply in the region of the celiac plexus. The eponym is now applied to the condition in which massive cecal and colonic dilatation is seen in the absence of mechanical obstruction. Other terms used to describe this condition are *acute colonic pseudo-obstruction, colonic ileus,* and *functional colonic obstruction.* It tends to occur in elderly patients in the setting of cardiopulmonary insufficiency, in other systemic disorders that require prolonged bed rest, and in the postoperative state. The diagnosis of Olgilvie's syndrome cannot be confirmed until mechanical obstruction of the distal colon is excluded by colonoscopy or contrast enema. Delay in decompressing the dilated cecum is inappropriate since colonic ischemia and perforation become a distinct hazard as the cecum reaches this degree of dilatation. Cautious endoscopic colonic decompression has been demonstrated recently to be a safe and effective form of treatment. Endoscopy should be combined with rectal tube placement, correction of metabolic abnormalities, and the discontinuation of medications that diminish gastrointestinal motility. The high complication rate in this population notwithstanding, a direct surgical approach to decompression becomes necessary when colonoscopic decompression fails since a perforated cecum is a catastsrophic event in such patients.

348. The answer is E (all). *(Schwartz, 6/e, pp 1078–1079.)* Premature contraction of the cricopharyngeus muscle on swallowing, which leads to partial obstruction, is believed to be the cause of this diverticulum of the pharyngoesophageal junction. High intraluminal pressure results in an outpouching of mucosa through the oblique fibers of the pharyngeal constrictors. Dysphagia is common and is the usual presenting symptom. The diagnosis is established by barium swallow. Treatment is surgical: diverticulectomy or suspension of the diverticulum is usually recommended. Because the diverticulum is located above the superior esophageal sphincter, no mechanism exists to prevent aspiration of the contents of the diverticulum. Pulmonary complications are common.

349. The answer is E (all). *(Merrell, West J Med 155:621–625, 1991.)* Quincke's classic triad of abdominal pain in the right upper quadrant, jaundice, and gastrointestinal bleeding is present in 30 to 40 percent of patients with hemobilia. With more frequent use of percutaneous liver procedures (e.g., transhepatic cholangiogram, transhepatic catheter drainage), iatrogenic injury has replaced other trauma as the most common cause of bloody bile. Other causes include spontaneous bleeding during anticoagulation, gallstones, parasitic infections/abscesses, and neoplastic lesions. Angiography and endoscopy are useful diagnostic studies and intrahepatic bleeding can be controlled by embolization in up to 95 percent of cases. Surgical treatment is advocated for bleeding from extrahepatic bile ducts or the gallbladder or in cases of penetrating trauma in which associated injuries might need attention.

350. The answer is A (1, 2, 3). *(Schwartz, 6/e, pp 1408–1413.)* Acute pancreatitis is usually treated by withholding administration of all fluids and foods by mouth and administering parenteral analgesics (meperidine is preferred) and fluids. Adjuncts to this therapy may include placement of a nasogastric tube and administration of anticholinergic agents, calcium gluconate, and antacids. In hemorrhagic pancreatitis, more aggressive therapy occasionally may be required, including blood transfusions and surgery. Although some workers still advocate the use of antibiotics, most now recommend their use only for specific indications in unusual cases. Use of the nasogastric tube is generally recommended, although several controlled studies cast doubt regarding its benefit, particularly in the presence of significant patient discomfort. Steroids are not recommended as they may cause pancreatitis.

351. The answer is A (1, 2, 3). *(Gibney, Br J Surg 77:368–372, 1990.)* The widespread use of diagnostic ultrasonography has led to the discovery of an increasing number of asymptomatic, or silent, gallstones. Current evidence suggests that most people with silent gallstones will remain asymptomatic. With the low mortality following cholecystectomy for symptomatic gallstones, awaiting the occurrence of symptoms in the majority of patients prior to performing cholecystectomy seems reasonable. However, the incidence of acute cholecystitis is more common in several subpopulations, including diabetics and patients with sickle cell anemia, and complications are frequent following emergency surgery among these patients. Therefore, routine gallstone screening and prophylactic cholecystectomy for diabetics and patients with sickle cell anemia may be desirable. Patients with stones detected incidentally at laparotomy also seem to be at greater risk of developing postoperative gallbladder symptoms and complications. This observation may be explained by the fact that anesthesia, narcotics, and fasting cause gallbladder stasis. Most studies of incidental cholecystectomy have concluded that adding cholecystectomy to another intraabdominal procedure does not increase morbidity or mortality. The availability of percutaneous endoscopic techniques for cholecystectomy does not change the basic indications for the operation. Most patients with asymptomatic gallstones should be managed by observation for symptoms. Gallbladder carcinoma occurs predominantly in elderly women and has a very poor prognosis. Although there is a strong association of gallbladder carcinoma with gallstones, only a small fraction of patients with chronic gallstones will develop gallbladder carcinoma. Therefore, cholecystectomy cannot be advocated as routine prophylaxis.

352. The answer is B (1, 3). *(Cameron, 4/e, pp 34–37.)* The condition demonstrated is a paraesophageal hernia. It is encountered much less frequently (approximately 5 percent) than is the sliding hiatal hernia and, as noted in the explanation to the previous question, it has completely different therapeutic implications. Paraesophageal hernias are acquired, rarely present before middle age, and are most common in patients in their seventh decade. The position of the gastroesophageal junction distinguishes the two types of hernias, which occur near the esophageal hiatus of the diaphragm. In the more common sliding hernia, the gastroesophageal junction protrudes above the diaphragm; in the paraesophageal hernia the anatomical junction between the esophagus and the stomach is anchored in its normal position below the diaphragm. The gastric cardia or fundus and occasionally other viscera herniate into the thorax within a true peritoneal sac alongside the gastroesophageal junction. Surgical repair is indicated as soon as the patient can be properly prepared for the procedure.

353. The answer is C (2, 4). *(Brooks, pp 263–279.)* The vast majority of pancreatic carcinomas are located in the head of the gland. Patients may present with painless jaundice by virtue of the carcinoma's obstruction of the intrapancreatic portion of the common bile duct. It is in this group of patients that resection is even possible—although most will be unresectable. Tumors in the body or tail of the gland are universally unresectable. The cause of pancreatic cancer is not known. There is a very strong association with diabetes mellitus but the nature of this relationship is not known. Prognosis is uniformly dismal whether resection is done or not and only an anecdotal survivor will be alive at 5-year follow-up.

354. The answer is C (2, 4). *(Schwartz, 6/e, pp 1701–1702.)* Intussusception is the result of invagination of a segment of bowel into distal bowel lumen. The most common type is ileocolic, which typically appears as a "coiled spring" on barium enema. Ileoileal and colocolic intussusceptions occur less commonly and are not easily diagnosed on barium enema. If bloody mucus, peritonitis, or systemic toxicity have not developed, hydrostatic reduction by barium enema is the appropriate initial treatment. Most patients are successfully managed this way and do not require surgical intervention. Immediate treatment should be instituted to avert the danger of bowel infarction. Recurrence is surprisingly uncommon after either surgical or nonsurgical treatment.

355. The answer is D (4). *(Schwartz, 6/e, pp 1177, 1316.)* Carcinoid tumors arise from the neuroectoderm and are a type of apudoma. The most common site of carcinoid tumors is the small bowel, although appendiceal carcinoids are also common. Carcinoid syndrome, which is characterized by flushing, diarrhea, and cardiac valvular disease, occurs in a small percentage of patients with carcinoid tumors; it is rarely seen with appendiceal carcinoids. The appropriate therapy for a small carcinoid (less than 2 cm) of the appendix is simple appendectomy.

356. The answer is C (2, 4). *(Schwartz, 6/e, pp 1518–1536.)* Direct inguinal hernias occur medial to the inferior epigastric vessels and are best repaired by reapproximating the transversalis fascia to Cooper's ligament and thus reconstructing the floor of the inguinal canal. The hernia sac is opened and ligated routinely during indirect hernia repair but not during direct hernia repair. The most common inguinal hernia in women is an indirect hernia.

357. The answer is C (2, 4). *(Cosentino, Surgery 112:740–748, 1992.)* Choledochal cysts are congenital cystic dilatations of the extrahepatic biliary ducts. Intrahepatic cystic dilatation can coexist (Caroli's disease), but it represents a distinct problem and is managed differently. Patients may present with symptoms at any age, but the classic triad of epigastric pain, abdominal mass, and jaundice is not frequently seen. Rather, most patients present with other conditions such as cholecystitis, cholangitis, or pancreatitis. Ultrasonography or endoscopic retrograde cholangiopancreatography (ERCP) is helpful in demonstrating cysts. Nonsurgical treatment of these cysts results in a high morbidity and mortality, and therefore surgery is advised in all cases. The present recommendation is for complete resection of the cyst and Roux-en-Y choledochojejunostomy. Since malignant changes in choledochal cysts have been frequently described, complete resection is preferred whenever the resection can be done safely rather than the performance of an internal drainage procedure.

358. The answer is D (4). *(Schwartz, 6/e, pp 1032–1033.)* Stress ulceration refers to acute gastric or duodenal erosive lesions that occur following shock, sepsis, major surgery, trauma, or burns. These lesions tend to be superficial and can involve multiple sites. McClelland and associates showed that patients subjected to trauma and subsequent hemorrhagic shock do not have increased gastric secretion, but rather show decreased splanchnic blood flow. Ischemic damage to the mucosa may therefore play a role. Unlike chronic benign gastric ulcers, which generally are found along the lesser curvature and in the antrum, acute erosive lesions usually involve the body and fundus and spare the antrum.

359. The answer is A (1, 2, 3). *(Schwartz, 6/e, pp 1383–1384.)* Cholangitis is suggested by the presence of Charcot's triad: fever, jaundice, and pain, of the right upper quadrant. These symptoms are usually caused by choledocholithiasis, but they can also occur in association with obstructing neoplasms and choledochal cysts. Therapy is aimed at decompression of the common bile duct. This is usually best accomplished by surgical placement of a T tube into the duct. Percutaneous transhepatic catheter drainage is an acceptable alternative in select patients. This procedure often can provide effective decompression during the acute septic phase of the disease. Cholecystostomy will be effective only if there is free flow of bile into the gallbladder via the cystic duct and in general should not be depended on to secure drainage of the common bile duct.

360. The answer is B (1, 3). *(Moertel, N Engl J Med 322:352–358, 1990. Schwartz, 6/e, pp 1259–1300.)* Chemotherapeutic agents have been of little benefit in treating patients with colorectal carcinomas for palliation of metastatic disease. Combination chemotherapy with levamisole and 5-FU has been shown to improve survival following resection of Dukes' C colon carcinomas. Radiotherapy is usually ineffective because colorectal carcinomas are not especially radiosensitive tumors and the gastrointestinal tract does not tolerate radiation very well.

361. The answer is D (4). *(Reilly, Dig Dis Sci 36:1702–1707, 1991.)* Dieulafoy's lesion has been identified more frequently recently as a source of gastrointestinal bleeding. It is characteristically located within 6 cm distal to the gastroesophageal junction. Dieulafoy's lesion typically consists of an abnormally large submucosal artery that protrudes through a small, solitary mucosal defect. The lesions may bleed spontaneously and massively for unclear reasons, in which case they require emergency intervention. Upper endoscopy is usually successful in localizing the lesion, and permanent hemostasis can be obtained endoscopically in most cases with injection sclerotherapy, electrocoagulation, or heater probe. If surgery is required, a gastrotomy and simple ligation or wedge resection of the lesion is adequate. Resection or acidreducing procedures play no role in preventing further bleeding from this lesion.

362. The answer is A (1, 2, 3). *(Schwartz, 6/e, pp 1416–1421.)* Pancreatic pseudocysts can develop in the setting of acute and chronic pancreatitis. They are cystic collections that do not have an epithelial lining. Most pseudocysts will spontaneously resolve. Therapy should not be considered for 6 weeks to allow for the possibility of spontaneous resolution as well as to allow for maturation of the cyst wall if the cyst persists. Complications of pseudocysts include gastric outlet and extrahepatic biliary obstructions as well as spontaneous rupture and hemorrhage. Pseudocysts can be excised, externally drained, or internally drained into the gastrointestinal tract (most commonly the stomach or a Roux-en-Y limb of jejunum).

363. The answer is D (4). *(Schwartz, 6/e, pp 1412, 1416–1419.)* Acute peritonitis generally mandates celiotomy. An important exception is the peritonitis that results from pancreatitis, which is usually treated by conservative measures because operative intervention increases mortality (acute hemorrhagic pancreatitis is often the exception). Whatever the degree of hypocalcemia associated with pancreatitis, it is treated medically. Pancreatic pseudocysts, which may be associated with either chronic or acute pancreatitis, are often symptomatic or lead to complications such as abscess formation. These may resolve spontaneously or be managed by percutaneous drainage. In some cases, surgical decompression is necessary. For patients with gallstone pancreatitis, removal of common duct stones surgically or endoscopically can reduce morbidity and mortality.

364. The answer is E (all). *(Schwartz, 6/e, p 1416.)* The metabolic consequences of total pancreatectomy are manifold. They include weight loss, malabsorption attended by hypocalcemia and hypophosphatemia, diabetes mellitus, diarrhea, and both iron deficiency and pernicious anemia. In theory, total pancreatectomy should provide good surgical treatment for pancreatic carcinoma; in reality, the severe metabolic problems that result from total removal of the pancreas make partial pancreaticoduodenectomy a frequently preferred treatment for most cases of pancreatic carcinoma that are resectable. Because of the frequently multicentric nature of pancreatic cancers, however, some surgeons would rather perform a total pancreatectomy and accept the more complicated postoperative metabolic management entailed by the loss of pancreatic endocrine function.

365. The answer is C (2, 4). *(Schwartz, 6/e, pp 1203–1207.)* Cecal diverticula must be differentiated from the more common variety of diverticula that are usually found in the left colon. Cecal diverticula are thought to be a congenital entity. The cecal diverticulum is often solitary and involves all layers of the bowel wall; therefore, cecal diverticula are true diverticula. Diverticula elsewhere in the colon are almost always multiple and are thought to be an acquired disorder. These acquired diverticula are really herniations of mucosa through weakened areas of the muscularis propria of the colon wall. The preoperative diagnosis in the case of cecal diverticulitis is "acute appendicitis" about 80 percent of the time. If there is extensive inflammation involving much of the cecum, an ileocolectomy is indicated. If the inflammation is well localized to the area of diverticulum, a simple diverticulectomy with closure of the defect is the procedure of choice. To avoid diagnostic confusion in the future, the appendix should be removed whenever an incision is made in the right lower quadrant, unless operatively contraindicated.

366. The answer is B (1, 3). *(Schwartz, 6/e, pp 1335–1337.)* Hepatic hemangiomata are the most common of all liver tumors. The infantile forms are highly vascular and occasionally cause hepatomegaly or congestive cardiac failure that requires angiographic or surgical interruption. The diagnostic incidence of incidental cavernous hemangiomata in adults has increased in this era of noninvasive imaging of organs with MRI, ultrasonography, and CT. When this lesion is suspected, the diagnosis can be confirmed with sensitive and more specific imaging techniques such as labeled red blood cell scanning. The mean age of presentation in adults is about 50 years and the vast majority of these lesions are asymptomatic. There is no evidence that they undergo malignant transformation. They may enlarge and become symptomatic more readily in women after multiple pregnancies or during the use of estrogen or oral contraceptives. The risk of rupture and severe hemorrhage into or from hemangiomata is extremely low; when it does occur it is usually iatrogenic (following attempted biopsy). Given their typically benign and static nature, management by angiographic embolization or resection should be reserved for the rare patient with symptomatic or complicated hemangioma.

367. The answer is A (1, 2, 3). *(Reilly, Dig Dis Sci 36:1702–1707, 1991.)* Polypoid lesions of the gallbladder are found most often in the third through fifth decades of life and are increasingly being detected by ultrasonography. Ninety percent of these lesions are benign lesions such as cholesterol polyps (pseudotumors). True adenomas constitute about 10 percent of these benign lesions, but they can undergo malignant transformation. The indications for operative intervention remain controversial. Recent reviews suggest that the vast majority of malignant polypoid lesions are solitary, larger than 1.0 cm, and much more common in patients greater than 50 years of age. There is also an increased incidence of malignancy if the lesions are associated with gallstones. Symptomatic lesions should be removed regardless of their size. Asymptomatic small lesions can probably be safely followed by ultrasonography.

368. The answer is D (4). *(Schwartz, 6/e, p 1298.)* Rectal carcinoids are slowly growing tumors, but they can be locally invasive and metastasize in up to 15 percent of patients. Patients manifest systemic signs of the carcinoid syndrome only in the rare circumstance where hepatic metastases have occurred. The malignant potential is low in carcinoid tumors when they are less than 2 cm in diameter, as is typically the case when diagnosed. The tumors are curable by wide, local, transanal resection that includes the muscle layer. Endoscopic treatment leaves tumor cells near the margin of resection and is felt to increase the risk of recurrence. Whether more aggressive resection (abdominoperineal or low anterior resection) improves the prognosis in larger tumors remains controversial. The prognosis is excellent for patients with local disease.

369. The answer is C (2, 4). *(Schwartz, 6/e, pp 1272, 1278, 1639.)* CEA is a tumor marker described in 1965 by Gold and Freedman. It is a nonspecific tumor marker that is elevated in only about one-half of patients with colorectal tumors and is often elevated in patients with lung, pancreatic, gastric, and gynecological malignancies. Patients in whom the primary colon tumor produced CEA and in whom the level falls below 2 to 3 ng/mL after resection have an excellent prognosis for disease control. In such patients, a subsequent rise in CEA has been demonstrated to be a very sensitive marker of the presence and extent of recurrent disease. Many surgeons follow CEA levels and perform "second-look" operations to resect local disease or possibly isolated metastatic disease if the levels become elevated postoperatively. Some surgeons recommend exploration in that circumstance even in the absence of other evidence (CT scan, colonoscopy) of recurrence. The long-term survival seems to be improved following this aggressive approach in some patients. Very high elevations of CEA, however, suggest extensive liver disease or peritoneal spread, which is unresectable.

370–373. The answers are 370-C, 371-C, 372-B, 373-B. *(Schwartz, 6/e, pp 1239–1245.)* Ulcerative colitis and Crohn's colitis are each forms of inflammatory bowel disease. Ulcerative colitis is a chronic inflammatory disease limited to the colonic mucosa. The rectum is almost always involved and the colon may be involved as well in a continuous distribution. Ulcerative colitis is a major risk factor for the development of carcinoma of the colon and approximately 5 percent of patients will develop a carcinoma after 10 years of ulcerative colitis. Crohn's colitis is a transmural inflammatory disease of the colon in which chronic inflammation (with granuloma formation) is seen in all layers of the colon. It frequently spares the rectum (50 percent of cases) and involves the remainder of the colon segmentally with skip areas. Crohn's colitis is also felt to be a precancerous lesion. Colonoscopy is commonly performed in both. Toxic megacolon may complicate either ulcerative colitis or Crohn's colitis. Sclerosing cholangitis is associated with both; however, perianal fistulas are generally seen only with Crohn's colitis.

374–377. The answers are 374-D, 375-A, 376-B, 377-E. *(Schwartz, 6/e, pp 212, 1378, 1438. Wilson, 12/e, pp 1303, 1366, 1374, 1384.)* Patients with splenic rupture may relate a history of pain at the tip of the left shoulder (Kehr's sign), which is caused by the irritation of the left hemidiaphragm by blood. This pain might only occur when the patient is in a supine or head-down position. It occurs in less than half of patients with splenic rupture.

In a patient with acute cholecystitis, deep inspiration with the examiner's hand on the right upper quadrant will cause the gallbladder to move caudad and strike the parietal peritoneum, which will thus cause pain (Murphy's sign).

Acute pancreatitis, if severe and hemorrhagic, may result in the tracking of blood through the tissue planes of the retroperitoneal space. Discoloration of the skin of the flanks (Turner's sign) and of the periumbilical region (Cullen's sign) may occur.

Patients with obstructive jaundice secondary to pancreatic cancer will often present with a dilated, palpable gallbladder (Courvoisier's sign). This is not always present because the gallbladder may be fibrotic and nondistensible owing to chronic inflammation from gallstones or because the cystic duct may be occluded by the tumor.

378–380. The answers are 378-D, 379-D, 380-E. *(Schwartz, 6/e, pp 1106–1112.)* Paraesophageal hernias, generally thought to be acquired, involve herniation of any portion or all of the stomach into the thoracic cavity via the esophageal hiatus. These hernias are usually repaired electively because of a high incidence of complications. In these dangerous hernias, the cardioesophageal junction is in its normal position below the diaphragm.

Diaphragmatic ruptures usually affect adults and result from blunt trauma to the abdomen. Unless such ruptures are repaired, the negative intrathoracic pressure associated with each respiratory effort tends to suck the abdominal contents into the chest with consequent loss of necessary space for lung expansion and substantial risk of damage to the intrathoracic bowel.

Sliding hiatal hernias, the most frequent type of hernia found in adults, generally are acquired. The significance of this type of hernia rests in its association with gastroesophageal reflux, a condition that may lead to reflux esophagitis. Because sliding hiatal hernias frequently do not exhibit significant gastroesophageal reflux, it is likely that other factors may be more important in the pathophysiology of that disorder.

The foramen of Bochdalek hernia is a congenital hernia of the posterolateral aspect of the diaphragm, in which abdominal viscera enter the thorax and cause acute respiratory distress in infants. This hernia requires emergency repair.

The foramen of Morgagni hernia, although also congenital, is not usually detected until adulthood. It is usually an incidental finding on chest x-ray, where it appears as a low anterior mediastinal mass. However, on rare occasions it can produce acute respiratory distress in infants.

Cardiothoracic Problems

DIRECTIONS: Each question below contains five suggested responses. Select the **one best** response to each question.

381. Among the cardiovascular anomalies of newborns, the one most likely to present with cyanosis is

(A) patent ductus arteriosus
(B) coarctation of the aorta
(C) atrial septal defect
(D) ventricular septal defect
(E) transposition of the great vessels

382. The superior vena cava syndrome is most frequently seen in association with

(A) histoplasmosis (sclerosing mediastinitis)
(B) substernal thyroid
(C) thoracic aortic aneurysm
(D) constrictive pericarditis
(E) bronchogenic carcinoma

383. During endoscopic biopsy of a distal esophageal cancer, perforation of the esophagus is suspected when the patient complains of significant new substernal pain. An immediate chest film reveals air in the mediastinum. You would recommend

(A) placement of a nasogastric tube to the level of perforation, antibiotics, close observation
(B) spit fistula (cervical pharyngostomy), gastrostomy
(C) left thoracotomy, pleural patch oversewing of perforation, drainage of mediastinum
(D) esophagogastrectomy via celiotomy and right thoracotomy
(E) transhiatal esophagogastrectomy with cervical esophagogastrostomy

Questions 384–385

384. A noncyanotic 2-day-old child has a systolic murmur along the left sternal border; the examination is otherwise normal. Chest x-ray and electrocardiogram are normal. These findings are most closely associated with which of the following congenital cardiac anomalies?

(A) Tetralogy of Fallot
(B) Ventricular septal defect
(C) Tricuspid atresia
(D) Transposition of the great vessels
(E) Patent ductus arteriosus

385. A 3-year-old child with congenital cyanosis most probably is suffering from

(A) tetralogy of Fallot
(B) ventricular septal defect
(C) tricuspid atresia
(D) transposition of the great vessels
(E) patent ductus arteriosus

386. A 4-year-old boy is seen 1 h after ingestion of a lye drain cleaner. No oropharyngeal burns are noted, but his voice is hoarse. Chest x-ray is normal. Of the following, which is the most appropriate therapy?

(A) Immediate esophagoscopy
(B) Parenteral steroids and antibiotics
(C) Administration of an oral neutralizing agent
(D) Induction of vomiting
(E) Rapid administering of a quart of water to clear remaining lye from the esophagus and dilute material in stomach

387. Each of the laboratory findings below is characteristic of a pleural transudate rather than an exudate EXCEPT

(A) pH 7.40
(B) lactic dehydrogenase (LDH) 150 IU
(C) white blood cell count 950/mm^3
(D) protein level 3.5 g/dL
(E) specific gravity 1.008

388. A 45-year-old woman was found at the wheel of her car after a high-speed motor vehicle accident. On arrival in the emergency room, she is in severe respiratory distress, with a systolic blood pressure of 90 mmHg. Examination reveals crepitus and paradoxical movement of a large segment of the right chest. A right-sided chest tube is placed without improvement in her respiratory status and the decision is made to intubate. She is now thrashing around in agitation. All the following are indicated EXCEPT

(A) cricoid pressure (Sellick maneuver)
(B) a left-sided chest tube
(C) administration of 2 mg/kg ketamine intravenously for sedation
(D) administration of 3 mg/kg of curare for muscle relaxation
(E) axial traction applied to the head

389. A stockbroker in his mid-forties consults you with complaints of episodes of severe, often incapacitating chest pain on swallowing. The diagnostic studies on the esophagus you have ordered yield the following: endoscopic examination and biopsy— mild inflammation distally; manometry—prolonged high amplitude contractions from the arch of the aorta distally, lower esophageal sphincter (LES) pressure 20 mmHg with relaxation on swallowing; barium swallow—2-cm epiphrenic diverticulum. You would recommend

(A) myotomy from level of aortic arch to distal sphincter; no disruption of LES
(B) diverticulectomy, myotomy from level of aortic arch to fundus, fundoplication
(C) diverticulectomy, cardiomyotomy of distal 3 cm of esophagus and proximal 2 cm of stomach with antireflux fundoplication
(D) a trial of calcium channel blockers
(E) pneumatic dilation of LES

Questions 390–391

A 26-year-old man is brought to the emergency room after being extricated from the driver's seat of a car involved in a head-on collision in which he was not wearing his seat belt. His ECG is shown below.

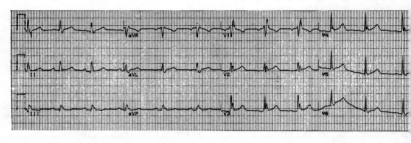

390. His ECG is most consistent with

(A) preexisting disease
(B) myocardial ischemia that caused the accident
(C) myocardial contusion that resulted from the accident
(D) Chagas' disease
(E) normal variant

391. The best test for establishing the diagnosis and the degree of myocardial dysfunction is

(A) serial ECGs
(B) creatine phosphokinase (CPK-MB) fractionation
(C) echocardiography
(D) radionuclide angiography
(E) coronary angiography

392. A previously healthy 20-year-old man is admitted to a hospital with acute onset of left-sided chest pain. The electrocardiographic findings are normal but chest x-ray shows a 40 percent left pneumothorax. Treatment consists of which of the following procedures?

(A) Observation
(B) Barium swallow
(C) Thoracotomy
(D) Tube thoracostomy
(E) Thoracostomy and intubation

393. A 50-year-old salesman is on a yacht with a client when he has a severe vomiting and retching spell punctuated by a sharp substernal pain. He arrives in your emergency room 4 h later and has a chest film in which the left descending aorta is outlined by air density. Optimum strategy for his care would be

(A) immediate thoracotomy
(B) serial ECGs and CPKs to rule out myocardial ischemia
(C) left chest tube and spit fistula (cervical esophagostomy)
(D) flexible esophagogastroscopy to establish diagnosis
(E) nasogastric tube, antibiotics, close monitoring

Questions 394–395

Several days following esophagectomy a patient complains of dyspnea and chest tightness. A large pleural effusion is noted on chest radiograph and thoracentesis yields milky fluid consistent with chyle.

394. Initial management of this patient consists of which of the following procedures?

(A) Immediate operation to repair the thoracic duct
(B) Immediate operation to ligate the thoracic duct
(C) Tube thoracostomy and low-fat diet
(D) Observation and low-fat diet
(E) Observation and antibiotics

395. Two weeks following the initial management of this patient's chylothorax there is persistent accumulation of chyle in the pleural space. Appropriate management at this time includes which of the following procedures?

(A) Neck exploration and ligation of the thoracic duct
(B) Subdiaphragmatic ligation of the thoracic duct
(C) Thoracotomy and repair of the thoracic duct
(D) Thoracotomy and ligation of the thoracic duct
(E) Thoracotomy and abrasion of the pleural space

396. An 89-year-old man has lost 30 pounds over the past 2 years. He reports that food frequently sticks when he swallows. He also complains of a chronic cough. Pulmonary function tests show a vital capacity of 60 percent of expected, and forced expiratory volume is 50 percent of predicted. Barium swallow is shown below. Which of the following statements is true?

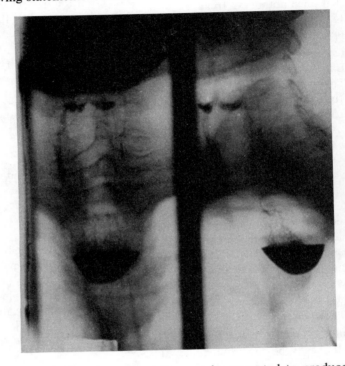

(A) Radiation therapy and stenting can be expected to produce the same long-term survival as would surgery
(B) Esophagoscopy and biopsy should be performed to confirm the x-ray findings
(C) This patient is atypical in that the lesion usually appears in the second or third decade of life
(D) The patient should be treated with antituberculous medications before any surgical intervention is considered
(E) The carotid bifurcation lies adjacent to the lesion

397. A full-term male newborn experiences respiratory distress immediately after birth. A prenatal sonogram had been read as normal. An emergency radiograph is shown below. The patient was intubated and placed on 100% O_2. The arterial blood gas revealed pH 7.24, P_{O_2} 60 torr, and P_{CO_2} 52 torr. The baby has sternal retractions and a scaphoid abdomen. Which of the following statements correctly refers to this condition?

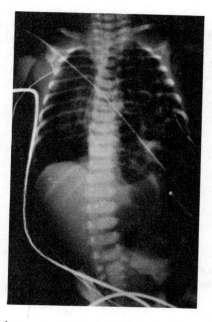

(A) The most likely cause of this problem is in utero traumatic rupture of the diaphragm
(B) The most important aspect in his management would be immediate exploration and repair of the defect
(C) The size of the defect directly correlates with severity of the disease
(D) The defect is usually anteromedial in location
(E) Any abdominal organ can be involved

398. A 56-year-old woman was treated for 3 years for wheezing on exertion, which was diagnosed as asthma. The chest radiograph below was obtained, which reveals a midline mass compressing the trachea. The most likely diagnosis is

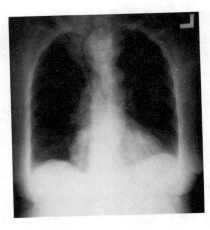

(A) lymphoma
(B) neurogenic tumor
(C) lung carcinoma
(D) goiter
(E) pericardial cyst

399. Esophageal atresia in combination with tracheoesophageal fistula is associated with all the following EXCEPT

(A) 80 percent survival rate following surgical repair
(B) excessive burping during feeding efforts
(C) air in the stomach
(D) copious mucus in the stomach
(E) regurgitation of feedings

DIRECTIONS: Each question below contains four suggested responses of which **one or more** is correct. Select

A	if	**1, 2, 3**	are correct
B	if	**1 and 3**	are correct
C	if	**2 and 4**	are correct
D	if	**4**	is correct
E	if	**1, 2, 3, and 4**	are correct

400. Correct statements concerning aortocoronary bypass grafting include which of the following?

1) It is indicated for crescendo (preinfarction) angina
2) It is indicated for congestive heart failure
3) It is indicated for chronic disabling angina
4) It is associated with a 10 percent operative mortality

401. Correct statements concerning the thoracic outlet syndrome include which of the following?

1) It may be difficult to distinguish from cervical spine disk disease
2) It is reliably diagnosed by positional obliteration of the radial pulse
3) If conservative measures fail, it is best treated by surgical decompression of the brachial plexus
4) It most commonly affects the median nerve

402. A 35-year-old man presents with a history of 4 days of severe substernal pain and fever to 38.89°C (102°F). He has a past medical history of peptic ulcer disease that resulted in a Billroth II procedure 5 years earlier. On admission, the chest film below is obtained. True statements regarding this patient's case include which of the following?

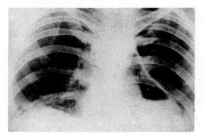

(1) Pneumopericardium is present
(2) The condition is a surgical emergency
(3) The condition could have resulted from recurrent peptic ulcer disease
(4) The condition could have resulted from spontaneous formation of gas from anaerobic bacteria

SUMMARY OF DIRECTIONS

A	B	C	D	E
1,2,3	1,3	2,4	4	All are
only	only	only	only	correct

403. Superior pulmonary sulcus carcinomas (Pancoast's tumors) are bronchogenic carcinomas that typically produce which of the following clinical features?

(1) Horner's syndrome
(2) Atelectasis of the involved apical segment
(3) Pain in the T1 and C8 dermatomes
(4) Nonproductive cough

404. A 2-year-old asymptomatic child is noted to have a systolic murmur, hypertension, and diminished femoral pulses. Correct statements about this child's disorder include which of the following?

(1) The life expectancy without surgery is about 30 years
(2) Immediate surgery is indicated
(3) Rib notching is often seen on x-ray
(4) Claudication is frequently noted

405. Correct statements concerning bronchial carcinoid tumors include that

(1) they infrequently metastasiz
(2) they most commonly arise i the major proximal bronchi
(3) they rarely produce the car noid syndrome
(4) they are radiosensitive

406. Currently accepted indications for insertion of a permane cardiac pacemaker include

(1) sick sinus syndrome with symptomatic bradycardic e sodes
(2) Mobitz type II AV block
(3) symptomatic bifascicular or trifascicular block
(4) carotid sinus syncope

407. Generally accepted indications that a lung carcinoma is in curable by surgery include

(1) bloody pleural effusion
(2) new-onset Horner's syndrome
(3) chest-wall extension
(4) superior vena cava syndrom

408. The condition shown in the x-rays below is compatible with which of the following manifestations?

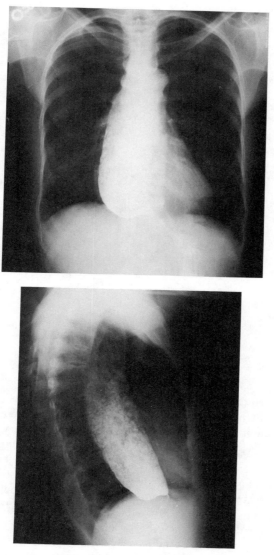

(1) Difficulty swallowing both solids and liquids
(2) Higher-than-normal incidence of esophageal carcinoma
(3) Failure of the lower esophageal sphincter to relax in response to swallowing
(4) Higher-than-normal pressure in the body of the esophagus

SUMMARY OF DIRECTIONS

A	B	C	D	E
1,2,3	1,3	2,4	4	All are
only	only	only	only	correct

Questions 409–410

Six months ago at the time of lumpectomy for breast cancer, a 60-year-old female attorney quit a 30-year smoking habit of two packs per day. She had a chest radiograph (below) as part of her routine follow-up examination.

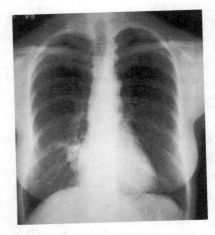

409. True statements about the lesion visualized on the film include which of the following?

(1) It is more apt to be a primary lung carcinoma than metastatic breast carcinoma

(2) There is a 90 percent chance that this mass is malignant

(3) Since the diagnosis can only be established with certainty by resection, the mass should be excised

(4) If the mass is malignant, the possibility for cure with excision is remote

410. At the time of operation on the patient in the preceding question, a firm, rubbery lesion in the periphery of the lung is discovered. It is sectioned in the operating room to reveal tissue that looks like cartilage and smooth muscle. Likely diagnoses include

(1) fibroma
(2) chondroma
(3) osteochondroma
(4) hamartoma

DIRECTIONS: Each group of questions consists of lettered headings followed by a set of numbered items. For each numbered item select the **one** lettered heading with which it is **most** closely associated. Each lettered heading may be used **once, more than once, or not at all.**

Questions 411–415

For each physical finding or group of physical findings below, select the cardiovascular disorder with which it is most likely to be associated.

(A) Massive tricuspid regurgitation
(B) Aortic regurgitation
(C) Coarctation of the aorta
(D) Thoracic aortic aneurysm
(E) Myocarditis

411. Argyll Robertson pupil

412. Exophthalmos

413. Quincke's pulse

414. Conjunctivitis, urethral discharge, and arthralgia

415. Short stature, webbed neck, low-set ears, and epicanthal folds

Questions 416–420

For each pathological sign below, select the mediastinal tumor with which it is most likely to be associated.

(A) Thymoma
(B) Hodgkin's disease
(C) Neuroblastoma
(D) Parathyroid adenoma
(E) Cystic teratoma

416. Increased urinary catecholamine level

417. Red blood cell aplasia

418. Renal stones

419. T-cell deficiency

420. Ectopic hair

Cardiothoracic Problems

Answers

381. The answer is E. *(Way, 9/e, pp 386–397.)* With the exception of coarctation, in which no shunt (or cyanosis) exists, the anomalies listed cause a shunting of blood between the systemic and lower pressure pulmonary circulation. Transposition of the great vessels is a right-to-left shunt that leads to cyanosis. Except where there is persistent congenital pulmonary hypertension, patent ductus arteriosus and atrial septal defects cause a shunting of oxygenated blood from the aorta and left atrium, respectively, back into the pulmonary artery and right atrium. These anomalies cause "recirculation" of oxygenated blood within the cardiopulmonary circuit but not cyanosis. When a ventricular septal defect is combined with pulmonary artery atresia (tetralogy of Fallot), the resulting undercirculation in the pulmonary system would join transposition as a cause of cyanosis. Other less common congenital lesions in which the pulmonary arterial blood flow is relatively decreased include tricuspid atresia, Ebstein's anomaly, and hypoplastic right ventricle.

382. The answer is E. *(Sabiston, 5/e, pp 503–504. Schwartz, 6/e, pp 921–922.)* Superior vena cava obstruction is almost always due to malignancy and, in three out of four cases, results from invasion of the vena cava by bronchogenic carcinoma. Lymphomas account for most of the remaining cases of the superior vena cava syndrome. Fibrosing mediastinitis as a complication of histoplasmosis or ingestion of methysergide may occur but is rare. Rarely a substernal thyroid or thoracic aortic aneurysm may be responsible for the obstruction. Although constrictive pericarditis may decrease venous return to the heart, it does not produce obstruction of the superior vena cava. Whatever the cause of the superior vena cava syndrome, the resultant increased venous pressure produces edema of the upper body, cyanosis, dilated subcutaneous collateral vessels in the chest, and headache. Cervical lymphadenopathy may also be present as a result of either stasis or metastatic involvement. When carcinoma is the cause of the superior vena cava syndrome, the treatment is usually palliative and consists of diuretics and radiation.

383. The answer is D. *(Schwartz, 6/e, pp 1101–1103.)* Perforation of the esophagus in the chest is a surgical catastrophe that requires aggressive intervention in virtually all circumstances. While that intervention can usually consist of efforts to patch the perforation and drain the mediastinum, concomitant obstructive esophageal disease, whether inflammatory stenosis or cancer, mandates removal or bypass of the obstruction if control of the leak and its consequent persisting mediastinal and pleural contamination is to be accomplished. For distal esophageal cancers, many thoracic surgeons would use the classic Ivor-Lewis operation, which consists of mobilizing the stomach in the abdomen and then performing a right thoracotomy with mediastinal cleanout, esophagectomy, and esophagogastrostomy. In some circumstances, and by some surgeons' preference, a left thoracotomy approach might be used. The transhiatal approach would probably be avoided in this situation where an unknown amount of mediastinal contamination has taken place.

384–385. The answers are 384-B, 385-A. *(Sabiston, 5/e, pp 1314–1331.)* Ventricular septal defect accounts for 20 to 30 percent of all congenital cardiac anomalies. It may lead to cardiac failure and pulmonary hypertension if the defect is larger than 1 cm; or it may be asymptomatic if the defect is small. Surgery is not indicated for the asymptomatic patient with a small defect since a substantial number of these anomalies close spontaneously during the first few years of life. Operation is indicated in infants with congestive heart failure or rising pulmonary vascular resistance (owing to the left-to-right shunt). When symptoms are mild and can be controlled medically, operation is usually delayed until age 4 to 6. Operative mortality ranges from less than 5 percent to more than 20 percent depending on the degree of pulmonary vascular resistance.

Tetralogy of Fallot, transposition, and tricuspid atresia are cyanotic lesions. Congenital cyanosis that persists beyond the age of 2 years is associated, in the vast majority of cases, with a tetralogy of Fallot. Patent ductus arteriosus is associated with the characteristic continuous machinery murmur.

386. The answer is B. *(Schwartz, 6/e, pp 1104, 1145–1146.)* Corrosive injuries of the esophagus most frequently occur in young children by accidental ingestion of strong alkaline cleaning agents. Significant esophageal injury occurs in 15 percent of patients with no oropharyngeal injury, while 70 percent of patients with oropharyngeal injury have no esophageal damage. Signs of airway injury or imminent obstruction warrant close observation and possibly tracheostomy. The risk of add-

ing injury, particularly in a child, makes esophagoscopy contraindicate
in the opinion of most surgeons. Administration of oral "antidotes" i
ineffective unless given within moments of ingestion; even then, the ad
ditional damage potentially caused by the chemical reactions of neu
tralization often makes use of them unwise. A barium esophagogram i
usually done within 24 h unless evidence of perforation is present. I
most reports, steroids in conjunction with antibiotics reduce the inci
dence of formation of strictures from about 70 to about 15 percent
Vomiting should be avoided, if possible, to prevent further corrosiv
injury and possible aspiration. It is probably wise to avoid all oral intak
until the full extent of injury is ascertained.

387. The answer is D. *(Schwartz, 6/e, pp 695–702.)* The protein level
in transudative fluid should be low since the intact capillary membrane
do not allow large molecules to leak. Transudates are seen in CHF, ne
phrosis, cirrhosis, and rheumatoid arthritis. Most of the transudativ
analyses will result in concentrations of components below those ex
pected in the serum. Exudates are found in pneumonia, empyema, ma
lignancy, and pancreatitis and characteristically have lower pH (<7.2)
higher specific gravity (>1.016), LDH levels above 200 IU, and bloo
cells.

388. The answer is D. *(Schwartz, 6/e, pp 674–676.)* Patients who hav
suffered blunt trauma sufficient to produce flail segments of the ches
often develop severe hypoxemia. Though some references suggest tha
the paradoxical movement of the flail segment produces mechanic
problems that impair pulmonary ventilation, it is more likely that th
underlying pulmonary contusion is the major cause of hypoxemia i
these patients. When hypoxemia occurs, the preferred treatment is er
dotracheal intubation and positive pressure ventilation. The applicatio
of positive pressure ventilation to a seriously injured chest should prob
ably be accompanied by the insertion of chest tubes into both pleur
spaces, particularly in a hypotensive, unstable patient. The hypotensio
in this patient is presumably the consequence of hypovolemia. Mo
anesthetic agents cause a peripheral vasodilation, which could be fat
in this case. Ketamine, with sympathomimetic properties, is a notabl
exception. Muscle blockers can also cause hypotension by histamin
release. The worst offender is curare; the safest is probably pancur
nium. All victims of deceleration injuries should be presumed to hav
unstable cervical fractures until proved otherwise. For this reason som
trauma surgeons prefer nasotracheal intubation. It is probably saf

however, to intubate the patient orally if axial traction is applied to the head during intubation.

389. The answer is A. *(Schwartz, 6/e, pp 1084–1086.)* The diagnostic studies listed reveal minimal reflux esophagitis, normal LES relaxation and pressure, and an incidental small epiphrenic diverticulum. None of these findings justifies treatment and none explains the patient's symptoms. On the other hand the finding of prolonged high amplitude contractions in the body of the esophagus in a highly symptomatic patient is diagnostic of diffuse esophageal spasm. The cause of this hypermotility disorder is unknown but its symptoms can be disabling. The recommended treatment for this relatively rare disorder is a long myotomy guided by the manometric evidence. If the LES is functioning properly, most surgeons would now recommend stopping the myotomy short of the normal lower sphincter. It should continue upward at least to the level of the aortic arch—higher if manometric findings of spasm are noted above that level. Eighty to ninety percent of patients treated in this fashion will experience acceptable relief of symptoms.

390–391. The answers are 390-C, 391-D. *(Sabiston, 5/e, p 396.)* The incidence of myocardial contusion is about 25 percent in patients with severe blunt injury to the chest. The injury occurs as a result of direct compression of the heart between the sternum and the vertebral column. The right ventricle, being the most anterior portion of the heart, is the most commonly injured portion. The blow causes extravasation of blood into the myocardium and results in a progressive loss of ventricular compliance and decreased cardiac output, which usually peaks by 8 to 24 h after the injury.

The most helpful ECG finding is the presence of a new right bundle branch block, which occurs because of damage to the anterior portion of the interventricular septum; ST-segment and T-wave changes and even the development of new Q waves may be seen. CPK-MB fractions are useful if they are positive; however, frequent false negatives may be seen because of the release of CPK-MM from other contused organs, such as the pectoralis muscles, which can dilute the cardiac CPK-MB to nondiagnostic levels. Echocardiography may be helpful but the right ventricle is often poorly visualized. Radionuclide angiography is most useful by suggesting the degree of myocardial impairment caused by decreased compliance.

Therapy of myocardial contusion is directed at inotropic support of the ventricle; usually, the coronary arteries are intact after the injury and so there is little role for coronary vasodilators and less for coronary artery bypass grafting.

392. The answer is D. *(Sabiston, 5/e, pp 455–458. Schwartz, 6/e, pp 704–707.)* Spontaneous pneumothorax usually results from the rupture of subpleural blebs in young men (age 20 to 40), which is often signaled by a sudden onset of chest and shoulder pain. Pneumothorax of more than 25 percent requires placement of a chest tube; thoracotomy with bleb excision and pleural abrasion is generally recommended if spontaneous pneumothorax is recurrent. Small pneumothoraxes in patients with minimal symptoms usually resolve and therefore can be observed. A spontaneous perforation of the esophagus (Boerhaave's syndrome) can result in hydropneumothorax as well as the more usual pneumomediastinum, but would not present with an isolated 40 percent pneumothorax. Barium swallow is an appropriate diagnostic test for evaluation of a suspected leaking esophagus.

393. The answer is A. *(Henderson, Am J Med 86:559–567, 1989.)* The presence of air in the mediastinum after an episode of vomiting and retching is virtually pathognomonic of spontaneous rupture of the esophagus (Boerhaave's syndrome). The evidence is overwhelming that without prompt surgical exploration of the mediastinum by left thoracotomy, the patient has little chance for a short-term outcome of low morbidity. The aspiration of highly acidic gastric contents into the mediastinum creates havoc in the tissues exposed to it. The surgical procedure must include extensive opening of the mediastinal pleura and removal of any particulate debris that might have been aspirated into the thorax from the stomach. Closure of the esophageal laceration with reinforcement by a pleural flap and secure chest tube drainage of the pleural space are mandatory. If the operation is delayed beyond the first 8 to 24 h, the mortality rises sharply and survival will only follow prolonged intensive care and multiple operations. This catastrophic event is one of the few in which prompt diagnosis and intervention is crucial to success. Because the findings are classic and the diagnosis is so important, Boerhaave's syndrome justifiably receives emphasis in educational programs for emergency physicians, internists, radiologists, and surgeons alike.

394–395. The answers are 394-C, 395-B. *(Schwartz, 6/e, pp 700–702.)* Chylothorax may occur after intrathoracic surgery, or it may follow malignant invasion or compression of the thoracic duct. Intraoperative recognition of a thoracic duct injury is managed by double ligation of the duct. Direct repair is impractical owing to the extreme friability of the thoracic duct. Injuries not recognized until several days after intrathoracic surgery frequently heal following the institution of a low-fat diet and either repeated thoracentesis or tube thoracostomy drainage. A low-fat, medium-chain triglyceride diet often reduces the flow of chyle. Failure of this treatment modality requires direct surgical ligation of the thoracic duct. This is best approached from below the diaphragm, regardless of the site of intrathoracic injury.

396. The answer is E. *(Schwartz, 6/e, pp 1078–1079.)* Pharyngoesophageal (Zenker's) diverticulum is an outpouching of mucosa between the lower pharyngeal constrictor and the cricopharyngeus muscles. It is thought to result from an incoordination of cricopharyngeal relaxation with swallowing. These diverticula occur in elderly patients and more commonly on the left. The typical patient will present with complaints of dysphagia, weight loss, and choking. Others present with the effects of repeated aspiration, pneumonia, or chronic cough. A mass is sometimes palpable and a gurgle may be heard. Treatment is excision and division of the cricopharyngeus muscle, which can be done under local anesthesia in a cooperative patient. Esophagoscopy is dangerous because the blind pouch is easily perforated. Even though the pouch may extend down into the mediastinum, the origin of the diverticulum is at the cricopharyngeus muscle near the level of the bifurcation of the carotid artery.

397. The answer is E. *(Schwartz, 6/e, pp 1686–1687.)* This radiograph of a child with a scaphoid abdomen and respiratory disease is characteristic of a congenital diaphragmatic hernia. These defects are posterolateral and occur from failure of the embryological diaphragm to fuse between the 8th and 12th weeks of intrauterine life. The size of the defect does not correlate with symptoms. Even a large diaphragmatic hernia can be missed on prenatal sonogram if the abdominal contents have slipped back into the abdomen at the time of the study. Hernias of Morgagni are anteromedial and do not present as emergencies at birth. Any abdominal organ—pancreas, kidney, small and large intestine, stomach, liver, and spleen—can herniate into the chest. The abdominal organ acts as a space-occupying lesion and retards growth of the lung, which results in pulmonary hypoplasia. Respiratory problems at birth stem from primary pulmonary hypertension, the consequence of hypoplasia, rather than from compression of the lung by abdominal contents. Most experts recommend stabilizing the pulmonary hypertensive crisis medically or with extracorporeal membrane oxygenation (ECMO) prior to attempting repair.

398. The answer is D. *(Sabiston, 5/e, pp 505–533.)* The boundaries of the mediastinum are the thoracic inlet, the diaphragm, the sternum, the vertebral column, and the pleura bilaterally. The mediastinum itself is divided into three portions delineated by the pericardial sac: the antero-superior and posterosuperior regions are in front of and behind the sac, respectively, while the middle region designates the contents of the pericardium. Mediastinal masses occur most frequently in the anterosuperior region (54 percent) and less often in the posterosuperior (26 percent) and middle (20 percent) regions. Cysts (either pericardial, bronchogenic, or enteric) are the most common tumors of the middle region; neurogenic tumors are the most common (40 percent) of the primary tumors of the posterior mediastinum. The primary neoplasms of the mediastinum in the anteroposterior region are thymomas (31 percent), lymphomas (23 percent), and germ-cell tumors (17 percent). More commonly, though, a mass in this area will represent the substernal extension of a benign substernal goiter. Diagnosis may be made by visualization of an enhancing structure on CT; radioactive iodine scanning is useful in management as it may make the diagnosis if the mediastinal tissue is functional and will also document the presence of functioning cervical thyroid tissue to prevent removal of all functional thyroid tissue during mediastinal excision.

399. The answer is B. *(Schwartz, 6/e, pp 1690–1693.)* Esophageal atresia in association with tracheoesophageal fistula, the most common esophageal anomaly, involves a blind upper esophageal segment and a lower segment that communicates with the trachea, usually a point just above the bifurcation. Because the upper pouch is blind, regurgitation occurs but the affected infant is unable to belch. Coughing, copious mucus, and large amounts of air in the gastrointestinal tract are signs of communication between the lower esophageal segment (LES) and the trachea. There is a high association with other congenital anomalies, including cardiovascular disease (over 20 percent) and imperforate anus (12 percent). Over the past decade a variety of surgical techniques has evolved to improve the outlook for these infants; indeed, the most recent studies report that in over 80 percent of cases surgery has accomplished successful reconstitution of the intestinal tract.

400. The answer is B (1, 3). *(Sabiston, 5/e, pp 1820–1838.)* Coronary artery bypass surgery was developed in the late 1960s and is now being regularly performed. Indications for surgery include chronic disabling angina and crescendo (or preinfarction) angina. Cardiac catheterization with selective coronary angiography defines the extent of disease, which generally is localized to the proximal segments of the vessels. Operative mortality is about 2 percent and relief of angina is obtained in most affected patients. Patients with left main coronary artery disease have an increased longevity following successful bypass. Data regarding extension of life in other groups are conflicting.

401. The answer is B (1, 3). *(Sabiston, 5/e, pp 536–553.)* The thoracic outlet syndrome designates a symptom complex whose precise cause is unknown. It is felt to result from compression of the brachial plexus or subclavian vessels, or both, in the anatomical space bounded by the first rib, the clavicle, and scalene muscles. Since objective determinants of disease may be lacking or imprecise, the diagnosis often is established by resectional surgery. The carpal tunnel syndrome—compression of the median nerve as it passes through the carpal tunnel of the wrist—and cervical disk disease are the two entities most commonly confused with the thoracic outlet syndrome, whose symptoms and signs include pain, paresthesias, edema, venous congestion, and digital vasospastic changes. Positional dampening or obliteration of the radial pulse is an unreliable finding since it is present in up to 70 percent of the normal population. Neurological abnormalities may be documented by nerve conduction studies. Angiographic studies are often negative. Conservative management, which generally should precede surgery, consists of an exercise program to strengthen shoulder girdle muscles and decrease shoulder droop. Operative treatment includes division of the scalenus anticus and medius muscles, first rib resection, cervical rib resection, or a combination of all three.

402. The answer is E (all). *(Cummings, Ann Thorac Surg 37:511–518, 1984.)* This x-ray demonstrates an air-fluid level in the pericardium. Pneumopericardium can result from penetrating or blunt chest trauma, spontaneous formation of gas from anaerobic bacteria, iatrogenic causes, or direct extension into the pericardium by diseased adjacent organs. In this case, a patient with a high gastrojejunostomy developed a recurrent ulcer that eroded through the diaphragm and into the pericardium and thus caused a pneumopyopericardium. Often these patients will have an unrecognized gastrinoma (Zollinger-Ellison syndrome) and therefore continue to have peptic ulcer disease despite aggressive surgical therapy. The presence of pneumopyopericardium as seen in this chest film should be treated as a surgical emergency in this setting. Inability to demonstrate a fistula on roentgenographic investigation should not preclude the diagnosis of this entity. If the cause of the pericardial fluid is not clearly diagnosed by available means, then a pericardial window should be performed for diagnostic as well as therapeutic reasons. The pericardial sac should be irrigated and adequate continuing drainage should be ensured.

403. The answer is B (1, 3). *(Sabiston, 5/e, pp 560, 573–574.)* Pancoast's tumors are peripheral bronchogenic carcinomas that produce symptoms by involvement of extrapulmonary structures adjacent to the cupula. These structures include the nerve roots of C8 and T1, as well as the sympathetic trunk. Interruption of the cervical sympathetic trunk leads to miosis, ptosis, and anhidrosis, the triad of signs that constitutes Horner's syndrome. Involvement of the nerve roots causes pain along the corresponding dermatomes. The peripheral location of the neoplasm makes pulmonary signs, such as atelectasis and cough, unlikely.

404. The answer is B (1, 3). *(Sabiston, 5/e, pp 1134–1146.)* Coarctation of the aorta is a congenital anomaly that usually causes aortic stenosis just distal to the left subclavian artery in the area of the ligamentum arteriosum. Collateral circulation develops around the obstruction by way of intercostal vessels and accounts for the classic x-ray appearance of rib notching. Without surgery, the average life span is about 30 to 40 years with eventual death from cardiac failure, rupture of aortic aneurysms or of a cerebral artery, and bacterial endocarditis. Surgery can be accomplished with less than a 1 percent mortality and should be performed around 5 years of age, when the aorta is sufficiently large to be operable but before it becomes fibrotic and calcified, conditions that increase the technical difficulty of the operation.

405. The answer is A (1, 2, 3). *Schwartz, 6/e, p 749.)* Bronchial carcinoid tumors rarely produce the carcinoid syndrome. They are slow-growing, infrequently metastatic tumors that histologically resemble the carcinoid tumors of the small intestine. Over 80 percent arise in the major proximal bronchi and their intraluminal growth is responsible for the frequent presentation of bronchial obstruction. The only therapy for this lesion is operative resection since neither the primary tumor nor the infrequent lymph node metastasis is radiosensitive. The low malignant potential for this lesion is reflected by a long-term survival rate that approaches 90 percent.

406. The answer is E (all). *(Sabiston, 5/e, pp 1604–1606.)* During the early years of pacemaker insertion, the chief indication for insertion was complete AV block associated with presyncope or near syncope. Recently, more permanent pacemakers have been inserted for treatment of sick sinus syndrome. Currently accepted indications for pacemaker insertion include the following:

Complete AV block with
  Syncope or presyncope
  Congestive heart failure
  Ventricular tachycardia
  Heart rate less than 40 or asystole greater than 3 s
  Cerebral hypoperfusion
Second-degree AV block with symptoms
Acute MI with persistent second-degree AV block or complete
  AV block
Chronic bifascicular or trifascicular block with symptomatic, in-
  termittent complete or second-degree AV block
Sinus bradycardia or sinus pauses with symptoms
Hypertensive carotid sinus syndrome with recurrent syncope
Atrial fibrillation with slow ventricular rate and symptoms

407. The answer is A (1, 2, 3). *(Sabiston, 5/e, p 563.)* Lung cancer that has extended beyond either the lung parenchyma or the tracheobronchial tree is generally held to indicate surgical incurability. Indications of this are distant metastases, a bloody pleural effusion, Horner's syndrome (miosis, anhidrosis, and ptosis) indicating involvement of the cervical sympathetic trunk by extension out of the lung apex (also known as a Pancoast tumor), vocal cord paralysis indicating involvement of the recurrent laryngeal nerves in the mediastinum, or phrenic nerve involvement suggested by elevation of a hemidiaphragm. Attempts have been made to resect the superior vena cava en bloc with tumors with a 30 percent 5-year survival in a very select group of patients, but in general, involvement of the superior vena cava indicates unresectability. En bloc resection of tumors with chest-wall resection can be performed with 50 percent survival at 5 years if there are neither regional lymph node nor distant metastases.

408. The answer is E (all). *(Sabiston, 5/e, pp 857–862.)* The x-rays presented in the question are consistent with a diagnosis of achalasia, a motility disorder of the esophagus that usually affects persons between 30 and 50 years of age. The x-rays show a classic beaklike narrowing of the distal esophagus and a large, dilated esophagus proximal to the narrowing. The diagnosis of achalasia is generally suspected on the basis of barium x-rays, but because other esophageal disorders may mimic the condition, an esophageal motility study is usually required to confirm the diagnosis. The characteristic findings on a motility study are small-amplitude, repetitive, simultaneous postdeglutition contractions in the body of the esophagus, failure of the lower esophageal sphincter to relax after deglutition, and a higher-than-normal pressure in the body of the esophagus. Carcinoma of the esophagus is approximately seven times more frequent in persons who have achalasia than in the general population.

409. The answer is B (1, 3). (*Sabiston, 5/e, pp 574, 605–614. Schwartz, 6/e, pp 746–749.*) "Coin lesions" have been defined as densities within the lung field of up to 4 cm, usually round, and free of signs of infections such as cavitation or surrounding infiltrates. Malignant solitary lesions may contain flecks of calcification, but heavy calcification or concentric rings of calcium generally suggest a benign etiology. The differential diagnosis for coin lesions includes primary pulmonary carcinomas, metastatic carcinomas to the lung, benign lung neoplasms such as chondromas and other benign lung processes such as granulomas, or vascular abnormalities such as arteriovenous malformations. The likelihood that a coin lesion is a primary lung malignancy increases linearly with age: 15 percent at age 40, 40 percent at age 55, 70 percent at age 75. With the diminishing frequency of granulomatous disease and the continued rise in lung cancers, such lesions should be removed because there is an excellent chance of cure if the lesion is a primary lung malignancy. If the patient has had a previous malignancy of tissue other than lung, the likelihood that the lesion represents a metastatic lesion depends on the tissue of origin of the previous malignancy. If all patients with a history of prior cancer are considered together, a lung nodule will be a new lung primary in 60 percent, a metastatic lesion in 25 percent, and a benign process in 15 percent of cases. However, 80 percent of solitary lesions in patients with melanoma represent metastatic disease, while only 40 percent of lesions in patients with breast cancer will represent metastasis, and solitary lesions in patients with colon carcinoma are equally likely to be metastatic or primary lung cancers.

410. The answer is D (4). (*Sabiston, 5/e, pp 588–598.*) The term *hamartoma* denotes a tumor that arises from the disorganized arrangemen of tissues normally found in an organ. Pulmonary hamartomas are solitary lesions of the pulmonary parenchyma and generally appear a asymptomatic peripheral nodules; they represent the most common benign epithelial and mesodermal elements. Pulmonary chondromas consist of mesodermal elements alone and arise centrally in major bronchi, where they produce signs and symptoms of bronchial obstruction. Fibromas are the most common benign mesodermal tumors found in the lung; they may occur either within the lung parenchyma or, more commonly, within the tracheobronchial tree. Osteochondromas are lesions of bone and are not found in the lung. Aspergillomas are due to infection with the fungus *Aspergillus* and most commonly appear in the upper lobes as oval, friable, necrotic gray or yellow masses often surrounded by evidence of preexisting parenchymal lung disease.

411–415. The answers are 411-D, 412-A, 413-B, 414-E, 415-C. *(Sabiston, 5/e, pp 1135–1136, 1182, 1505, 1573–1574.)* Myocarditis, aortitis, and pericarditis all have been described in association with Reiter's syndrome; the original description included conjunctivitis, urethritis, and arthralgias. Although its cause is unknown, Reiter's syndrome is associated with HLA-B27 antigen, as are aortic regurgitation, pericarditis, and ankylosing spondylitis.

Short stature, webbed neck, low-set ears, and epicanthal folds are the classic features of patients who have Turner's syndrome. Persons affected by the syndrome, which is commonly linked with aortic coarctation, are genotypically XO. However, females and males have been described with normal sex chromosome constitutions (XX, XY) but with the phenotypic abnormalities of Turner's syndrome. Additional cardiac lesions associated with Turner's syndrome include septal defects, valvular stenosis, and anomalies of the great vessels.

The Argyll Robertson pupil, a pupil that constricts with accommodation but not in response to light, is characteristic of central nervous system syphilis and is associated with vascular system manifestations of this disease. *Treponema pallidum* invades the vasa vasorum and causes an obliterative endarteritis and necrosis. The resulting aortitis gradually weakens the aortic wall and predisposes it to aneurysm formation. Once an aneurysm has formed, the prognosis is grave.

Massive *isolated* tricuspid regurgitation produces a markedly elevated venous pressure, usually manifested by a severely engorged (often pulsating) liver. If the venous pressure is sufficiently elevated, exophthalmos may result. Tricuspid regurgitation of rheumatic origin is almost never an isolated lesion, and the major symptoms of patients who have rheumatic heart disease usually are attributable to concurrent *left* heart lesions. Bacterial endocarditis from intravenous drug abuse is becoming an increasingly important cause of isolated tricuspid regurgitation.

Quincke's pulse, which consists of alternate flushing and paling of the skin or nail beds, is associated with aortic regurgitation. Other characteristic features of the peripheral pulse in aortic regurgitation include the water-hammer pulse (Corrigan's pulse—caused by a rapid systolic upstroke) and pulsus bisferiens, which describe a double systolic hump in the pulse contour. The finding of a wide pulse pressure provides an additional diagnostic clue to aortic regurgitation.

416–420. The answers are 416-C, 417-A, 418-D, 419-B, 420-E. (*Sabiston, 5/e, pp 506–508.*) Neuroblastoma, a highly malignant tumor of children, occurs along the distribution of the sympathetic nervous system. It is derived from ganglion cell precursors and thus usually causes an increased excretion of catecholamines and their metabolites. Because of its propensity to metastasize to bone and its histological resemblance to Ewing's sarcoma, its association with elevated catecholamine levels is a major factor in differential diagnosis.

Renal stones occur in about half the cases of hyperparathyroidism. Other disorders sometimes associated with hyperparathyroidism include peptic ulcers, pancreatitis, and bone disease; central nervous system symptoms also may arise in connection with hyperparathyroidism. Occasionally, parathyroid adenomas occur in conjunction with neoplasms of other endocrine organs, a condition known as multiple endocrine adenomatosis.

Cystic teratomas, or dermoid cysts, include endodermal, ectodermal, and mesodermal elements. They characteristically are cystic and contain poorly pigmented hair, sebaceous material, and occasionally teeth. Dermoid cysts occur in the gonads and central nervous system, as well as in the mediastinum. With rare exceptions, the lesion is benign.

Thymomas are associated with myasthenia gravis, agammaglobulinemia, and red blood cell aplasia. These tumors are typically cystic and occur in the anterior mediastinum. Most thymic lesions associated with myasthenia gravis are hyperplastic rather than neoplastic.

Persons afflicted with Hodgkin's disease have impaired cell-mediated immunity and are particularly susceptible to mycotic infections and tuberculosis. The severity of the immune deficiency correlates with the extent of the disease. The nodular sclerosing variant of primary mediastinal Hodgkin's disease is the most common type.

Peripheral Vascular Problems

DIRECTIONS: Each question below contains five suggested responses. Select the **one best** response to each question.

421. Patients with phlebographically confirmed deep vein thrombosis of the calf

(A) can expect asymptomatic recovery if treated promptly with anticoagulants

(B) may be effectively treated with low-dose heparin

(C) may be effectively treated with pneumatic compression stockings

(D) may be effectively treated with acetylsalicyclic acid

(E) are at risk for significant pulmonary embolism

422. Following aortic reconstruction, the viability of the sigmoid colon can most reliably be evaluated by

(A) intraoperative measurement of inferior mesenteric artery stump pressure

(B) intraoperative Doppler arterial signal in the sigmoid mesentery

(C) intraoperative observation of bowel peristalsis

(D) postoperative sigmoidoscopy

(E) postoperative barium enema

423. A 25-year-old woman presents to the emergency room complaining of redness and pain in the right foot up to the level of the midcalf. She reports that her right leg has been swollen for at least 15 years, but her left leg has been normal. On physical examination she has a temperature of 39°C (102.2°F). Her left leg is normal. The right leg is not tender, but it is swollen from the inguinal ligament down and she has an obvious cellulitis of her foot. Her underlying problem is

(A) popliteal entrapment syndrome

(B) acute arterial insufficiency

(C) primary lymphedema

(D) deep venous thrombosis

(E) none of the above

424. For the first 6 h following surgical repair of a leaking abdominal aortic aneurysm in a 70-year-old man, oliguria (total urinary output of 25 mL since the operation) has become a concern. Of most diagnostic help would be

(A) renal scan
(B) aortogram
(C) left heart preload pressures
(D) urinary sodium concentration
(E) creatinine clearance

425. A 76-year-old woman is admitted with back pain and hypotension. A CT scan (shown below) is obtained, and the patient is taken to the operating room. Three days after resection of a ruptured abdominal aortic aneurysm, she complains of severe, dull left flank pain and passes bloody mucus per rectum. The diagnosis that must be immediately considered is

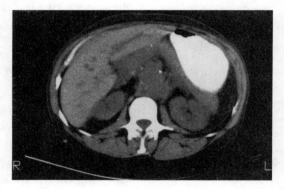

(A) staphylococcal enterocolitis
(B) diverticulitis
(C) bleeding AV malformation
(D) ischemia of the left colon
(E) bleeding colonic carcinoma

426. The angiogram depicted below is most typical of the patient whose history includes

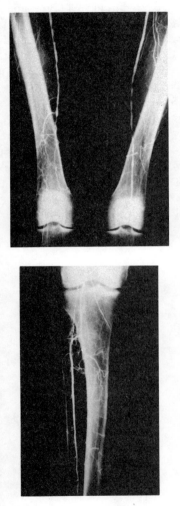

427. An 80-year-old man is found to have an asymptomatic abdominal mass and an arteriogram is obtained, which is pictured below. This patient should be advised that

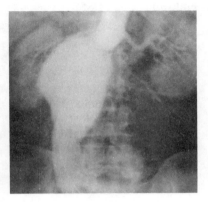

(A) surgery should be performed, but a mortality of 20 percent is to be anticipated
(B) surgery should be performed only if symptoms develop
(C) surgery will improve his 5-year survival
(D) surgery this extensive should not be performed in a patient of his age
(E) surgery should be performed only if follow-up ultrasound demonstrates increasing size

(A) cigarette smoking
(B) alcoholism
(C) hypertension
(D) diabetes
(E) type I hyperlipoproteinemia

428. A 55-year-old man with recent onset of atrial fibrillation presents with a cold, pulseless left lower extremity. He complains of left leg paresthesia and is unable to dorsiflex his toes. Following a successful popliteal embolectomy, with restoration of palpable pedal pulses, he is still unable to dorsiflex his toes. The next step in his management should be

(A) electromyography (EMG)
(B) measurement of anterior compartment pressure
(C) elevation of the left leg
(D) immediate fasciotomy
(E) application of a posterior splint

429. Reconstructive arterial surgery rather than conservative management is generally recommended for patients with all the following symptoms or signs of arterial insufficiency EXCEPT

(A) ischemic ulceration
(B) ischemic neuropathy
(C) claudication
(D) nocturnal foot pain
(E) toe gangrene

430. While evaluating a patient for the repair of an expanding abdominal aortic aneurysm, he is discovered to have a horseshoe kidney. The optimum surgical approach would be

(A) midline abdominal incision, preservation of the renal isthmus
(B) midline abdominal incision, division of the renal isthmus
(C) retroperitoneal approach, implantation of anomalous renal arteries
(D) nephrectomy, repair of aneurysm, chronic dialysis
(E) repair of aneurysm after autotransplantation of the kidney into the iliac fossa

DIRECTIONS: Each question below contains four suggested responses of which **one or more** is correct. Select

A	if	**1, 2, and 3**	are correct
B	if	**1 and 3**	are correct
C	if	**2 and 4**	are correct
D	if	**4**	is correct
E	if	**1, 2, 3, and 4**	are correct

431. A 55-year-old man is scheduled to undergo elective coronary artery bypass, and during evaluation an asymptomatic right carotid bruit is discovered. An aortic arch angiogram is obtained, which is pictured below. This patient should be informed that

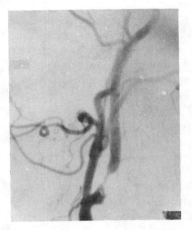

(1) he has a stenosis of the right internal carotid artery
(2) he should undergo carotid endarterectomy just prior to coronary artery bypass surgery in order to prevent an intraoperative stroke
(3) he may eventually develop transient ischemic attacks because of emboli from this stenotic, irregular internal carotid artery
(4) about 50 percent of patients suffer a stroke as the first symptom of carotid artery disease

SUMMARY OF DIRECTIONS

A	B	C	D	E
1,2,3	1,3	2,4	4	All are
only	only	only	only	correct

432. A 50-year-old male construction worker in relatively good health complains of severe pain of the left hip and lower extremity that limits his walking radius to 100 feet. The angiogram pictured below was obtained. Therapeutic options in this patient include

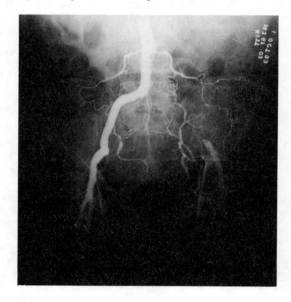

(1) femorofemoral bypass
(2) aortobifemoral bypass
(3) aorto–left-femoral bypass
(4) femoropopliteal bypass

433. Correct statements concerning antiplatelet therapy include

(1) aspirin has been shown to be an effective antiplatelet agent
(2) most antiplatelet agents work by inhibiting prostaglandin synthesis
(3) antiplatelet agents are used clinically in an attempt to increase patency rates of coronary artery bypass grafts
(4) it can be used to treat deep venous thrombophlebitis

434. The subclavian steal syndrome is associated with which of the following hemodynamic abnormalities?

(1) Reversal of flow through a vertebral artery
(2) Occlusion of a vertebral artery
(3) Occlusion of the subclavian artery
(4) Venous congestion of upper extremities

435. Symptoms of atherosclerotic occlusive disease of the bifurcation of the abdominal aorta (Leriche's syndrome) include

(1) claudication of the buttock and thigh
(2) claudication of the calf
(3) sexual impotence
(4) gangrene of the feet

436. Among patients with suspected (occult) coronary artery disease, the occurrence of postoperative ischemic cardiac events following peripheral vascular surgery correlates closely with abnormal preoperative

(1) exercise stress testing
(2) gated blood pool studies
(3) coronary angiography
(4) dipyridamole-thallium imaging

SUMMARY OF DIRECTIONS

A	B	C	D	E
1,2,3	1,3	2,4	4	All are
only	only	only	only	correct

437. A 60-year-old man is admitted to the coronary care unit with a large anterior wall myocardial infarction. On his second hospital day he begins to complain of the sudden onset of numbness in his right foot and an inability to move his right foot. On physical examination the right femoral, popliteal, and pedal pulses are no longer palpable. Vascular consultation is obtained. Diagnosis of acute arterial embolus is made. Correct statements concerning this condition include

(1) appropriate management would be embolectomy of the right femoral artery under general anesthesia
(2) noninvasive hemodynamic testing is required
(3) prophylactic exploration of the contralateral femoral artery should be done despite the presence of a normal pulse
(4) the source of the embolus is most likely the left ventricle

438. True statements concerning the condition depicted on the arteriogram shown below include which of the following?

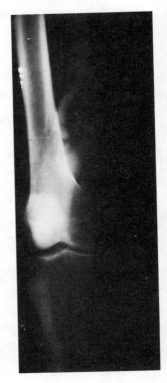

(1) Surgery should be performed even if the patient is asymptomatic
(2) Limb loss is a definite risk in the untreated patient
(3) The contralateral limb is often similarly affected
(4) Embolization is unlikely

439. A 65-year-old male cigarette smoker reports onset of claudication of his right lower extremity approximately 3 weeks previously. His walking radius is limited to three blocks before the onset of claudication. Physical examination reveals palpable pulses in his entire left lower extremity, but no pulses are palpable below the right groin level. Noninvasive flow studies are obtained, which are pictured below. Correct statements regarding this patient's condition include which of the following?

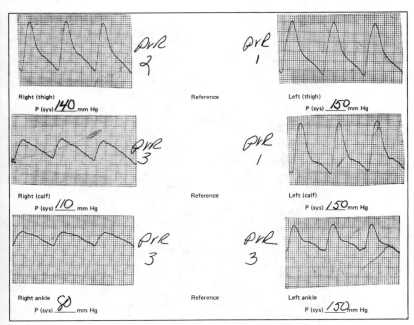

(1) Operative therapy (i.e., femoropopliteal bypass) is indicated on a relatively urgent basis in order to salvage the right leg
(2) The occlusive process is in the right superficial femoral artery with flow to the right foot supplied by the profunda femoris artery
(3) About one-half of patients with similar symptoms will ultimately require amputation
(4) The occlusive process is most likely caused by atherosclerotic disease

SUMMARY OF DIRECTIONS

A	B	C	D	E
1,2,3	1,3	2,4	4	All are
only	only	only	only	correct

440. Indications for placement of the device pictured in the abdominal x-ray shown below include

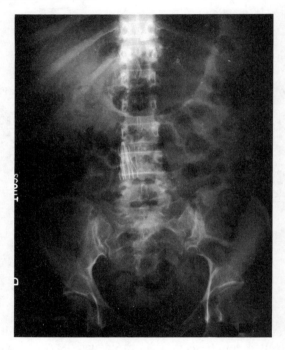

(1) recurrent pulmonary embolus despite adequate anticoagulation therapy
(2) axillary vein thrombosis
(3) pulmonary embolus in a patient with a bleeding duodenal ulcer
(4) pulmonary embolus due to deep vein thrombosis of the lower extremity that occurs 2 weeks postoperatively

441. A 64-year-old man is admitted 14 months following a femoropopliteal bypass graft procedure with a cold foot and no graft pulse. Urokinase infusion is begun. True statements regarding his management include

(1) clot lysis is accomplished in 75 percent of patients
(2) after successful clot lysis, surgical revision of the opened graft should be considered only if early reocclusion occurs
(3) with optimal treatment, a 20 percent reocclusion rate is expected within 1 year
(4) urokinase is less successful in lysing acute thromboses of prosthetic grafts than those of vein grafts

442. Two days after admission to the hospital for a myocardial infarction, a 65-year-old man complains of severe, unremitting midabdominal pain. His cardiac index is 1.6. Physical examination is remarkable for an absence of peritoneal irritation or distention despite the patient's persistent complaint of severe pain. Serum lactate is 9 (normal less than 3). In managing this problem you should

(1) perform computed tomography
(2) perform mesenteric angiography
(3) perform laparoscopy
(4) defer decision to explore the abdomen until cardiac function is optimized

443. True statements regarding pulmonary thromboembolism include which of the following?

(1) It is associated with clinically apparent deep vein thrombosis in less than 33 percent of patients
(2) It is believed to originate in deep vein thrombosis of the lower extremities in 85 to 90 percent of cases
(3) It causes hypoxemia owing to a ventilation-perfusion imbalance
(4) It must occlude more than 20 percent of the pulmonary vascular bed to produce symptoms in a previously healthy patient

444. Correct statements regarding Raynaud's disease include which of the following?

(1) The cause is unknown
(2) It more commonly affects women
(3) Vasoconstriction is usually precipitated by exposure to cold
(4) The upper extremities are almost always symmetrically involved

445. A 19-year-old man is admitted to the hospital following a gunshot wound to the left thigh. An arteriogram demonstrates an intimal flap of the left superficial femoral artery. Acceptable treatment plans include

(1)   close observation and follow-up arteriogram
(2)   femoropopliteal bypass graft with a synthetic conduit
(3)   femoropopliteal bypass graft with saphenous vein from the contralateral leg
(4)   femoropopliteal bypass graft with saphenous vein from the ipsilateral leg

Peripheral Vascular Problems

Answers

421. The answer is E. *(Bergqvist, pp 69–77, 89–111, 120–123. Cameron, 4/e, pp 776–780.)* Low-dose heparin and pneumatic compression stockings have been shown to be effective prophylaxis against deep vein thrombosis; however, they are not effective against established thrombosis, the treatment for which is therapeutic heparinization. Salicylate has not been convincingly shown to have either a prophylactic or therapeutic role in the treatment of deep vein thrombosis. Even following prompt, aggressive treatment of deep vein thrombosis of the calf as many as half of affected patients will develop symptoms of chronic venous hypertension, and a larger number will have abnormal venous hemodynamic findings. Untreated vein thrombosis of the calf may propagate into the larger popliteal veins and cause life-threatening pulmonary embolism.

422. The answer is D. *(Schroeder, Surg Gynecol Obstet 160:299–303, 1985.)* Viability of the colon can be evaluated intraoperatively by Doppler auscultation of the bowel mesentery and serosa, observation of bowel peristalsis, and measurement of the IMA stump pressure. A strong pulsatile Doppler signal in the mesentery, active sigmoid peristalsis, a chronically occluded IMA, or a patent IMA with stump pressure greater than 40 mmHg presage viability of the sigmoid colon postoperatively. However, none of these observations excludes the possibility of late sigmoid ischemia. Serial postoperative sigmoidoscopic examination is the best predictor of ischemic colitis and in experienced hands allows assessment of the depth of ischemic injury before frank perforation has occurred. Barium enema is not as accurate as sigmoidoscopy in determining depth of injury and carries grave risks of contamination by barium and feces if perforation occurs.

423. The answer is C. *(Schwartz, 6/e, pp 1011–1013.)* This patient is at high risk for developing cellulitis of her right foot because her underlying problem is unilateral primary lymphedema. Hypoplasia of the lymphatic system of the lower extremity accounts for greater than 90 percent of patients with primary lymphedema. If edema is present at birth it is referred to as *congenital*, but if it starts early in life (as in this woman) it is called *praecox*, and if it appears after age 35 it is *tarda*. The inadequacy of the lymphatic system accounts for the repeated episodes of cellulitis that these patients experience. Swelling is not seen with acute arterial insufficiency or with popliteal entrapment syndrome. Deep venous thrombophlebitis will result in tenderness and is generally not a predisposing factor for cellulitis of the foot.

424. The answer is C. *(Hall, pp 323, 1394–1395.)* By far the most likely cause of the oliguria observed in this patient is hypovolemia. Volume status would be best assessed by floating a Swan-Ganz catheter to measure the preload pressures in the left atrium (by inference from the pulmonary capillary wedge pressures). Patients who have had a leaking aneurysm and then a long, usually difficult operation with large surgical fields that collect "third-space" fluids may be intravascularly depleted despite large volumes of intravenous fluid and blood replacement. The proper management usually involves titrating the cardiac output by providing as much fluid as necessary to keep the wedge pressures near 15 mmHg. The other studies listed might become useful if urinary flow remains depressed after optimal cardiac output has been achieved, but in view of the probability of hypovolemia, they are not indicated as a first diagnostic study.

425. The answer is D. *(Brewster, Surgery 109:447–457, 1991.)* The CT scan reveals a fractured ring of calcification in the abdominal aorta with significant density in the para-aortic area. The inferior mesenteric artery (IMA) is always at risk in patients with the changes in the vessel wall characteristic of abdominal aneurysms, but particularly so in the presence of rupture and retroperitoneal dissection of blood under systemic arterial pressures. The incidence of ischemic colitis following abdominal aortic resection is about 2 percent. Blood flow to the left colon normally derives from the IMA with collateral flow from the middle and inferior hemorrhoidal vessels. The superior mesenteric artery (SMA) may also contribute via the marginal artery of Drummond. If the SMA is stenotic or occluded, flow to the left colon will be primarily dependent on an intact IMA. The IMA is usually ligated at the time of aneurysmorrhaphy. Those patients at highest risk for diminished flow through collateral vessels are those with a history of visceral angina, those found to have a patent IMA at the time of operation, patients who have suffered an episode of hypotension following rupture of an aneurysm, those in whom preoperative angiograms reveal occlusion of the

IMA, and those in whom Doppler flow signals along the mesenteric border cease following occlusion of the IMA. Recognition of bowel ischemia at the time of operation should be treated by reimplantation of the IMA into the graft to restore flow.

126. **The answer is A.** *(Schwartz, 6/e, pp 955–956.)* The angiogram presented in the question demonstrates an isolated segment of atherosclerotic occlusion of the superficial femoral artery. Patients who have isolated femoropopliteal disease tend to be smokers, whereas those who have isolated tibioperoneal disease frequently are diabetic. Hypertension and hyperlipidemia predispose to accelerated atherosclerosis. On the other hand, type I hyperlipoproteinemia (hyperchylomicronemia), which is associated with dramatic levels of plasma triglyceride and formation of xanthomas, does not cause accelerated vascular disease.

127. **The answer is C.** *(Schwartz, 6/e, pp 933–940.)* Most abdominal aortic aneurysms are asymptomatic and are discovered on palpation by a physician. A radiograph of the abdomen is useful in demonstrating the aneurysm if there is calcification in the walls. Ultrasound is generally the first diagnostic procedure in confirming the presence of an aneurysm with arteriography performed if the aneurysm is considered large enough to require resection (greater than 5 cm in diameter). Recently CT scan has been useful as a preoperative study in patients suspected of having aneurysms. Surgery should be performed despite the absence of symptoms and can be carried out with a mortality of less than 5 percent. With leaking or ruptured aneurysms, the operative mortality associated with this emergency situation is upwards of 75 percent. The patient's age is not a contraindication to surgery since several studies have demonstrated a low mortality (less than 5 percent) and satisfactory long-term survival and quality of life in elderly, even octogenarian patients.

128. **The answer is D.** *(Schwartz, 6/e, pp 1863, 1880–1881.)* This case illustrates two (among many) conditions that lead to the anterior compartment syndrome, namely, acute arterial occlusion without collateral inflow, and rapid reperfusion of ischemic muscle. Treatment for a compartment syndrome is prompt fasciotomy. Assessing a compartment syndrome and proceeding with fasciotomy are generally based on clinical judgment. Inability to dorsiflex the toes is a grave sign of anterior compartment ischemia. EMG studies and compartment pressure measurements would probably be abnormal, but are unnecessary in view of the known findings and would delay treatment. Mere elevation of the leg would be an ineffective means of relieving compartment pressure although elevation should accompany fasciotomy. Application of splint has no role in the acute management of this problem.

429. The answer is C. *(Schwartz, 6/e, pp 929–930.)* The major threat i patients with arterial occlusive disease is limb loss. Ischemic ulceration neuropathy, rest pain, and gangrene represent advanced stages of arte rial insufficiency and warrant reconstructive surgery whenever clin cally feasible. Claudication, in most cases, reflects mild ischemia; th majority of affected patients are successfully managed without surger (only 2.5 percent develop gangrene). Most will stabilize or improve wit development of increased collateral blood flow following institution a program of daily exercise, cessation of smoking, and weight loss. Va sodilator drugs have been shown to have little benefit in the conserva tive management of intermittent claudication.

430. The answer is C. *(O'Hara, J Vasc Surg 17:940–947, 1993.)* horseshoe kidney is a fused kidney that occupies space on both sides the vertebral column. The fusion is ordinarily at the lower poles wi the isthmus anterior to the aorta. The ureters run anterior to the isthmu and the kidney frequently has an anomalous blood supply. The arteri supply to the kidney is highly variable with vessels arising not only fro the normal position in the aorta but also from a variable number of a cessory segmental end-arteries from the lower aorta and iliac arterie Most cases of abdominal aortic aneurysm associated with a horsesho kidney can be successfully resected, but these anomalies make the r pair challenging. When the horsehoe kidney is recognized preoper tively, an arteriogram helps to define the vascular anatomy. The pr ferred operative approach is then via a retroperitoneal dissection. Th allows the kidney and its collecting system to be swept anteromedial and provides relatively unobstructed access to the aneurysm. All anor alous renal arteries should be implanted into the graft after the ane rysm sac is opened since the proportionate contribution from each ma be hard to determine.

The renal isthmus and collecting system restrict access to the ane rysm and make the anterior approach less desirable. Though division the isthmus can be accomplished, there is high risk of calyceal or ur teral injury. Given the numerous arterial, venous, and collecting syste anomalies, autotransplantation of the kidney is not a good option. Th presence of the fresh intravascular foreign body (aortic graft) contrai dicates dialysis because of the excessive risk of infecting the graft.

431. The answer is B (1, 3). *(Barnes, Stroke 12:497–500, 1981. Davis, pp 2096–2103.)* The treatment of the asymptomatic carotid bruit remains controversial. Agreement is fairly complete that patients with transient ischemic attacks (TIAs) caused by extracranial vascular disease (i.e., internal carotid artery stenosis or plaque ulceration) should undergo carotid endarterectomy to reduce the probability of stroke. Most patients with carotid disease experience a TIA as the first symptom rather than a stroke. A study by Barnes and Marszalek has suggested that the presence of an asymptomatic carotid bruit does not increase the risk of intraoperative stroke during cardiac surgery, and therefore there is no urgent need to perform carotid endarterectomy in this asymptomatic patient prior to coronary bypass surgery.

432. The answer is A (1, 2, 3). *(Schwartz, 6/e, pp 950–956.)* This patient has a total occlusion of the left common iliac artery. His symptoms are severe and limit his lifestyle and ability to earn a living, and therefore surgery is indicated. Therapeutic options include bypass from the aorta to the left common femoral artery or bypass to both common femoral arteries in the expectation that progression of disease will eventually cause problems on the currently uninvolved side. Femorofemoral bypass is also a reasonable option with an excellent long-term patency rate and the added advantage of not disturbing sexual function in this relatively young man. Dissection around the aorta will frequently result in a disturbance of the ejaculatory mechanism, which produces retrograde ejaculation. Femoropopliteal bypass or profundaplasty without correction of the iliac occlusion would be of no benefit to this patient.

433. The answer is A (1, 2, 3). *(Willerson, Am J Cardiol 67:12A–18A, 1991.)* Aspirin exerts an antiplatelet effect that will last for the life of the platelet. Patients who take aspirin will experience its effect for 7 to 10 days after stopping the medication. Aspirin interferes with platelet function by inhibiting the synthesis of thromboxane A_2 and the subsequent production of prostaglandins. The platelet does not have a nucleus and thus cannot remanufacture the prostaglandins necessary for its functioning. Antiplatelet agents are generally used to prevent thrombotic and embolic events on the arterial side of the circulation. The Canadian Cooperative Study has shown antiplatelet therapy to be effective in preventing strokes in men with carotid artery disease, but it is not used to treat thrombophlebitis in the deep venous system. Antiplatelet therapy has been shown to increase graft patency rates following coronary artery bypass grafting if the medication is started preoperatively and continued postoperatively.

434. The answer is B (1, 3). *(Schwartz, 6/e, pp 963–964.)* Atherosclerotic occlusion of the subclavian artery proximal to the vertebral artery is the anatomical situation that results in the subclavian steal syndrome. On being subjected to exercise the involved extremity (usually left) develops relative ischemia, which gives rise to reversal of flow through the vertebral artery with consequent diminished flow to the brain. The upper extremity symptom is intermittent claudication. Venous occlusive disease is not a feature of the syndrome. The operative procedure for treating the subclavian steal syndrome consists of delivering blood to the extremity by creating either a carotid-subclavian or axillo-axillary bypass.

435. The answer is A (1, 2, 3). *(Schwartz, 6/e, pp 950–956.)* The slow progression of aortoiliac atherosclerotic occlusive disease is usually associated with the development of collateral flow through the lumbar branches of the aorta, anastomosing via retroperitoneal branches of the gluteal arteries with the profunda femoris arteries in the legs. This network of collateral vessels provides sufficient blood flow to nourish the extremities at rest but cannot prevent claudication of the upper and lower muscle groups of the leg during exercise. Sexual impotence is believed to be a result of bilateral stenosis or occlusion of the hypogastric (internal iliac) arteries. Gangrene of the feet or toes is rarely seen unless distal embolization of atherosclerotic material from the aorta occludes the pedal or digital arteries.

436. The answer is C (2, 4). *(Boucher, N Engl J Med 312:389–394, 1985. Pasternack, Circulation 72:13–17, 1985.)* The occurrence of perioperative ischemic cardiac events among patients undergoing peripheral vascular reconstruction has been found to correlate with gated blood pool ejection fractions of 35 percent or less and with reversible perfusion defects (thallium redistribution) on dipyridamole-thallium imaging. Ischemic rest pain on early onset of claudication after minimal exercise limits the effectiveness of stress testing as a screening procedure for occult coronary artery disease in this group of patients. Screening coronary angiography, followed by angioplasty or bypass of asymptomatic lesions, had an adverse effect on patient survival in a large prospective study of patients who had peripheral vascular surgery.

437. The answer is D (4). *(Schwartz, 6/e, pp 943–946.)* The heart is the most common source of arterial emboli and accounts for 90 percent o cases. Within the heart, sources include diseased valves, endocarditis, the left atrium in patients with unstable atrial arrhythmias, and mural thrombus on the wall of the left ventricle in patients with a myocardial infarction. The diagnosis in this patient is clear, and therefore noninvasive testing is not indicated. Arteriography is also not necessary and may prove to be too stressful for a patient undergoing an acute myocardial infarction. Embolectomy of the femoral artery can be performed under local anesthesia with minimal risk to the patient. Emboli typically lodge in one femoral artery and contralateral exploration is not indicated in the absence of signs or symptoms.

438. The answer is A (1, 2, 3). *(Schwartz, 6/e, pp 941–943.)* Popliteal aneurysms are usually due to atherosclerosis, are bilateral 25 percent of the time, and require excision even if asymptomatic. Because of the risk of embolization (60 to 70 percent) and thrombosis with resultant gangrene, as well as the lesser risk of rupture, all of which lead to substantial likelihood of limb loss, even relatively small, asymptomatic aneurysms should be excised when discovered.

439. The answer is C (2, 4). *(Schwartz, 6/e, pp 949–957.)* This patient has occlusion of the right superficial femoral artery caused by atherosclerosis, and this is confirmed by both physical examination and the flow study findings, which indicate a sharp decrease in the blood pressure below the level of the common femoral artery. Less than 10 percent of patients with claudication progress to gangrene and the need for amputation. Operative therapy would not be suggested at this time as it is quite likely that with cessation of cigarette smoking and adherence to an exercise program he could markedly improve his walking radius as collateral vessels enlarge to deliver more blood to the affected tissues. Operative therapy (femoropopliteal bypass) would be indicated at this time in this patient only if symptoms of rest pain or ischemic ulceration were present. Since physical examination and flow studies indicate disease distal to the aortoiliac distribution, aortoiliac reconstruction is not likely to be indicated in this patient.

440. The answer is B (1, 3). *(Cameron, 4/e, pp 791–794.)* The Greenfield filter pictured on the x-ray is used to interrupt migration of emboli to the lungs from the veins below the level of the filter. It is indicated in patients who sustain a recurrent pulmonary embolus despite adequate anticoagulant therapy or in patients with pulmonary emboli who cannot receive anticoagulants because of a contraindication (e.g., bleeding ulcer, intracranial hemorrhage). The filter is not used in patients who sustain a single pulmonary embolus. The filter is placed in the inferior vena cava just below the renal veins and therefore would not be effective for emboli that arise cephalad to its position.

441. The answer is B (1, 3). *(Belkin, Surgery 212:769–773, 1986. Eisbud, Am J Surg 160:160–165, 1990.)* Management of acute graft occlusion must include both reestablishment of peripheral perfusion and correction of any underlying hemodynamic problem. Urokinase is associated with fewer allergic reactions than streptokinase and is the preferred thrombolytic agent. Treatment results in total clot lysis in 75 percent of patients. However, high reocclusion rates are observed (20 percent within 1 year) even if angioplasty or anastomotic revision is performed after successful lysis. Without surgical revision following clot lysis, a 50 percent reocclusion rate is expected within 3 months. Urokinase has proved equally successful in opening both vein and prosthetic graft thromboses.

442. The answer is C (2, 4). *(Cameron, 4/e, pp 757–761.)* Abdominal pain out of proportion to findings on physical examination is characteristic of intestinal ischemia. The etiology of ischemia may be embolic or thrombotic occlusion of the mesenteric vessels or nonocclusive ischemia due to a low cardiac index or mesenteric vasospasm. Differentiation among these etiologies is best made by mesenteric angiography. While not without serious risks, angiography also offers the possibility of direct infusion of vasodilators into the mesenteric vasculature in the setting of nonocclusive ischemia. This patient, with a recent myocardial infarction and a low cardiac index, is at risk for embolism of clot from a left ventricle mural thrombus as well as "low-flow" mesenteric ischemia. If embolism or thrombosis is found angiographically (usually involving the superior mesenteric artery), operative embolectomy or vascular bypass is indicated to restore flow. If occlusive disease cannot be demonstrated, efforts should be made to simultaneously increase cardiac output with inotropic agents and dilate the mesenteric vascular bed by angiographic instillation of papaverine, nitrates, or calcium channel blockers. Computed tomography is not helpful in delineating the cause of intestinal ischemia since it does not provide a sufficiently detailed image of the mesenteric vessels. Laparoscopy might secure the diagnosis of intestinal ischemia, but requires administering general anesthesia and would shed no light on the etiology of this patient's problem.

443. The answer is E (all). *Cameron, 4/e, pp 785–791. Hardy, 2/e, pp 1002–1015.)* Although the vast majority of pulmonary emboli are believed to originate in deep vein thrombosis of the legs (the remainder originating in the pelvic veins, right heart, and deep veins of the upper extremities), emboli in more than two-thirds of patients have clinically occult origins. A variety of diagnostic studies using impedance plethysmography, ^{125}I-fibrinogen scanning, contrast venography, radionuclide (blood pool) venography, ultrasonography, and computed tomography have been employed to identify the source of pulmonary emboli. While arteriovenous shunting in the lungs appears to play a role in the hypoxemia of pulmonary embolism, an increase in the ventilation-perfusion ratio of the affected areas, followed by reflex and, possibly, serotonin-mediated bronchoconstriction, is the main physiological derangement. An otherwise healthy patient who has less than 20 percent of the pulmonary vascular bed occluded would remain asymptomatic, and therefore the occlusion would not be discovered without screening studies.

444. The answer is E (all). *(Cameron, 4/e, pp 751–753.)* Vasospasm in the upper extremities initiated by exposure to cold or stress was described by Raynaud in 1862. It is now known that the condition can exist as a primary disorder (Raynaud's disease) or may be secondary to another disease (Raynaud's phenomenon). Associated conditions seen with Raynaud's phenomenon are thromboangiitis obliterans (Buerger's disease), scleroderma, cervical rib, atherosclerosis, disseminated lupus erythematosus, or periarteritis nodosa. The condition affects mainly women (sex ratio of 5:1) and appears before age 40 in over 90 percent of patients. In the majority of patients, the episodes of vasoconstriction are precipitated by exposure to cold, but intense emotion has been noted as an inciting factor in some patients. The condition affects the upper extremities symmetrically, though in the minority of patients the lower extremities may also be affected. The findings of physical examination are usually normal in the early stages of the condition with ulcerations and punctate scars from healed ulcerations noted later as the disease progresses. When the condition is first noted, a thorough search for an underlying condition should be undertaken and the patient should be labeled as having primary Raynaud's disease only if no associated condition is discovered within 2 to 3 years after onset of symptoms. Treatment consists of avoidance of cold exposure and tobacco and the selective use of vasodilating drugs or intraarterial reserpine. Cervical dorsal sympathectomy with removal of the first, second, and third thoracic ganglia (preserving the cervical portion of the stellate ganglion to avoid a Horner's syndrome) has given excellent early results, but relapses are common. For this reason, sympathectomy is the therapy of last resort when symptoms are very severe and all other approaches have proved ineffective.

445. The answer is B (1, 3). *(Stain, Arch Surg 124:1136–1141, 1989.)* For a penetrating injury to a major artery of an extremity that causes an intimal flap seen on arteriogram, management has historically been (1) direct suture repair of the flap or (2) excision of the involved segment and placement of a venous interposition graft harvested from the contralateral leg. Obtaining the vein graft from the wounded (ipsilateral) leg is discouraged because of the possibility of compromising venous outflow of the involved leg and increasing the risk of amputation. Recently, selective management of these injuries with serial arteriograms or noninvasive duplex scans has yielded acceptable results. Placement of synthetic grafts, especially in young patients, should be avoided, since foreign graft material is more susceptible to infection and is more likely to occlude than an autologous vein graft.

SPECIALTIES

Urology

DIRECTIONS: Each question below contains five suggested responses. Select the **one best** response to each question.

446. A patient who has a flaccid neurogenic bladder may benefit initially from all the following measures EXCEPT

(A) being trained to void at timed intervals
(B) self-catheterization
(C) administration of bethanechol chloride (Urecholine)
(D) limiting fluid intake to less than 300 mL/day
(E) transurethral resection of the bladder neck

447. All the following statements regarding hypospadias are correct EXCEPT

(A) it is often associated with chordee (ventral curvature of the penis)
(B) it is associated with undescended testes
(C) it is the most frequent fusion defect of the male urethra
(D) it is a hereditary disorder
(E) the most common location is penoscrotal

448. The recommended treatment for stage A (superficial and submucosal) transitional cell carcinoma of the bladder is

(A) local excision
(B) radical cystectomy
(C) radiation therapy
(D) topical (intravesicular) chemotherapy
(E) systemic chemotherapy

449. A 36-year-old man presents to the emergency room with renal colic. A radiograph reveals a 1.5-cm stone. Which of the following statements regarding his disorder is correct?

(A) Conservative treatment including hydration and analgesics will not result in a satisfactory outcome
(B) Serial KUB (kidney, ureter, bladder) radiographs should be used to follow this patient
(C) The urinalysis will nearly always reveal microhematuria
(D) When the acute event is correctly treated, this disease seldom recurs
(E) Elevated BUN and creatinine are expected

450. Optimal management of bilateral undescended testicles in an infant is

(A) immediate surgical placement into the scrotum
(B) chorionic gonadotropin therapy for 1 month; operative placement into the scrotum before age 1 if descent has not occurred
(C) observation until the child is 2 years old because delayed descent is common
(D) observation until age 5; if no descent by then, plastic surgical scrotal prostheses before the child enters school
(E) no therapy; reassurance of the parent that full masculinization and normal spermatogenesis are likely even if the testicle does not fully descend

DIRECTIONS: Each question below contains four suggested responses of which **one or more** is correct. Select

A	if	**1, 2, and 3**	are correct
B	if	**1 and 3**	are correct
C	if	**2 and 4**	are correct
D	if	**4**	is correct
E	if	**1, 2, 3, and 4**	are correct

451. A 15-year-old boy presents to the emergency room with testicular pain of 5 h duration. His pain was of acute onset and woke him from sleep. On physical examination, he is noted to have a high-riding, indurated, and markedly tender left testis. Pain is not diminished by elevation. Urinalysis is unremarkable. Correct statements regarding the patient's diagnosis and treatment include which of the following?

(1) There is a strong likelihood that this patient's father or brother has had or will have a similar event

(2) Operation should be delayed until a technetium scan clarifies the diagnosis

(3) The majority of testicles that have undergone torsion can be salvaged if surgery is performed within 24 h

(4) If torsion is found, both testes should undergo orchiopexy

452. Seminoma is accurately described by which of the following statements?

(1) It is the most common type of testicular cancer

(2) Metastases to liver and bone are frequently found

(3) It is a very radiosensitive tumor

(4) The 5-year survival rate approaches 50 percent

453. True statements regarding benign prostatic hyperplasia (BPH) include which of the following?

(1) The fibrostromal proliferation of BPH occurs mainly in the outer portion of the gland

(2) Assuming a voided volume greater than 100 mL, a peak urine flow rate less than 10 mL/h is good evidence of outflow obstruction

(3) Suprapubic prostatectomy for BPH involves enucleation of the entire prostate and eliminates the risk of future prostate cancer

(4) Indications for surgery include acute urinary retention and recurrent urinary tract infections (UTIs)

SUMMARY OF DIRECTIONS

A	B	C	D	E
1,2,3	1,3	2,4	4	All are
only	only	only	only	correct

454. True statements regarding carcinoma of the prostate include

(1) it has a higher incidence among American blacks than other American ethnic groups
(2) a single microscopic focus of prostate cancer discovered on transurethral resection of the prostate (TURP) is indication for radical prostatectomy
(3) it arises initially in the gland's periphery
(4) it commonly produces osteoclastic bony metastases

455. During the course of an operation on an unstable, critically ill patient, the left ureter is lacerated through 50 percent of its circumference. If the patient's condition is felt to be too serious to allow time for definitive repair, alternative methods of management include

(1) ligation of the injured ureter and ipsilateral nephrostomy
(2) ipsilateral nephrectomy
(3) placement of a catheter from the proximal ureter through an abdominal wall stab wound
(4) placement of a suction drain adjacent to the injury without further manipulation that might convert the partial laceration into a complete disruption

456. Genitourinary tuberculosis in a male patient is suggested by which of the following findings?

(1) Microscopic hematuria
(2) Pyuria without bacteriuria
(3) Unilateral renal calcification
(4) Painless swelling of the epididymis

457. A pedestrian is hit by a speeding car. Radiological studies obtained in the emergency room, including a retrograde urethrogram, are consistent with a pelvic fracture with a rupture of the urethra superior to the urogenital diaphragm. Management should consist of

(1) immediate placement of a suprapubic cystostomy tube
(2) immediate placement of a Foley catheter through the urethra into the bladder to align and stent the injured portions
(3) reconstruction of the ruptured urethra after 3 to 6 months to allow for resorption of the pelvic hematoma
(4) immediate exploration of the pelvis for control of hemorrhage from pelvic fracture and drainage of the pelvic hematoma

Urology
Answers

446. The answer is D. *(Schwartz, 6/e, pp 1737–1739.)* Patients who have a lower motor neuron lesion (flaccid neurogenic bladder) can usually be managed by conservative measures that prevent the development of a large residual urine volume in the bladder. These measures include intermittent self-catheterization and scheduled voiding with increased abdominal pressure provided by Valsalva's maneuver or manual pressure on the abdomen. Detrussor contractions can sometimes be strengthened by parasympathomimetic agents. Bladder neck resection may reduce outlet obstruction, but ureteral diversion is indicated only in the presence of gross ureterocalyxectasis that resists the foregoing measures. Severely restricting fluid intake is impractical and may promote formation of calculi.

447. The answer is E. *(Schwartz, 6/e, pp 1778–1780.)* Hypospadias is a congenital anomaly of the penis resulting from incomplete development of the anterior urethra. It occurs in about 1/300 live births and is believed to have a multifactorial genetic mode of inheritance. Of those with hypospadias, about 7 percent will have a father with the disorder 14 percent a brother, and 20 percent a second family member. Hypospadias occurs in the corona in about 75 percent of cases, where it is often accompanied by chordee. Undescended testes occur in about 10 percent of cases of hypospadias, as do inguinal hernias. Hypospadias in the scrotal area is associated with bilateral undescended testes and infertility and must be differentiated from pseudohermaphroditism and adrenogenital syndrome.

448. The answer is D. *(Way, 9/e, pp 929–932.)* Bladder cancer represents 2 percent of all cancers, and 90 percent of the bladder cancers are of transitional cell origin. It is most prevalent among men with a heavy smoking history and is usually multifocal and superficial, even when recurrent. When the disease is still superficial, transurethral resection of visible lesions and intravesicular chemotherapy are most often recommended. More radical surgical extirpation is reserved for advanced stages of the disease.

449. The answer is A. *(Schwartz, 6/e, pp 1743–1752.)* Initial management should include hydration and analgesics. However, as the stone is larger than 1 cm, it is unlikely to pass spontaneously, though stones less than 0.5 cm usually do pass spontaneously. The size of the stone also makes a high-grade obstruction more likely; therefore an intravenous pyelogram (IVP) must be urgently performed. A high-grade obstruction will require nephrostomy of the passage of a ureteral stent. If the stone is completely occluding the lumen of the ureter, the urinalysis may not show microhematuria and thus may be misleading. Approximately 15 percent of patients will have a recurrence within 1 year, and almost 50 percent may have a recurrence within 4 years. Elevated BUN and creatinine are expected only in the setting of an obstructed *single* functioning kidney.

450. The answer is B. *(Schwartz, 6/e, pp 1711–1712, 1777.)* By the second year, a testicle not in the cooler environment of the scrotal sac will begin to undergo histological changes characterized by reduced spermatogonia. Testicles left longer in the undescended state not only have a higher incidence of malignant degeneration, but are inaccessible for examination. If a malignancy should occur, diagnosis will be delayed. There is also a substantial psychological burden when children reach school age or are otherwise subjected to exposure of their deformed genitalia. Gel-filled prostheses are generally inserted when a testicle cannot be placed in the scrotum. Close follow-up by a physician until the late teens is indicated in all patients who have had an undescended testicle. Since these patients may be at increased risk for malignancy throughout their life, careful training should be given in self-examination.

451. The answer is D (4). *(Schwartz, 6/e, pp 1731–1732.)* Testicular torsion occurs commonly in adolescents. The underlying pathology is secondary to an abnormally narrowed testicular mesentery with tunica vaginalis surrounding the testis and epididymis in a "bell-clapper" deformity. As the testis twists, it comes to lie in a higher position within the scrotum. Urinalysis is usually negative. Elevation will not provide a decrease in pain (negative Prehn's sign); a positive Prehn's sign might indicate epididymitis. A technetium 99m pertechnetate scan may be helpful in clarifying a confusing case; however, operation should not be delayed beyond 6 h from the time of onset of symptoms in order to maximize testicular salvage. This patient's presentation warrants immediate operation. The salvage rate for delay greater than 12 h is less than 20 percent. Both the affected and unaffected testes should undergo orchiopexy. Epididymitis usually occurs in sexually active males. Urinalysis is usually positive for inflammatory cells, and urethral discharge is often present.

452. The answer is B (1, 3). *(Schwartz, 6/e, pp 1731, 1764–1765.)* Seminomas tend to grow slowly and metastasize late. They represent about 40 percent of malignant testicular tumors; embryonal cell carcinoma and teratocarcinoma each represents about 25 percent. Since most tumors have mixed elements, they are usually classified according to the most malignant cell type encountered, whatever the predominant cell type. When metastases occur, they are usually along the regional lymphatic drainage pathways to the iliac, aortic, and renal lymph nodes. Because of their slow growth and radiosensitivity, seminomas are associated with a 90 percent 5-year survival rate. Therapy generally consists of removing the affected testis and sampling the lymph nodes (usually external iliac) for evidence of metastasis. If metastases are present, radiation therapy is given locally to areas of known involvement. Radiation therapy is highly effective in seminoma, and metastatic disease may be palliated for extended periods.

453. The answer is C (2, 4). *(Schwartz, 6/e, pp 1728–1729.)* In contrast to prostate cancer, BPH arises first in the periurethral prostate tissue as a fibrostromal proliferation. As the periurethral prostate grows, the outer prostate glands are compressed against the true prostatic capsule, which results in a thick pseudocapsule. As the prostate enlarges, it encroaches on the urethra and causes urinary outflow obstruction. Obstructive symptoms include decreased force of stream, hesitancy, recurrent UTIs, and occasionally acute urinary retention; the latter two are indications for surgery. Uroflow is the best noninvasive method of estimating the degree of outlet obstruction. Flow less than 10 mL/h is good evidence of significant obstruction. The major treatments for BPH are surgical. Simple prostatectomy involves shelling out prostate adenoma and leaving the pseudocapsule (true prostate) behind. Therefore these patients are still at risk of developing prostate cancer.

454. The answer is B (1, 3). *(Schwartz, 6/e, pp 1762–1794.)* One of the most frequent causes of male cancer deaths, prostate cancer has an incidence of more than 75,000 new cases per year in the U.S. American blacks appear to have a 50 percent higher incidence and mortality. Prostate cancer (adenocarcinoma) arises initially in the periphery of the gland. Therefore, the best screening test is careful rectal examination. Spread is by direct local extension and by lymphatic and vascular cha nels. The most common locations of distant metastases are in the axial skeleton with osteoblastic bony lesions. A single focus of disease discovered on TURP or simple prostatectomy is considered stage A_1. Only 2 percent of patients will have unsuspected nodes (i.e., only 2 percent 5- to 10-year mortality). Therefore, no definitive therapy is required except possibly in patients less than 60 years old. Follow-up should be undertaken and progression of disease may be treated as necessary. Several foci or diffuse disease is considered stage A_2 and surgery or radiation therapy is generally indicated.

455. The answer is B (1, 3). *(Shires, 3/e, pp 354–355.)* If time and the patient's condition permit, primary ureteral reconstruction should be carried out. In the middle third of the ureter, this will usually consist of ureteroureterostomy using absorbable sutures over a stent. If the injury involves the upper third, ureteropyeloplasty may be necessary. In the lower third, ureteral implantation into the bladder using a tunneling technique is preferred. If time does not permit definitive repair, suction drainage adjacent to the injured segment alone is inadequate; either ligation and nephrostomy or placement of a ureteral catheter is an acceptable alternative that would allow reconstruction to be performed later. The creation of a watertight seal is difficult and nephrectomy may be required if the injury occurs during a procedure in which a vascular prosthesis is being implanted (e.g., resection of an aortic aneurysm, aortoiliac bypass procedures) and contamination of the foreign body by urine must be avoided.

456. The answer is E (all). *(Schwartz, 6/e, pp 1743–1745.)* Genitourinary tuberculosis develops from reactivation of foci in the renal cortex or prostate that were hematogenously seeded during the primary (usually asymptomatic) pulmonary infection. Local spread from the renal and prostatic sites can lead to involvement of the calyx, ureter, bladder, vas deferens, epididymis, and (rarely) the testis. A low-grade inflammatory response results in pyuria or hematuria. Whenever pus cells are seen on routine urine culture without bacteria on smear or culture plate, genitourinary tuberculosis should be considered. The end result of focal caseation necrosis in the kidney may be scarring and dystrophic calcification. Genital tract infection often causes an asymptomatic swelling in the epididymis; secondary infection or formation of a sinus tract to the scrotal skin may cause more dramatic signs and symptoms.

457. The answer is B (1, 3). *(Shires, 3/e, pp 358–361.)* If a rupture of the urethra is suspected, a retrograde urethrogram should be obtained *before* any attempts are made to place a Foley catheter, as efforts to do so may result in the creation of multiple false passages or conversion of a partial laceration into complete rupture. Previously, treatment had included attempts to realign the urethra immediately through the placement of interlocking sounds and traction using either a catheter passed over the sounds or perineal traction sutures through the bladder neck. Preferred treatment currently avoids both dissection into the pelvic hematoma surrounding the disruption and manipulation of the urethra; instead, only a suprapubic tube is placed immediately with delayed reconstruction after 3 to 6 months, at which time the hematoma will have resolved and the prostate will have descended into the proximity of the urogenital diaphragm.

Orthopedics

DIRECTIONS: Each question below contains five suggested responses. Select the **one best** response to each question.

458. Meniscal tears usually result from which of the following circumstances?

(A) Hyperextension
(B) Flexion and rotation
(C) Simple hyperflexion
(D) Compression
(E) Femoral condylar fracture

459. Volkmann's ischemic contracture is associated with

(A) intertrochanteric femoral fracture
(B) supracondylar fracture of the humerus
(C) posterior dislocation of the knee
(D) traumatic shoulder separation
(E) Colles' "silver-fork" fracture

460. In an uncomplicated dislocation of the glenohumeral joint, the humeral head usually dislocates primarily in which of the following directions?

(A) Anteriorly
(B) Superiorly
(C) Posteriorly
(D) Laterally
(E) Medially

461. The most severe epiphyseal growth disturbance is likely to result from which of the following types of fracture?

(A) Fracture dislocation of a joint adjacent to an epiphysis
(B) Fracture through the articular cartilage extending into the epiphysis
(C) Transverse fracture of the bone shaft on the metaphyseal side of the epiphysis
(D) Separation of the epiphysis at the diaphyseal side of the growth plate
(E) Crushing injury compressing the growth plate

462. All the following are associated with postmenopausal osteoporosis EXCEPT

(A) Colles' fracture
(B) femoral neck fracture
(C) intertrochanteric fracture
(D) clavicular fracture
(E) vertebral compression fracture

463. Which nerve is most at risk in the injury in the accompanying radiograph?

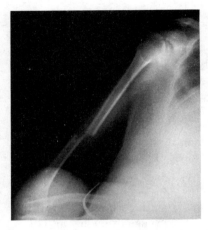

(A) Median nerve
(B) Radial nerve
(C) Posterior interosseous nerve
(D) Ulnar nerve
(E) Ascending circumflex brachial nerve

464. In a failed suicide gesture, a depressed student severs her radial nerve at the wrist. The expected disability is

(A) loss of ability to extend wrist
(B) loss of ability to flex wrist
(C) wasting of the intrinsic muscles of the hand
(D) sensory loss over the thenar pad and the thumb web
(E) palmar insensitivity

DIRECTIONS: Each question below contains four suggested responses of which **one or more** is correct. Select

A	if	**1, 2, and 3**	are correct
B	if	**1 and 3**	are correct
C	if	**2 and 4**	are correct
D	if	**4**	is correct
E	if	**1, 2, 3, and 4**	are correct

465. True statements regarding compartment syndromes following orthopedic injuries include which of the following?

(1) The first sign is usually loss of pulse in the extremity
(2) Passive flexion of the distal extremity will aggravate the pain
(3) Surgical decompression (fasciectomy) is necessary only as a last resort
(4) They are most commonly associated with supracondylar fractures of the humerus and tibial shaft

466. Correct statements concerning congenital dysplasia and dislocation of the hip (CDH) include

(1) children of both sexes require a physical examination for CDH at birth
(2) radiographic examinations are usually diagnostic
(3) a harness or abduction splint is the first line of treatment
(4) most children with CDH will eventually require surgery

467. In contrast with closed reduction, open reduction of a fracture causes

(1) a longer healing time
(2) increased trauma to the fracture site
(3) a higher incidence of non-union
(4) a greater risk of infection

DIRECTIONS: The group of questions below consists of four lettered headings followed by a set of numbered items. For each numbered item select

A	if the item is associated with	(A) **only**
B	if the item is associated with	(B) **only**
C	if the item is associated with	**both** (A) and (B)
D	if the item is associated with	**neither** (A) nor (B)

Each lettered heading may be used **once, more than once, or not at all.**

Questions 468–470

(A) Osteoarthritis
(B) Rheumatoid arthritis
(C) Both
(D) Neither

468. Often associated with systemic abnormalities

469. Treated initially with nonsteroidal anti-inflammatory medication

470. More common in women

DIRECTIONS: Each group of questions below consists of lettered headings followed by a set of numbered items. For each numbered item select the **one** lettered heading with which it is **most** closely associated. Each lettered heading may be used **once, more than once, or not at all.**

Questions 471–474

For each description below, select the type of fracture or dislocation with which it is most likely to be associated.

(A) Navicular fracture
(B) Monteggia's deformity
(C) Greenstick fracture
(D) Spiral fracture
(E) Posterior shoulder dislocation

471. Seen after epileptiform convulsion

472. Avascular necrosis not uncommon

473. Dislocation of the radial head and fracture of the proximal third of the ulna

474. Tenderness in the anatomist's snuffbox

Questions 475–477

For each description below, select the type of fracture or dislocation with which it is most likely to be associated.

(A) Osteoid osteoma
(B) Osteochondroma
(C) Osteosarcoma
(D) Aneurysmal bone cyst
(E) Unicameral bone cyst

475. Arises from the cartilaginous elements of developing bone; frequently asymptomatic

476. X-ray may show a round or oval defect in bone without adjacent reactive bone formation; the most common presenting symptom is pathological fracture

477. Proliferation of vascular tissue in bone destroys the overlying bone cortex

Orthopedics
Answers

458. The answer is B. *(Schwartz, 6/e, pp 1925–1926.)* Most meniscal tears are produced by flexion and rapid rotation. A classic example ("football knee") involves a player who is hit while running. The knee, supporting all the player's weight, usually is slightly flexed and the foot is anchored to the ground by cleats. Impact from an opposing player usually causes rotation almost entirely restricted to the knee. The injury involves rapid rotation of the flexed femoral condyles about the tibial plateau, which most frequently tears the medial, or, less frequently, the lateral meniscus. A tear in the inner free border of the cartilage is also common whenever excessive rotation without flexion or extension occurs. Early surgical removal of the displaced menisci is usually recommended to prevent further damage to the cartilage or ligaments.

459. The answer is B. *(Tintinalli, 3/e, p 975.)* Compromise of blood supply to the muscles of the forearm can lead to a compartment syndrome and permanent serious functional deformity of the arm. Any patient with a compressive dressing or cast of the upper extremity can experience this potential catastrophe. Whenever a patient has increasing pain in the presence of a circular dressing around the arm or forearm, the dressing should be removed immediately. If there is tenderness in the forearm on either the ulnar or dorsal aspect, a fasciotomy should be considered.

460. The answer is A. *(Schwartz, 6/e, pp 1910–1911.)* The glenohumeral joint is bounded posteriorly by the teres minor and infraspinatus muscles and partially by the long head of the triceps. It is bounded laterally by the powerful deltoid muscle; superiorly, the acromion process precludes upward dislocation. However, anteriorly and inferiorly the pectoralis major and the long head of the biceps do not completely stabilize the glenohumeral joint; in this region the articular ligaments and joint capsule provide the major structural support. Thus, the joint is not strongly supported in its anteroinferior aspect, and consequently anterior (or anteroinferior) dislocations are the most common glenohumeral dislocations. The humeral head is driven anteriorly, which tears the shoulder capsule, detaches the labrum from the glenoid, and produces a compression fracture of the humeral head. Most glenohumeral dislocations result from a posteriorly directed force on an arm that is partially abducted. Posterior dislocation is much rarer and should raise the possibility of a seizure as the precipitating cause.

461. The answer is E. *(Schwartz, 6/e, p 1906.)* Longitudinal growth of bone follows ossification of cartilage that forms at the epiphyseal plate. Fractures that involve separation of the growth plate (type I) (almost always on the diaphyseal side) may be realigned; normal growth usually follows epiphyseal separation because the proliferative cells are still attached to their blood supply in the bone epiphysis. Fractures that extend perpendicular to and through the epiphysis (types II, III, IV) may result in the formation of bony bridges across the epiphysis that can disrupt later growth. Though all the fractures listed in the question place the epiphyseal growth plate in some jeopardy, crushing injuries to the epiphysis (type V) have the worst prognosis; numerous bony bridges may form and prevent longitudinal growth.

462. The answer is D. *(Schwartz, 6/e, pp 1896–1897.)* Postmenopausal osteoporosis is responsible for a large number of fractures in elderly women. Though laboratory studies are normal in osteoporosis, the total amount of bone is decreased, which leads to osteopenia and weaker bones. Vertebral compression fractures are often sustained even without trauma. A minor fall on the outstretched hand can lead to a Colles' fracture. Either a femoral neck fracture or an intertrochanteric fracture can follow a fall on the hip. Clavicular fractures are common in children and young adults after violent falls onto an outstretched hand.

463. The answer is B. *(Schwartz, 6/e, pp 1911–1914.)* The radiograph demonstrates a transverse fracture of the distal half of the humeral shaft. The radial nerve runs in a groove on the posterior aspect of the humerus as it courses into the forearm compartment and is therefore at high risk of injury. If the nerve injury is apparent before any manipulation has been done, the fracture should be reduced; the nerve injury should be observed since the nerve function will likely improve with time. If the nerve injury is only present after reduction, immediate surgical exploration is warranted because the nerve might be trapped in the fracture site. At this level of the arm, the ulnar and median nerves are well protected by muscle. The posterior interosseous nerve is a distal branch of the radial nerve and may be injured in fractures near the radial head, but it is in no danger from injuries at the level seen in this radiograph. There is no "ascending circumflex brachial nerve."

464. The answer is D. *(Way, 9/e, pp 1140–1141.)* An injury to the radial nerve at the wrist would cause primarily sensory abnormalities. The dorsum of the hand from the radial aspect of the fourth digit over the thumb, including the thenar pad and thumb web, becomes insensate after severance of the radial nerve at the wrist. Radial injuries more proximally would impair extension of the wrist and digits as well as forearm supination.

465. The answer is D (4). *(Schwartz, 6/e, pp 1902, 2008–2009.)* Compartment syndromes result from increasing pressures in the fascial compartments of the arm or leg. When the pressure in the muscles is greater than that of the capillaries, ischemia and necrosis of the muscles occur even though the arterial pressure is still high enough to produce pulses; pulselessness is an unreliable sign. Extreme pain (out of proportion to the injury), pain on passive extension of the fingers or toes, pallor of the extremity, motor paralysis, and paresthesias are all components of the syndrome. The patient will usually hold the injured part in a position of flexion to maximally relax the fascia and reduce the pain; passive extension will usually produce severe pain. The diagnosis can be confirmed by measuring intracompartmental pressures, but whenever physical findings or symptoms are suspicious, immediate surgical decompression by fasciectomy is indicated since delay is likely to lead to irreversible damage.

466. The answer is B (1, 3). *(Schwartz, 6/e, pp 1883–1885.)* Because CDH is so common—approximately 1 in 800 white females—all children should have a physical examination to elicit signs of CDH at birth and throughout the first year. Repeated examinations have markedly decreased the number of missed cases with long-term sequelae. Though the physical examination is the gold standard in diagnosis, radiographs can provide clues to dysplasia despite the presence of the unossified cartilaginous femoral head. Most cases of CDH are adequately treated in a harness or splint that keeps the hips in a reduced position for a period of time. Only if this treatment is unsuccessful does the child require further intervention with some combination of open or closed reduction or surgical procedures on the acetabulum or femur.

467. The answer is E (all). *(Schwartz, 6/e, p 1906.)* Open reduction of a fracture involves the restoration of normal bone alignment under direct observation at surgery. In effect, open reduction converts a simple fracture into a compound (or open) fracture and thereby increases the risk of infection. Operative manipulation also increases trauma at the fracture site and may consequently add to the probability of infection. Hematomas at the site of fracture may be important for early healing; open reduction, which usually involves removing the clots in the field, could contribute to a delay in bone healing and to nonunion. The major advantage of open reduction is the shorter period of immobilization it allows, an advantage that often outweighs all the disadvantages previously mentioned, as in the open reduction of femoral neck fractures in the elderly. This allows these patients to get out of bed much sooner than if they were treated with several weeks of traction.

468–470. The answers are 468-B, 469-C, 470-C. *(Schwartz, 6/e, pp 1940–1946.)* Rheumatoid arthritis primarily affects joints but may also affect multiple other organ systems with damage to the eyes, liver, heart, lungs, blood vessels, and nerves. Osteoarthritis destroys only joints; it may be a primary disease or may be secondary to trauma, infection, congenital anomaly, or acquired deformity. Women are more commonly affected in both diseases with peak age of incidence in middle age for rheumatoid arthritis and over age 60 for osteoarthritis. Initial medical management consists of aspirin or a nonsteroidal medication. Patients with rheumatoid arthritis may progress to alternative medication including gold, penicillamine, or immunosuppressive agents like steroids; none of these agents are indicated in osteoarthritis. Reconstructive surgical procedures are used in both diseases when medical management fails to control pain, deformity, or loss of function.

471–474. The answers are 471-E, 472-A, 473-B, 474-A. *(Schwartz, 6/e, pp 1900–1934.)* Fractures of the navicular bone of the wrist should be suspected in anyone, particularly a young person, who falls on an outstretched hand. Although x-rays are mandatory, it is important to realize that the fracture may not be seen on the initial x-ray and that a presumptive diagnosis can and should be made on clinical grounds alone. Typically, there will be tenderness to palpation over the navicular tuberosity and limitation of wrist flexion and extension. Immobilization of the wrist for about 16 weeks and sometimes up to 6 months is required. Nonunion or avascular necrosis is not uncommon and may require bone grafting for correction.

Dislocation of the radial head with a fracture of the proximal third of the ulna is known as Monteggia's deformity. Usually, the radial head is dislocated anteriorly. The injury is usually caused by forced pronation. The injury can be treated by reduction and stabilization of the ulna followed by reduction of the radial head via supination and direct pressure.

Anterior shoulder dislocations occur more frequently than posterior dislocations. However, posterior dislocations are seen in special situations, such as during an epileptiform convulsion and during electroshock therapy. Closed reduction followed by immobilization is usually sufficient therapy.

A spiral fracture, frequently seen in the tibia in skiers, results from the application of torque to a long bone. Greenstick fractures are common in children. The bones of young children are able to bend to a greater degree than those of adults; the fracture may occur only at the site of maximal cortical stress but not at the opposite cortex, the site of maximal longitudinal compression.

475–477. The answers are 475-B, 476-E, 477-D. *(Schwartz, 6/e, pp 1881–1883, 1954–1956.)* Osteosarcomas arise from osteoblasts and usually cause death within 2 years of diagnosis. They generally arise in long bones—particularly the femur—and initially cause pain. Later, local swelling and tenderness may appear. Overlying bone is irregularly eroded; the tumor may break the cortex and expand into adjacent soft tissue. Osteosarcomas may arise in bones affected by Paget's disease.

Osteoid osteoma also arises from osteoblasts but is usually seen in males in their teens or twenties. Night pain, which responds only to aspirin, is the classic presenting symptom. Treatment is resection of the lesion, which is usually in the lower extremity or the spine.

Osteochondromas, which are benign projections of bone covered by a cartilaginous cap, usually develop at the end of a long bone, most frequently from the tibia or femur near the knee. Arising during the second decade of life, they cease growing upon closure of the epiphyses and are asymptomatic unless they are subjected to trauma or impinge on sensitive tissue. Osteochondromas occasionally undergo malignant transformation.

Unicameral bone cysts are single-chambered, benign lesions that most frequently occur as solitary lesions in the proximal humerus or femur. They frequently are associated with pathological fractures because of thinning of adjacent bone cortices. The cysts do not undergo malignant transformation. Treatment consists of scraping the cyst walls and packing with bone chips or removal of the entire segment of bone that contains a cyst (subperiosteal resection).

Aneurysmal bone cysts, thought to arise from vascular tissue in bone, frequently cause local pain. Pathological fractures are commonly associated with these cysts and may be accompanied by heavy bleeding. Preferred surgical treatment consists of curettage and packing with bone chips. Radiation may induce vascular sclerosis in surgically inaccessible cysts.

Neurosurgery

DIRECTIONS: Each question below contains five suggested responses. Select the **one best** response to each question.

478. All the following statements regarding the Glasgow coma scale are true EXCEPT

(A) it serves as a scale to assess severity of head trauma
(B) a high score correlates with a high mortality
(C) it measures eye opening
(D) it measures motor response
(E) it measures verbal response

479. Controlled hyperventilation (induced hypocapnia) is frequently recommended following head trauma. The therapeutic consequences of this therapy include

(A) reduction of endogenous catecholamines
(B) reduction of intracellular potassium levels
(C) increase in cerebrovascular resistance
(D) induction of compensatory metabolic alkalosis
(E) requirement of monitoring the intracranial pressure

480. A 25-year-old man is brought to the emergency room and gives a history of sudden onset of excruciating headache. There is no history of loss of consciousness. Physical examination does not disclose any evidence of focal neurological deficit. The most likely diagnosis is

(A) subdural hematoma
(B) epidural hematoma
(C) meningioma
(D) ruptured berry aneurysm
(E) carotid artery occlusion

481. A 60-year-old woman presents to her physician with a 3-week history of severe headaches. A contrast CT scan reveals a small, circular, hypodense lesion with ringlike contrast enhancement. The most likely diagnosis is

(A) brain abscess
(B) high-grade astrocytoma
(C) parenchymal hemorrhage
(D) metastatic lesion
(E) toxoplasmosis

482. All the following statements regarding skull fractures are true EXCEPT that

(A) depressed fractures are those in which the cranial vault is displaced inward
(B) compound fractures are those in which the bone and the overlying skin are broken
(C) any bone fragment displaced more than 1 cm inwardly should be elevated surgically
(D) drainage of cerebrospinal fluid via the ear or nose requires prompt surgical treatment
(E) most skull fractures do not require surgical treatment

483. A 39-year-old man presented to his physician with the complaint of loss of peripheral vision. The subsequent magnetic resonance imaging (MRI) scan below demonstrates

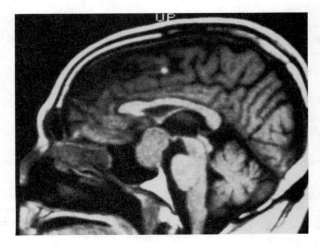

(A) cerebral atrophy
(B) pituitary adenoma
(C) optic glioma
(D) pontine hemorrhage
(E) multiple sclerosis plaque

484. An 18-year-old man is admitted to the emergency room following a motorcycle accident. He is alert and fully oriented but witnesses to the accident report an interval of unresponsiveness following the injury. Skull films disclose a fracture of the left temporal bone. Following x-ray the patient suddenly loses consciousness and dilatation of the left pupil is noted. This patient should be considered to have

(A) a ruptured berry aneurysm
(B) acute subdural hematoma
(C) epidural hematoma
(D) intraabdominal hemorrhage
(E) ruptured arteriovenous malformation

485. Which of the following statements regarding the cerebral angiogram below is true?

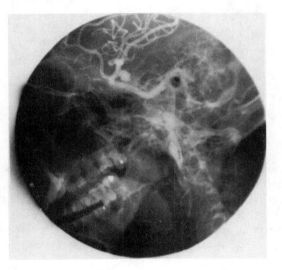

(A) The aneurysm arises from an arteriovenous malformation
(B) The lesion is a giant aneurysm
(C) There is a basilar artery lesion
(D) Initial treatment includes aggressive fluid hydration
(E) Surgical clipping of this lesion is curative

DIRECTIONS: Each question below contains four suggested responses of which **one or more** is correct. Select

A	if	**1, 2, and 3**	are correct
B	if	**1 and 3**	are correct
C	if	**2 and 4**	are correct
D	if	**4**	is correct
E	if	**1, 2, 3, and 4**	are correct

486. Correct statements regarding the condition suggested by the CT scan shown below include which of the following?

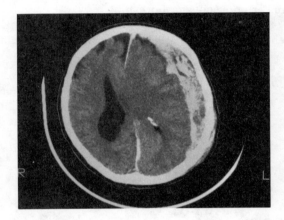

(1) It is caused by rupture of the veins traversing the subdural space
(2) Symptoms may occur at any time up to 2 months after injury
(3) Without treatment, the brainstem will be compressed by hemorrhage and edema with herniation and death will result
(4) The condition should be suspected in the presence of progressive change in mentation and a fluctuating level of consciousness

487. True statements regarding schwannomas include

(1) they represent peripheral nerve tumors
(2) the vestibulocochlear nerve is often affected
(3) they arise most frequently in sensory nerves
(4) they often degenerate to malignancy

488. Correct statements concerning craniopharyngiomas include which of the following?

(1) The tumors are frequently cystic
(2) The tumors are nearly always benign
(3) The tumors may cause compression of optic tracts and visual symptoms
(4) The tumors may cause ventricular obstruction and hydrocephalus

489. Correct statements regarding cerebral contusions include which of the following?

(1) They occur most frequently in the frontal lobes
(2) They may occur opposite the point of skull impact
(3) They are usually accompanied by parenchymal bleeding
(4) They may cause subsequent neurological disorders

490. A posterolateral herniation at the interspace between L4 and L5 may produce

(1) weakness of dorsiflexion of the great toe
(2) sensory deficit on the lateral aspect of the foot
(3) hyperesthesia on the dorsum of the foot
(4) weakness on plantar flexion

491. An acute increase in intracranial pressure is characterized by which of the following clinical findings?

(1) Respiratory irregularities
(2) Increased blood pressure
(3) Bradycardia
(4) Papilledema

492. True statements regarding glioblastoma multiforme include

(1) it is a neuronal cell tumor
(2) it arises from the malignant degeneration of an astrocytoma
(3) radiotherapy is curative in 20 percent of cases
(4) it is the most common primary intracranial neoplasm

Neurosurgery
Answers

478. The answer is B. *(Youmans, 3/e, pp 2206–2207.)* The Glasgow coma scale was developed to enable an initial assessment of the severity of head trauma. It is also now used to standardize serial neurological examinations in the early postinjury period. It measures the level of consciousness using three parameters: verbal response (5 points), motor response (6 points), and eye opening (4 points). The score is the sum of the highest number achieved in each category. The fully oriented and alert patient will receive a maximum score of 15. A score of less than 5 is associated with a mortality of over 50 percent.

479. The answer is C. *(Hall, pp 104–105.)* Controlled hyperventilation to a Pa_{CO_2} of 25 torr raises tissue pH, increases cerebrovascular resistance, decreases cerebral blood flow, and consequently reduces intracerebral pressure (ICP). In the effort to avoid brain swelling by lowering cerebral blood flow and ICP, the clinician must be wary of causing ischemic brain damage through hypoperfusion. The metabolic compensation to induced hypocapnia leads to normalization of the pH by loss of bicarbonate (metabolic acidosis), and over 8 to 24 h the beneficial effects of the hypocapnia will have been lost. The partial pressures of carbon dioxide should be allowed to slowly return to normal and held in reserve in case unanticipated increases in ICP require another pulse of short-term reduction. It is important to monitor the patient while the Pa_{CO_2} is rising because untoward or rapid increases in ICP may occur in response to the rising cerebral blood flow.

480. The answer is D. *(Youmans, 3/e, pp 1644–1689.)* In the absence of trauma, a subarachnoid hemorrhage (SAH) is the most likely diagnosis. The most common cause of an SAH is a ruptured berry aneurysm (51 percent). Other less frequent causes include hypertensive hemorrhage, trauma, and bleeding from an arteriovenous malformation. The most characteristic symptom of an SAH is a sudden, severe headache. Associated with this symptom may be nausea and vomiting, neck stiffness, dizziness, photophobia, depressed consciousness, hypertension, and temperature elevation. The majority of intracranial aneurysms arise from the arteries composing the circle of Willis and at the origin of large vessels from the vertebrobasilar system. Roughly 40 percent of people with an aneurysmal SAH die before entering a hospital. Approximately 60 percent of those admitted recover to their premorbid state. Surgical clipping of the aneurysm neck is the standard treatment. Early surgical management of these patients (within 72 h of SAH) allows for prevention of aneurysmal rebleeding and aggressive management of posthemorrhage vasospasm.

481. The answer is D. *(Youmans, 3/e, pp 3204–3223.)* The CT findings are consistent with any of the suggested lesions. However, the most likely diagnosis is metastatic disease. Almost 50 percent of intracranial neoplasms are metastatic lesions. Roughly 20 to 25 percent of cancer patients develop intracranial metastases during the course of their disease. Cancers of the lung and breast and melanomas frequently metastasize to the brain parenchyma. Leukemia shows a predilection for the leptomeninges. A large majority of these lesions become symptomatic owing to mass effect from white matter edema. Palliation is the primary goal for most patients and involves corticosteroids and radiation. Surgery is employed for the 25 percent of patients with a solitary brain metastasis and cured or arrested systemic disease.

482. The answer is D. *(Schwartz, 6/e, pp 1833–1834.)* Most skull fractures do not require surgical treatment unless they are depressed or compound. A general rule is that all depressed skull fractures should be surgically elevated, especially if they are depressed more than 1 cm, if a fragment is over the motor strip, or if small, sharp fragments are seen on x-ray (as they may tear the underlying dura). Compound fractures must be cleansed and debrided and the wound closed. When a skull fracture occurs in an area of the paranasal sinuses, mastoid air cells, or the middle ear, a tear in the meninges may result in cerebrospinal fluid drainage from the ear or nose. The presence of rhinorrhea or otorrhea requires observation and prophylactic antibiotics, as meningitis is a serious sequela. Otorrhea usually heals within a few days. Persistent cerebrospinal fluid from the nose or ear for more than 14 days requires surgical repair of the torn dura.

483. The answer is B. *(Grossman, pp 254–280. Youmans, 3/e, pp 3447–3499.)* This T1-weighted sagittal MRI scan reveals a dumbbell-shaped homogeneous mass involving the sella turcica and the suprasellar region. This lesion is most consistent with a pituitary adenoma, a benign tumor arising from the adenohypophysis. Pituitary adenomas are the most common sellar lesion and constitute 10 to 15 percent of all intra-

cranial neoplasms. Macroadenomas (> 10 mm) are generally nonsecret-
ing tumors. Microadenomas (< 10 mm) become clinically apparent from
hormonal secretion. They may secrete prolactin (amenorrhea or galactorrhea), growth hormone (gigantism or acromegaly), or ACTH (Cushing's syndrome). The tumor pictured is a macroadenoma. Its dumbbell
shape results from impingement on the adenoma by the diaphragm of
the sella turcica. The suprasellar extension seen here makes a frontal
craniotomy rather than a transsphenoidal approach more appropriate.

484.   The answer is C. *(Youmans, 3/e, pp 2017–2149.)* Epidural hematomas are typically caused by a tear of the middle meningeal artery or
vein, or a dural venous sinus. Ninety percent of epidural hematomas are
associated with linear skull fractures, usually in the temporal region.
*Only 2 percent of patients admitted with craniocerebral trauma suffer
epidural hematomas.* The lesion appears as a hyperdense biconvex
mass between the skull and brain on CT scan. Clinical presentation is
highly variable and outcome largely depends on promptness of diagnosis and surgical evacuation. The typical history is one of head trauma
followed by a momentary alteration in consciousness and then a lucid
interval lasting for up to a few hours. This is followed by a loss of consciousness, dilatation of the pupil on the side of the epidural hematoma,
and then compromise of the brainstem and death. Treatment consists of
temporal craniectomy, evaluation of the hemorrhage, and control of the
bleeding vessel. The mortality of epidural hematoma is approximately
50 percent.

485.   The answer is E. *(Osborn, pp 143–165.)* This digital subtraction
cerebral angiogram is an oblique view of the anterior circulation of the
brain. Dye injected in the internal carotid reveals an aneurysm at the
bifurcation of the internal carotid and the posterior communicating artery. A giant aneurysm is generally regarded as a lesion greater than 24
mm in cross-section. Surgical clipping of this aneurysm would be curative. Only after the risk of rebleeding is eliminated by clipping can the
patient undergo volume expansion if vasospasm arises. The vertebrobasilar system is not visualized here.

486.   The answer is E (all). *(Youmans, 3/e, pp 2046–2049.)* Subdural hematoma is caused by rupture of the veins traversing the subdural space
from the brain to the dural sinuses. The symptoms may occur within a
few minutes or as long as 8 weeks after injury. With acute subdural
hematoma, significant progressive neurological deficit is noted within
48 h of injury. Without treatment, the brainstem is compressed by hem-

orrhage and edema until herniation occurs and death results. Computerized axial tomography is accurate in defining the site of recent intracranial hemorrhage. Treatment consists of craniotomy with removal of the hematoma and relaxation of the compressing dura. Mortality in this acute form of the condition is very high (up to 80 percent) if the condition is not treated. Subacute subdural hematomas are defined as those that cause significant neurological deficits more than 48 h but less than 2 weeks after injury. Chronic subdural hematomas are those that cause symptoms 2 weeks or more after injury. They are most commonly seen in infants or elderly patients and are suggested by a change in mental faculties or a fluctuating or decreasing level of consciousness.

487. The answer is A (1, 2, 3). *(Youmans, 3/e, pp 3667–3676.)* Peripheral nerve tumors include lesions of peripheral nerves, the adrenal gland nerve tissue, and the sympathetic chain. Schwannomas are peripheral nerve sheath tumors that arise from perineural fibroblasts (Schwann cells). Intracranial schwannomas most frequently originate in the vestibular branch of the eighth cranial nerve and represent 10 percent of all intracranial neoplasms. Symptoms include hearing loss, tinnitus, and vertigo. Malignant schwannomas are rare. Neurofibromas are also Schwann cell tumors but are histologically distinguishable from schwannomas. Neurofibromatosis (von Recklinghausen's disease) involves multiple peripheral nerve neoplasms. Neuronal tumors of peripheral nerves include ganglioneuroma, neuroblastoma, chemodectoma, and pheochromocytomas.

488. The answer is E (all). *(Youmans, 3/e, pp 2970–2972, 3223–3238.)* Craniopharyngiomas are cystic tumors with areas of calcification and originate in the epithelial remnants of Rathke's pouch. These usually benign tumors are found in the sellar and suprasellar region and lead to compression of the pituitary, optic tracts, and third ventricle. As a result they can present with symptoms of visual disturbance, endocrine dysfunction, headache, or even hydrocephalus. Craniopharyngiomas are most commonly found in children but may also present in adulthood. Treatment consists of subfrontal or transsphenoidal excision with adjuvant radiotherapy if total removal is not possible.

489. The answer is E (all). *(Youmans, 3/e, pp 1960–1961, 1970–1972.)* Cerebral contusions are bruises of neural parenchyma that most commonly involve the convex surface of a gyrus. The most frequent sites of cerebral contusion are the orbital surfaces of the frontal lobes and the anterior portion of the temporal lobes. The etiology of the contusion is always traumatic and subsequent neurological impairment, such as epilepsy, is common if the original injury was significant. Patients deemed to have a substantial contusion should receive anticonvulsive medication in the early posttraumatic period.

490. The answer is B (1, 3). *(Youmans, 3/e, pp 2664–2694.)* The intervertebral disk is susceptible to degenerative changes especially in the lower cervical and lower lumbar spine. This can lead to a thinning of the annulus fibrosis and loss of its fibrocartilage. Marked mechanical stresses are another means of damage when they cause tears in the annulus. Herniation of a portion of the nucleus pulposus can result from either problem. Not all such herniations are symptomatic, but those in the lumbar region most often lead to numbness or pain or both. *Ninety-five percent of lumbar herniations are at L4–L5 or L5–S1.* A posterolateral herniation in the lumbar region impinges on the anterior and posterior nerve roots of the *inferior* intervertebral foramen. Thus, a herniation at the L4–L5 interspace will compress the fifth lumbar roots. The anterior roots of L5 serves the anterior crural and peroneal muscles. The most common sequela of compression is weakness of dorsiflexion of the great toe. The L5 posterior root serves the dermatome from the anterolateral aspect of the leg to the dorsum and the medial aspect of the foot. Compression here can result in pain on the dorsum of the foot. Weakness on plantar flexion and sensory deficit on the lateral aspect of the foot are symptoms associated with compression of the first sacral roots common with posterolateral herniations at L5–S1.

491. The answer is A (1, 2, 3). *(Youmans, 3/e, pp 661–696.)* The onset of irregular respirations, bradycardia, and finally increased blood pressure with increasing intracranial pressure (ICP) is termed the *Cushing response.* These physiological alterations are caused by brainstem compression. Slow rises in ICP are, by contrast, autoregulated by the brain's compensatory mechanisms and lead to a late onset of neurological sequelae. A mass lesion is more apt to compromise local cerebral blood flow and increase cerebral edema and ICP. The vector of the mass effect may lead to herniation of brain parenchyma through the tentorial incisura or foramen magnum with resultant brainstem compression. Herniation usually causes compression of the third cranial nerve and thus leads to a fixed and dilated pupil on that side. Papilledema is a finding with chronic increases in ICP.

492. The answer is C (2, 4). *(Youmans, 3/e, pp 2975–2981.)* Glioblastoma multiforme is the most common form of primary intracranial neuroepithelial tumor. It represents 25 percent of all intracranial tumors and 50 percent of tumors originating in the central nervous system. It is a heterogeneous glial cell tumor derived from the malignant degeneration of an astrocytoma or anaplastic astrocytoma. These tumors are most commonly found in the cerebral hemispheres during the fifth decade of life. CT and MRI scans typically reveal an irregular lesion with hypodense central necrosis, peripheral ring enhancement of the highly cellular tumor tissue, and surrounding edema and mass effect. Curative resections are rare. Therapy consists of diagnostic biopsy followed by radiotherapy to slow the tumor growth. The course of the disease progresses rapidly after presentation with few patients living more than 2 years.

Otolaryngology

493. Which of the following statements concerning nasopharyngeal cancer is true?

(A) It has an unusually high incidence among Chinese
(B) It occurs primarily after the sixth decade of life
(C) It undergoes early metastasis to the lungs
(D) The treatment of choice is wide surgical excision of the primary tumor
(E) Initial evaluation should involve a biopsy of the primary tumor and neck nodes

494. Severe maxillofacial trauma is often the result of high-velocity impact sustained in automobile or motorcycle accidents. Regarding these injuries, all the following statements are true EXCEPT

(A) evaluation of the cervical spine is a first-line priority
(B) severe hemorrhage from the nasopharynx often occurs with Le Fort's fractures
(C) direct oral or nasotracheal intubation should be performed promptly to prevent airway obstruction
(D) computed tomography is preferable to the standard tomographic "facial series" to assess the facial fractures
(E) definitive management of fractures of facial bones should be delayed until swelling subsides

495. All the following statements regarding chemotherapy for squamous cell carcinoma of the head and neck are true EXCEPT

(A) preoperative (induction) chemotherapy can be expected to produce responses in over 75 percent of patients

(B) when a "complete" response to induction chemotherapy occurs, there is a high probability of local control and cure

(C) if there is no response to induction chemotherapy, surgical resection should probably be avoided

(D) patients with complete responses to chemotherapy do not require surgery or irradiation

(E) the combination of chemotherapy, radiation, and surgery has not been shown to improve the cure rate for squamous cell cancers of the head and neck

DIRECTIONS: Each question below contains four suggested responses of which **one or more** is correct. Select

A	if	**1, 2, and 3**	are correct
B	if	**1 and 3**	are correct
C	if	**2 and 4**	are correct
D	if	**4**	is correct
E	if	**1, 2, 3, and 4**	are correct

496. Correct statements about branchial cleft anomalies include which of the following?

(1) A fistula that lies between the external auditory canal and the submandibular region originates from the first branchial cleft

(2) The course of the first branchial cleft fistula is through the bifurcation of the carotid artery

(3) Injury to the hypoglossal nerve may occur during excision of a second branchial cleft fistula

(4) The internal opening of the second branchial cleft fistula is usually found in the maxillary sinus

497. True statements regarding symptomatic thyroglossal duct cysts include

(1) they almost always manifest themselves before age 12

(2) treatment includes resection of the hyoid bone

(3) they usually present as a painful swelling in the lateral neck

(4) they may contain malignant elements

498. Pleomorphic adenomas (mixed tumors) of the salivary glands are characterized by which of the following?

(1) They occur most commonly on the lips, tongue, and palate

(2) They grow rapidly

(3) They tend to recur if simply enucleated

(4) They present as rock-hard masses

499. True statements regarding cancer of the tongue include which of the following?

(1) Carcinomas at the base of the tongue are best treated by irradiation alone rather than surgery

(2) Stage I and stage II cancers of the mobile tongue may be treated equally well by irradiation or surgery

(3) Tongue cancers are relatively rare tumors of the oral cavity and are usually advanced to stage III by the time they are diagnosed

(4) Prophylactic irradiation of the neck nodes is indicated in patients whose primary cancer of the tongue is treated by irradiation.

500. Verrucous carcinoma of the buccal mucosa is identified with which of the following characteristics?

(1) It is slower growing than the epidermoid form

(2) It is associated with tobacco chewing

(3) It has a predilection for the gingivobuccal gutter

(4) It rarely extends to the mandible

Otolaryngology
Answers

493. The answer is A. *(Schwartz, 6/e, pp 637–639.)* There is an unusually high incidence of carcinoma of the nasopharynx among Chinese. In the early stages of the disease, metastases remain confined to the neck. Diagnosis of nasopharyngeal cancer, which tends to arise in relatively young people, should be made by biopsy of the primary tumor. Biopsy of the neck nodes should be avoided because implantation of the tumor in skin and subcutaneous tissue may occur. Radiation therapy is the treatment of choice for the primary nasopharyngeal cancer. Cervical metastases that remain clinically evident should be removed by a radical neck dissection.

494. The answer is C. *(Trunkey, 2/e, pp 181–223.)* In patients with severe facial or mandibular trauma, airway difficulties may develop secondary to the effects of massive hemorrhage, tissue swelling, or associated laryngeal trauma. A cricothyroidotomy is preferred over direct oral or nasotracheal intubation because it can be performed quickly without manipulation of the cervical spine or injured parts. If prolonged postoperative airway problems are anticipated, the cricothyroidotomy may convert to a tracheostomy. Evaluation of the cervical spine is a top priority and should be performed in any patient with head trauma prior to further facial studies. Although most facial fractures can be diagnosed easily with a standard "facial series," computed tomography (CT) is extremely accurate, exposes the patient to less radiation, and allows assessment of areas (e.g., intracerebral contents) that cannot be evaluated by conventional techniques. Therefore, in most major centers, CT is presently the preferred method of evaluation for patients with severe maxillofacial trauma. Maxillary fractures are categorized by the Le Fort classification and unlike other facial fractures are frequently associated with severe nasal and nasopharyngeal hemorrhage. This may be treated with head elevation and ice compresses. Nasal packing also affords good control of hemorrhage, and in extreme cases ligation or embolization of the internal maxillary artery may be necessary. Definitive reduction and fixation of fractures may be delayed while other injuries and medical problems are addressed. In addition to control of hemorrhage, initial management of facial fractures may include temporary stabilization, wound closure, and oral lavage with solutions containing antibiotics.

495. The answer is D. *(Erwin, Semin Oncol 12:71–82, 1985.)* Induction (preoperative) chemotherapy can be expected to result in response rates at or above 75 percent. Variously reported clinical trials have found complete responses in 25 to over 50 percent. Evidence also suggests that those patients with a complete response to either chemotherapy or combined synchronous chemoradiotherapy are likely to have long-term local control ("cure"). Conversely, those who respond poorly to induction chemotherapy have a bad prognosis whatever subsequent therapy is provided. Many workers now urge that surgical efforts be avoided in patients who do not respond to pretreatment since even heroic palliative surgery will not prevent early relapse. It seems clear that with currently used chemotherapeutic agents, there is an accelerated rate of relapse if the chemotherapy is not followed by surgical or irradiation extirpation of the primary site; chemotherapy should be considered adjunctive, not definitive, treatment.

496. The answer is B (1, 3). *(Schwartz, 6/e, pp 1683–1685.)* Branchial cleft cysts, sinuses, and fistulas are remnants of the first and second branchial pouches. The internal opening of the first is the external auditory canal; for the second, it is the posterolateral pharynx below the tonsillar fossa. The facial nerve may be injured during dissection of the first fistula. The second fistula passes between the carotid bifurcation and adjacent to the hypoglossal nerve. In childhood most branchial cleft anomalies present as a painless nodule along the lateral border of the sternocleidomastoid muscle. In adults, superinfection of the cyst or fistulous drainage via an orifice in the supraclavicular region may occur. Treatment is surgical excision.

497. The answer is C (2, 4). *(Schwartz, 6/e, pp 595–596, 1683–1684.)* Thyroglossal duct cysts result from retention of an epithelial tract between the thyroid and its embryological origin in the foramen cecum at the base of the tongue. This tract usually penetrates the hyoid bone. There is no sex predilection, and although these cysts are more frequently detected in children, up to 25 percent do not become symptomatic until adulthood. The most common presentation is a painless swelling in the midline of the neck that moves with protrusion of the tongue or swallowing. The cysts are prone to infection and progressive enlargement. Although rare (less than 1 percent), epidermoid or papillary carcinomas do occur within thyroglossal duct cysts. Surgical resection is the standard therapy. The Sistrunk procedure, which involves local resection of the cyst and the central portion of the hyoid bone, is the operation of choice. Simple excision of the cyst results in an unacceptably high recurrence rate.

498. The answer is B (1, 3). *(Schwartz, 6/e, pp 650–655.)* There are approximately 400 to 700 minor salivary glands in the oral cavity. Pleomorphic adenomas (mixed tumors) can occur in any of them. These round tumors have a rubbery consistency and are slow-growing; all are potentially malignant. Unless adequately excised, they tend to recur locally in a high percentage of cases. The sites most commonly affected by pleomorphic adenomas of the salivary glands are the lips, tongue, and palate.

499. The answer is C (2, 4). *(Schwartz, 6/e, pp 630–631.)* Cancer of the tongue is the most common malignant tumor in the oral cavity and accounts for slightly less than a third of the malignancies in the area. About two-thirds of cases will present as early lesions in the mobile anterior portion of the tongue. Most workers in the field agree that for these stage I and stage II lesions, surgery and irradiation give equivalent results (45 percent 5-year survival) and the treatment, therefore, should be tailored to the patient. Failures are almost always due to supraclavicular recurrence and many recommend excision of the radiation scar and prophylactic irradiation of the neck nodes, particularly in the poorer prognosis stage II and stage IV tumors in the base of the tongue.

500. The answer is A (1, 2, 3). *(Schwartz, 6/e, pp 623–626.)* Verrucous carcinoma is a less aggressive form of locally invasive buccal cancer than the usual epidermoid form. Its frequency is increased in people who chew tobacco. The tumor usually grows very slowly, occurs chiefly in the gingivobuccal gutter, and has a tendency to invade bone. It is identified by its characteristic exophytic, white, shaggy appearance. Wide excision is the best initial treatment for this neoplasm. Even though the tumor may regress in response to radiation, it tends to recur in a more malignant form with metastases. Cervical metastases usually are not present when the lesion is first diagnosed; it is only for the most highly malignant grades of verrucous carcinoma that radical neck dissection and block excision of the cheek are indicated.

Bibliography

Anderson RJ, et al: Unrecognized adult salicylate intoxication. *Ann Intern Med* 85:745–748, 1976.

Barnavon Y, Wallack MK: Management of the pregnant patient with carcinoma of the breast. *Surg Gynecol Obstet* 171:347–352, 1990.

Barnes RW, Marszalek PB: Asymptomatic carotid disease in the cardiovascular surgical patient: Is prophylactic endarterectomy necessary? *Stroke* 12:497–500, 1981.

Belkin M, et al: Intra-arterial fibrinolytic therapy. Efficacy of streptokinase vs urokinase. *Arch Surg* 121:769–773, 1986.

Berci G, Sackier JM, Paz-Partlow M: Emergency laparoscopy. *Am J Surg* 161:332–335, 1991.

Bergqvist D: *Postoperative Thromboembolism: Frequency, Etiology, Prophylaxis.* New York, Springer-Verlag, 1983.

Blumberg HM, Stephens DS: Pyomyositis and human immunodeficiency virus infection. *South Med J* 83:1092–1095, 1990.

Boland G, Lee MJ, Mueller PR: Acute cholecystitis in the intensive care unit. *New Horizons* 2:246–260, 1993.

Boucher CA, et al: Determination of cardiac risk by dipyridamole-thallium imaging before peripheral vascular surgery. *N Engl J Med* 312:389–394, 1985.

Brewster DC, Franklin DP, Cambria RP, et al: Intestinal ischemia complicating abdominal aortic surgery. *Surgery* 109:447–454, 1991.

Brooks J: *Surgery of the Pancreas.* Philadelphia, WB Saunders, 1983.

Bunt TJ, et al: Frequency of vascular injury with blunt trauma-induced extremity injury. *Am J Surg* 160:226–228,1990.

Cameron JL: *Current Surgical Therapy,* 4/e. St. Louis, Mosby, 1992.

Case Records of the Massachusetts General Hospital. Weekly Clinicopathological Exercises. Case 45–1987:A 16-year-old girl with hepatic and pulmonary masses. *N Engl J Med* 317:1209–1218, 1987.

Cass AS: Renovascular injuries from external trauma. Diagnosis, treatment, and outcome. *Urol Clin North Am* 16:213–220, 1989.

Cerilli GJ: *Organ Transplantation and Replacement*. Philadelphia, JB Lippincott, 1988.

Charlson ME, et al: The preoperative and intraoperative hemodynamic predictors of postoperative myocardial infarction or ischemia in patients undergoing noncardiac surgery. *Ann Surg* 210:637–648, 1989.

Civetta JM, Taylor RW, Kirby RR (eds): *Critical Care, 2/e*. Philadelphia, JB Lippincott, 1992.

Collins PW, Newland AC: Treatment modalities of autoimmune blood disorders. *Semin Hematol* 29:64–74, 1992.

Copeland EM III: *Surgical Oncology*. New York, Wiley, 1983.

Cosentino CM, et al: Choledochal duct cyst: Resection with physiologic reconstruction. *Surgery* 112:740–748, 1992.

Cummings RA, et al: Pneumopericardium resulting in cardiac tamponade. *Ann Thorac Surg* 37:511–518, 1984.

Davis JH, et al (eds): *Clinical Surgery*. St. Louis, CV Mosby, 1987.

Diettrich NA, et al: A growing spectrum of surgical disease in patients with human immunodeficiency virus/acquired immunodeficiency syndrome. Experience with 120 major cases. *Arch Surg* 126:860–866, 1991.

Dubrow TJ, et al: Myocardial contusion in the stable patient. *Surgery* 106:267–273, 1989.

Dutky PA, Stevens SL, Maull KI: Factors affecting rapid fluid resuscitation with large-bore introducer catheters. *J Trauma* 29:856–860, 1989.

Eisbud DE, et al: Treatment of acute vascular occlusions with intraarterial urokinase. *Am J Surg* 160:160–165, 1990.

Erwin TJ, Clark JR, Weichselbaum RR: Multidisciplinary treatment of advanced squamous carcinoma of the head and neck. *Semin Oncol* 12:71–82, 1985.

Feliciano DV, et al: Splenorrhaphy: The alternative. *Ann Surg* 211:569–582, 1990.

Fidler TJ, Nicolson GL: The process of cancer invasion and metastasis. *Cancer Bull* 39:126–131, 1987.

Flint L, et al: Definitive control of mortality from severe pelvic fracture. *Ann Surg* 211:703–707, 1990.

Friesen SR, Thompson NW: *Surgical Endocrinology: Clinical Syndromes.* Philadelphia, JB Lippincott, 1990.

Gajraj H, Young AE: Adrenal incidentaloma. *Br J Surg* 80:422–426, 1993.

Gibney EJ: Asymptomatic gallstones. *Br J Surg* 77:368–372, 1990.

Goodnough LT, Shuck JM: Risks, options, and informed consent for blood transfusion in elective surgery. *Am J Surg* 159:602–609, 1990.

Graham DY, Go MF: Helicobacter pylori: Current status. *Gastroenterology* 105:279–282, 1993.

Grossman CB: *Magnetic Resonance Imaging and Computed Tomography of the Head and Spine.* Baltimore, Williams & Wilkins, 1990.

Hall JB, Schmidt GA, Wood LDH: *Principles of Critical Care.* New York, McGraw-Hill, 1992.

Hall EJ: Radiation biology. *Cancer* 55:2051–2057,1985.

Hardy JT (ed): *Hardy's Textbook of Surgery, 2/e.* Philadelphia, JB Lippincott, 1988.

Henderson JA, Peloquin AJ: Boerhaave revisited: Spontaneous esophageal perforation as a diagnostic masquerader. *Am J Med* 86:559–567, 1989.

Heys SD, et al: Nutrition and malignant disease: Implications for surgical practice *Br J Surg* 79:614–623, 1992.

Khuroo MS, et al: Ascaris-induced acute pancreatitis. *Br J Surg* 79:1335–1338, 1992.

Kohn HI, Fry RJM: Radiation carcinogenesis. *N Engl J Med* 310:504–511, 1984.

Landercasper J, et al: Perioperative stroke risk in 173 consecutive patients with a past history of stroke. *Arch Surg* 125:986–989, 1989.

Larew RE: Malignant hyperthermia: Quick recognition and treatment to avoid death. *Postgrad Med* 85:117–118, 128–129, 1989.

Mahmoodian S: Appendicitis complicating pregnancy. *South Med J* 85:19–24, 1992.

McQuaid KR, Isenberg JI: Medical therapy of peptic ulcer disease. *Surg Clin North Am* 72:285–316, 1992.

Melton AT, et al: Malignant hyperthermia in humans. *Anesth Analg* 69:437–443, 1989.

Merrell SW, Schneider PD: Hemobilia: Evolution of current diagnosis and treatment. *West J Med* 155:621–625, 1991.

Miller FB, Shumate CR, Richardson JD: Myocardial contusion. When can the diagnosis be eliminated? *Arch Surg* 124:805–808, 1989.

Miller RD: *Anesthesia,* New York, Churchill Livingstone, 1990.

Mizrahi S, et al: Posttraumatic autotransplantation of spleen tissue *Arch Surg* 124:863–865, 1989.

Moertel CG, et al: Levamisole and fluorouracil for adjuvant therapy of resected colon carcinoma. *N Engl J Med* 322:352–358, 1990.

Moosa AR, Mayer AD, Stabile B: Iatrogenic injury to the bile duct: Who, how, where? *Arch Surg* 125:1028–1031, 1990.

Norton JA: Controversies and advances in primary hyperparathyroidism. *Ann Surg* 215:297–299, 1992.

O'Hara PJ, Hakaim AG, Hertzer NR, et al: Surgical management of aortic aneurysm and coexistent horseshoe kidney: Review of a 31 year experience. *J Vasc Surg* 17:940–947, 1993.

Osborn AG: *Introduction to Cerebral Angiography.* New York, Harper & Row, 1980.

Osther PJ, Balslev E, Blichert-Toft M: Paget's disease of the nipple. A continuing enigma. *Acta Chir Scand* 156:343–352, 1990.

Pasternack PF, et al: The value of the radionuclide angiogram in the prediction of perioperative myocardial infarction in patients undergoing lower extremity revascularization procedures. *Circulation* 72:13–17, 1985.

Potts JT, et al: Diagnosis and management of primary hyperparathyroidism: Consensus development conference statement. *Ann Intern Med* 114:593–597, 1991.

Pruitt BA Jr, et al: Evaluation and management of patients with inhalation injury. *J Trauma* 30 (suppl):S63–68, 1990.

Recommendations for prevention of HIV transmission in health care settings. *N Y State J Med* 88:25–31, 1988.

Reilly HF, al-Kawas FH: Dieulafoy's lesion. Diagnosis and management. *Dig Dis Sci* 36:1702–1707, 1991.

Rhame FS: Preventing HIV transmission. Strategies to protect clinicians and patients. *Postgrad Med* 91:144, 147–152, 1992.

Robinson T, et al: Body smuggling of illicit drugs: Two cases requiring surgical intervention. *Surgery* 113:709–711, 1993.

Sabiston DC Jr, Spencer FC: *Gibbon's Surgery of the Chest,* 5/e. Philadelphia, WB Saunders, 1990.

wyers JL: Management of postgastrectomy syndromes. *Am J Surg* 159:8–14, 1990.

chirmer BD, Dix J, Edge SB, et al: Laparoscopic cholecystectomy in the obese patient. *Ann Surg* 216:146–152, 1992.

chroeder T, et al: Ischemic colitis complicating reconstruction of the abdominal aorta. *Surg Gynecol Obstet* 160:299–303, 1985.

chwartz SI, Ellis H: *Maingot's Abdominal Operations,* 9/e. Norwalk, CT, Appleton & Lange, 1989.

chwartz SI, Shires GT, Spencer FC (eds): *Principles of Surgery,* 6/e, New York, McGraw-Hill, 1993.

hires GT (ed): *Principles of Trauma Care,* 3/e. New York, McGraw-Hill, 1985.

hoemaker WC, Thompson WL, Holbrook PR: *The Society of Critical Care Medicine: Textbook of Critical Care,* 2/e. Philadelphia, WB Saunders, 1988.

tain SC, et al: Selective management of nonocclusive arterial injuries. *Arch Surg* 124:1136–1141, 1989.

Thoren T, Wattwil M: Effects on gastric emptying of thoracic epidural analgesia with morphine or bupivacaine. *Anesth Analg* 67:687–694, 1988.

Tintinalli JE, Ruiz E, Krome RL: *Emergency Medicine: A Comprehensive Study Guide,* 3/e. New York, McGraw-Hill, 1992.

Trunkey DD: *Current Therapy of Trauma,* 2/e. Philadelphia, BC Decker, 1986.

Trunkey DD: Shock trauma. *Can J Surg* 27:479–486, 1984.

von Schilfgaarde R, Hardy MA (eds): *Transplantation of the Endocrine Pancreas in Diabetes Mellitus.* New York, Elsevier, 1989.

Walt AJ: *Early Care of the Injured Patient,* 3/e. Philadelphia, WB Saunders, 1982.

Walters HL, et al: Peritoneal lavage and the surgical resident. *Surg Gynecol Obstet* 165:496–502, 1988.

Way LW: *Current Surgical Diagnosis and Treatment,* 9/e. Norwalk, CT, Appleton & Lange, 1991.

Weissman C: The metabolic response to stress: An overview and update *Anesthesiology* 73:308–327, 1990.

West JB: *Respiratory Physiology: The Essentials,* 4/e. Baltimore, Williams & Wilkins, 1990.

Wilkening GM, Sutton CH: Health effects of nonionizing radiatic
    Med Clin North Am 74:489–507, 1990.

Willerson JT, et al: Role of new antiplatelet agents as adjunctive ther
    pies in thrombolysis. *Am J Cardiol* 67:12A–18A, 1991.

Wilmore DW, Brennan MF, Harken AH, et al (eds): *Care of the Su*
    gical Patient. New York, Scientific American Books, 1990.

Wilson JD, Braunwald E, Isselbacher KJ, et al: *Harrison's Principle*
    of Internal Medicine, 12/e. New York, McGraw-Hill, 1991.

Wilson SE, et al: Acquired immune deficiency syndrome (AIDS). Ir
    dications for abdominal surgery, pathology, and outcome. *Ann Sur*
    210:428–434, 1989.

Wilson SE, Williams RA, Robinson G: Operating on HIV-positive pa
    tients. What are the risks to healthcare workers? To patients? *Post*
    grad Med 88:193–194, 199–201, 1990.

Wiot JF: The radiologic manifestations of blunt chest trauma. *JAM,*
    231:500–503, 1975.

Youmans JR (ed): *Neurological Surgery,* 3/e. Philadelphia, WB Saun
    ders, 1990.

Zuidema GD, Rutherford RB, Ballinger WF II: *The Management o*
    Trauma, 4/e. Philadelphia, WB Saunders, 1985.